exercise physiology

exercise physiology

DAVID H. CLARKE
University of Maryland

Prentice-Hall, Inc., Englewood Cliffs, New Jersey

Library of Congress Cataloging in Publication Data

CLARKE, DAVID H
    Exercise physiology.

    Includes bibliographies and index.
    1. Exercise—Physiological effect.   I. Title.
[DNLM: 1. Physical education and training.
2. Physiology.   QT255 C597e]
QP301.C585   612'.76   75-9735
ISBN 0-13-294967-9

10   9   8   7   6   5   4   3   2   1

Printed in the United States of America

PRENTICE-HALL INTERNATIONAL, INC., *London*
PRENTICE-HALL OF AUSTRALIA, PTY. LTD., *Sydney*
PRENTICE-HALL OF CANADA, LTD., *Toronto*
PRENTICE-HALL OF INDIA PRIVATE LIMITED, *New Delhi*
PRENTICE-HALL OF JAPAN, INC., *Tokyo*
PRENTICE-HALL OF SOUTHEAST ASIA (PTE.), *Singapore*

To my Wife
Louise Terani Clarke
and Children
Stephen, Gregory, and Meredith

contents

preface

Exercise Physiology presents the material essential for understanding relevant changes in various mechanisms of the body that occur during the onset of exercise. A second equally important objective of this book is to explore the long-term effects of exercise, as one engages in systematic physical training. Both aspects of the physiology of exercise are necessary to an understanding of the mechanisms that account for human physical fitness. To realize these objectives a knowledge of basic human physiology is also necessary, and for that purpose relevant physiological mechanisms are presented along with those related to exercise. Thus, the text is designed to be useful to the upper division undergraduate student with a moderate background in basic anatomy and physiology. Extensive prerequisites in chemistry and physics are not required to understand the concepts presented.

To make the concepts presented more readily understood, the text is liberally illustrated. There is an appropriate use of references, but an attempt has been made to document only the most pertinent matters, not to try to be exhaustive. At the end of each chapter a summary of the most important features is provided along with a brief list of selected references.

The first four chapters contain material on the neuromuscular system. Chapter 1, Nervous Integration, considers the manner in which the nerve impulse originates and is transmitted, as well as the characteristics of the action potential. Also presented are the essential elements of the sarcotubular system. The structure of muscle and the sliding filament model of contraction are presented in Chapter 2, Skeletal Muscle, in addition to a molecular theory that describes the events associated with contraction. Chapter 3, Mechanical and Dynamic Properties of Muscle, brings together a number of the diverse elements that describe the manner in which muscles function. Muscular fatigue is considered in some depth, and a new concept, the *muscular strength debt*, is proposed. Also, muscular training is examined and the most current techniques are presented, along with the newest concepts of hypertrophy. Chapter 4,

Proprioception, focuses on the muscle spindle and the gamma efferent system as they function in reflex activity. In addition, contrasting action of the Pacinian corpuscle and Golgi tendon organ are presented.

The next three chapters describe aerobic capacity, the metabolic activities of the cell, and corresponding factors of nutrition. In Chapter 5 both aerobic and anaerobic metabolism are presented, along with extensive descriptions of glycolysis, the Krebs cycle, and respiratory chain oxidation. Concepts of training, including the new techniques of glycogen loading are discussed. Submaximal and maximal work capacity are considered in Chapter 6. Chapter 7 considers diet, mechanical efficiency, and body composition, in addition to the concept of exercise and weight control and athletic performance.

The factors associated with gas transfer and respiration are considered in detail in Chapters 8 and 9. Chapter 8 discusses gas exchange at the lungs and the tissues, as well as gas transport and oxygen and carbon dioxide dissociation. In Chapter 9 the mechanics of breathing are explained, with special emphasis on the reflex and humoral regulation of respiration. Of particular concern is the "mysterious hyperpnea of exercise," the mechanisms that control ventilation in exercise, and training.

The next two chapters deal with circulation. Chapter 10, Central Circulation, discusses cardiac output, coronary circulation, and the mechanisms that control heart function. In addition, the effects of exercise and training on cardiac output are presented. In Chapter 11, Peripheral Circulation, the characteristics of systemic circulation are presented, along with various local and reflex control mechanisms. The effects of exercise and training on peripheral resistance and blood pressure are considered.

Chapter 12, Environmental Physiology, includes studies of altitude physiology, the physiology of diving, temperature regulation, and warm-up. Chapter 13, Physiology of Physically Handicapping Conditions, is a unique attempt in a book of this sort to relate the physiological mechanisms previously discussed with certain disabilities often seen in adapted physical education. These are presented under such categories as neuromuscular and metabolic disorders, and cardiovascular and coronary heart disease. The final chapter, Measurement and Evaluation, discusses the testing of muscular and cardiovascular aspects of exercise physiology, and gives examples of various tests that can be employed.

DAVID H. CLARKE

exercise
physiology

chapter 1

nervous integration

Muscles are so completely subservient to the nerve impulse for activation that any successful patterning of muscular activity in performing coordinated motor acts must be preceded by an appropriate train of motor-nerve impulses. Thus, coordinated behavior must arise initially as a nervous-system decision, then pass along in rather predictable ways to the skeletal muscles for action. The fact that complicated skills are performed imperfectly on initial trials attests to the well-known dictum that simply knowing what has to be done holds no guarantee for successful execution. Even simple and isolated movements reflect improvement over trials, so apparently any number of factors are responsible for effecting coordinated action. When one compares simple tasks with some of the more complicated ones involved in athletic endeavor, he senses that the nervous integration required, both planned and reflexive, must be of considerable magnitude.

A complete description of the nervous system is beyond the scope of this text, and the reader is encouraged to consult current accounts of neurophysiology and neurology for an in-depth analysis of the foundation for motor learning. The various functions of the higher nervous centers, where movement is ultimately originated, are interconnected, coordinated, and directed toward the periphery, where eventually the muscles receive a motor message which results in purposeful movement. The muscles in turn respond, not only with contraction, but with appropriate sensory feedback to the central nervous system, permitting the neuromuscular apparatus to adjust to any changing set of circumstances. Some aspects of this response will be discussed later. The present chapter, however, will deal primarily with the lower nervous centers, principally the peripheral nerve and the excitation-contraction coupling process between motor neuron and muscle fiber membrane.

THE MOTOR NEURON

The term *neuron* is employed to represent the nerve cell accompanied by its processes, the *dendrites* and the *axon*. Its special function is to transmit a *nerve impulse*. Neurons vary in size and shape in different parts of the body, being only 5 μ (microns) in diameter in certain portions of the brain, and 120 μ in diameter in some of the large nerves of the spinal cord. Lengths also vary considerably, extending from a few microns to as long as 90 cm. The *motor neuron* is uniquely designed to convey nerve impulses from the central nervous system to other cells, such as muscle cells. The essential features of a motor neuron are presented in Figure 1. The motor neuron is made up of a *cell body*, containing a *nucleus*, with a number of branching projections called *dendrites*. One very long branch is the *axon*, which is the peripheral nerve fiber. The axon arises at the *axon hillock* and travels to the muscle fiber. It contains intracellular fluid, *axoplasm*, and is enclosed by a fatty sheath, the *myelin sheath*, which is white and gives rise to the pale appearance of nerves and the white matter of the brain and spinal cord. Myelin serves as an insulator, but is interrupted at intervals of about one millimeter by *nodes of Ranvier*, which permit the *axon cylinder* to come into contact with the intercellular fluids, so that ions can flow during nerve conduction. Outside the myelin is a fine sheath which contains a nucleus called the *Schwann cell*, which serves a very important function in the regeneration of peripheral nerves that have been damaged. Since the brain and spinal cord have no Schwann cells,

Figure 1. The Motor Neuron.

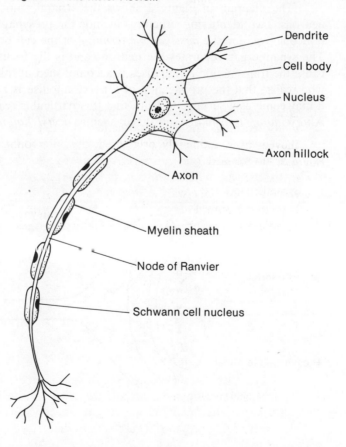

nerve tissue in these areas is not repaired. This is a rather vital difference and explains the permanent nature of brain and spinal cord injuries as compared with lesions of peripheral nerves.

THE SYNAPSE

The nerve cell functions as a separate nervous system by itself, in the sense that it receives sensory messages from other neurons through the use of *synapses*, or terminal contacts, which can be found on the cell body and the dendrites. It sorts out the messages so as to make a suitable response, and sends the messages out along an axon to some receptor organ. Large numbers of small *presynaptic terminals* are present on the cell body and dendrites of the neuron, which are themselves the ends of other neurons that originated elsewhere. While it is typical to think of synapses as *excitatory*—that is, as receiving an impulse and conducting it across the *synaptic gap*—it should be kept in mind that some of these presynaptic terminals are *inhibitory* and thereby prevent the transmission of an impulse.

The diagram in Figure 2 shows the synaptic junction between two neurons. Two identifying structures include the presynaptic terminal, mentioned above, and the *postsynaptic terminal* of the cell body of the neuron. The synaptic gap separates the neurons and is the focus of attention, because the transmission of impulses is accomplished at this point. For those who realize that the propagation of a nerve impulse is basically electrical, it may come as a surprise to learn that this particular reaction is chemical. An *excitatory transmitter* substance, such as *acetylcholine*, is released from

Figure 2. The Synapse.

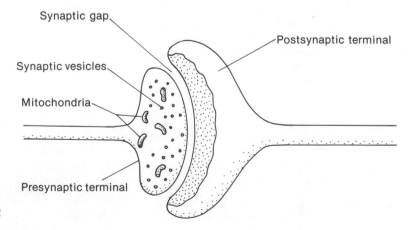

4

synaptic vesicles, permitting inflow of sodium ions and subsequent outflow of potassium ions which depolarize the postsynaptic terminal, thus propagating the impulse along the axon. If the chemical liberated is insufficient to depolarize the postsynaptic terminal, it may still give rise to a local change, an *excitatory postsynaptic potential* (EPSP), making it possible for the neuron to fire more readily in the event the next stimulus arrives soon after the first. This condition is known as *temporal summation*, and refers to repeated activity in the same presynaptic terminal, usually taking place within a period of 15 milliseconds. However, *spatial summation* occurs when a number of excitatory presynaptic terminals are excited at the same time, resulting in a progressive increase in postsynaptic potential, causing propagation of the nerve impulse.

Inhibition results from the secretion at the synaptic vesicles of an *inhibitory transmitter* substance which increases the permeability of the neuron, not to sodium ions, as would be necessary for facilitation, but to potassium and chloride ions instead. This leads to what is known as an *inhibitory postsynaptic potential* (IPSP). For the effective inhibition of impulses in the central nervous system, short *interneurons* are employed; their importance cannot be overemphasized, because they permit the elimination of unwanted stimuli and the selection of purposeful ones from the great bombardment of incoming nerve impulses. An attractive example— covered in more detail in Chapter 4—involves the concept of *reciprocal inhibition* (or reciprocal innervation). In the process of completing a stretch reflex, collateral impulses are transmitted to an interneuron whose function is to cause inhibition of those impulses that would travel to antagonistic muscles. The reader can quickly envision the confusion that would ensue if, in the course of purposeful movement, unwanted muscle activity were not screened out. Further thought will reveal that coordination must be intimately involved in such concepts, that learning to perform a motor act lies not only in obtaining effective muscle innervation, but also in eliminating extraneous and even harmful actions.

TRANSMISSION OF THE NERVE IMPULSE:
THE SPIKE POTENTIAL

The primary function of neurons is to convey changes in electrical potential across the cell membrane and to bring the wave of excitation to a receptor organ. This receptor organ may be a muscle or a gland, or it may be the central nervous system (CNS) itself. The *peripheral nervous system* is composed of sensory and motor nerves. The former, called *afferent* neurons, conduct impulses toward the CNS, while the latter, *efferent* neurons, conduct information outward. Still others, referred to previously as interneurons, remain within the central nervous system, operating as relay systems to connect various levels and portions of the intricate electrical system that controls human nervous function.

Active Transport

Before we consider the actual details of ion distribution and depolarization, it may be helpful to know something about *active transport*. We know from physics and chemistry, for example, that gas molecules diffuse from a point of high pressure to one of low and that the reverse of this would be highly unlikely, so that when it comes to respiratory gases, one can usually predict the direction of movement. This is not always true of the components of the *intracellular fluid*, the fluid inside the cells of the body, and the *extracellular fluid*, the fluid outside the cells. Two substances of importance to cell-membrane transport are *sodium* and *potassium*, and their concentrations are vital to this discussion. For example, the extracellular fluid contains large quantities of sodium, but the intracellular fluid contains only small amounts. The opposite is true for potassium, the intracellular fluid containing the largest amount, the extracellular fluid less. Also present in abundance outside the cell is *chloride*, with smaller concentrations inside. Chloride ions are not freely diffusible through the cell membrane. As we shall see, the resting state in nerve cells requires that sodium ions (Na^+) be continuously extruded from the cell against a rather large concentration gradient. The process that the cell employs in moving molecules against an electrochemical gradient is called active transport, a process which requires the expenditure of energy.

Resting Membrane Potential

When a microelectrode is placed inside the axon, its potential can be compared with one placed in the extracellular fluid. This will reveal that the interior of the axon is some 70 to 90 millivolts (mv) negative with respect to the exterior. The cause is the concentration of ions on either side of the cell membrane. This relative distribution, illustrated in Figure 3, shows that the outside contains relatively large amounts of sodium (Na^+) and chloride ions (Cl^-), but a small amount of potassium (K^+). The reverse is true for the inside, where additional large numbers of anions (A^-) are also present as well. These anions (negatively charged ions), which include phosphate ions, sulfate ions, and protein ions, are not freely diffusible through the nerve membrane, and so their function is rather passive. So-called sodium and potassium pumps actively extrude sodium to the exterior

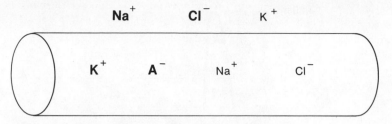

Figure 3. Resting Membrane Potential.

and potassium to the interior against their concentration gradients, a process described above as one of active transport. The net resting membrane potential averages approximately —85 mv and is known as the *resting potential*. Figure 4 illustrates the position of charges across the membrane, with positive charges on the exterior and negative charges on the inside.

The Action Potential

The resting cell membrane is said to be polarized. When the axon is stimulated, its surface potential reverses in polarity and a nerve impulse is propagated. The membrane quickly returns to its resting state, but the sequence has produced an *action potential*, sometimes called a *spike potential*, which is the nerve impulse. The action potential is represented in Figure 5. The resting potential is suddenly reversed so that it becomes positive, then quickly returns. The entire duration probably is no longer than .5 msec. The process results in uneven phases, called *negative* and *positive after-potentials*, which will be described below. The outcome is that by means of a succession of *local circuits* the action potential is propagated along the length of the axon at speeds of up to 100 meters per second in some nerves.

The specific ionic events that accompany the action potential are reflected in Figure 6. The arrival of the nerve impulse causes a rapid in-

Figure 4. Arrangement of Charges on the Membrane of an Axon.

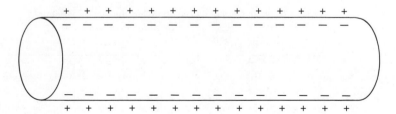

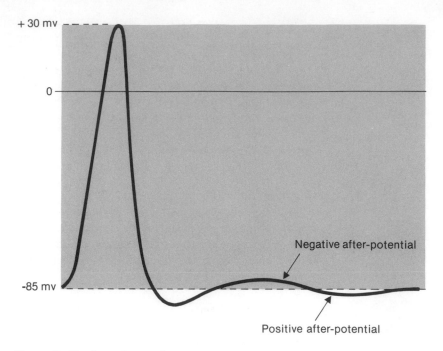

Figure 5. The Action Potential.

crease in *sodium conductance* across the membrane barrier, which increases the number of positive ions inside the axon, a factor which is monitored electrically by the rising portion of the spike (Figure 5). There is a gradual decrease in the influx of sodium and a gradual outflow of potassium, which soon takes over and becomes dominant. Thus, the spike descends as the outside of the membrane becomes positive once again. During the neuron's inactive period the sodium and potassium are restored to their appropriate locations by the sodium and potassium pumps.

The *negative after-potential*, shown in Figure 5, a condition in which the membrane is less negative than normal, follows directly after the spike and results from a deposition of K^+ outside the membrane, leaving their concentration inside the cell slightly less than normal. During this brief period the membrane is somewhat hyperexcitable. Subsequently, there is

Figure 6. Ionic Changes Accompanying the Action Potential.

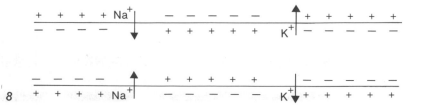

a period of *positive after-potential*, caused by the sodium pump's putting Na⁺ to the outside of the nerve cell, and the membrane becomes subnormal in excitability.

In this manner the wave of excitability passes along the axon cylinder from one node of Ranvier to the next, as in Figure 7. This method of propagation, in which the active process leaps from node to node, is termed *saltatory conduction*, and is appropriate for description of nerve conduction in myelinated fibers. This mode of activity helps explain why the nerve impulse in myelinated fibers is faster than in unmyelinated fibers, since it can skip along the axon in greater steps. Actually, the wave of excitation may pass in both directions along the axon, but if stimulation is given somewhere along the motor nerve and passes back toward the central nervous system, synapses there will prevent further action. Action potentials, however, can be caused by various mechanisms, including such things as heat, cold, chemical changes, or mechanical pressures.

Characteristics of the Action Potential

Once the exciting stimulus reaches a threshold of intensity for that nerve fiber, it creates an action potential. Further increase in the intensity of stimulus fails to increase the size of the deflection. Either the single fiber does not respond with a spike or it does so to its maximum ability. This phenomenon is known as the *all-or-none law*. The magnitude of current that is just sufficient to excite either a nerve or a muscle is called the *rheobase*; the length of time a current twice the rheobase must be applied to produce a response is known as the *chronaxie*. This relationship is presented in Figure 8. Chronaxie studies are widely used in physical therapy as a means for evaluating the excitability of tissue, and this measure has been used as a clinical index of denervation and reinnervation of muscle in human patients.

During a short interval following the passage of an action potential, no stimulus, no matter how strong, can initiate a new impulse. This is known as the *absolute refractory period*. For the next few milliseconds there is a *relative refractory period*, during which it is possible for a second action potential to be obtained. However, there is a greater than normal threshold for this new stimulus, and the response that is obtained is smaller than usual. The refractory periods occur as a result of the temporary disruption of the sodium and potassium carrier mechanism, caused by the

Figure 7. Local Circuit Theory in Myelinated Fibers.

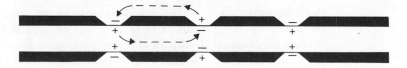

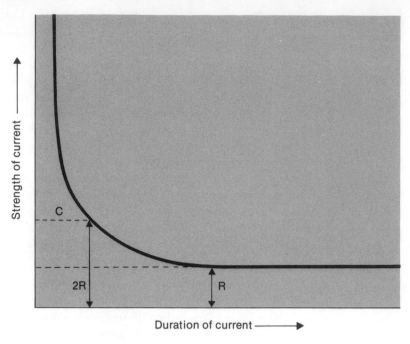

Figure 8. Strength-Duration Curves.

first action potential. Gradually, the fiber returns to full capability. The size of this capability may be realized when one considers that some large-diameter fibers can conduct 1,000 impulses per second, performing their task intermittently so as to reduce fatigue.

EXCITATION-CONTRACTION COUPLING

The primary task of the motor nerve is to cause a muscular contraction, yet we must consider the process only half complete with a successful excitation of the neuron. The next stage is to learn how the action potential can exert its influence on the muscle fiber membrane. This process is called *excitation-contraction coupling.*

The Neuromuscular Junction

The motor nerve fiber loses its myelin sheath as it approaches a striated muscle fiber to form a *motor end plate*, or *neuromuscular junction.* A single motor axon divides into several branches to innervate a number of muscle fibers (multiple innervation), but essentially the same sequence of events occurs with each of the neuromuscular junctions. The terminal branch of the axon becomes somewhat enlarged as it makes contact with the muscle fiber membrane, as shown in Figure 9. The muscle fiber is

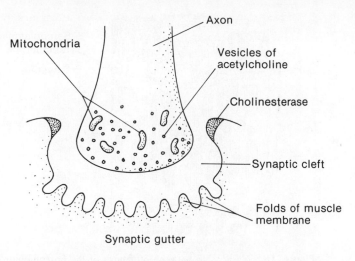

Figure 9. The Neuromuscular Junction.

actually separated from the axon by a space called the *synaptic cleft*, at the bottom of which are folds constituting the *postsynaptic membrane*. This terminal branch of the axon contains a large number of vesicles.

The arrival of the nerve impulse causes the release of *acetylcholine* (ACh), which diffuses to the motor end plate and depolarizes the surface membrane of the muscle fiber, setting up a *muscle action potential*. This in turn leads to muscle contraction. Acetylcholine is rapidly destroyed by the enzyme *cholinesterase*, which is located on the postsynaptic membrane. Thus, ACh remains in contact with the membrane of the muscle fiber for only about 2 milliseconds, but this is sufficient for it to change the permeability of the sarcolemma, the muscle cell membrane.

The arrival of the nerve impulse across the neuromuscular junction causes a *wave of excitation* to pass the length of the muscle fiber. This electrical activity can be monitored by an instrument known as an *electromyograph*—an especially valuable tool in the biomechanics field for obtaining quantitative measures of action potentials resulting from the excitation process.

The Sarcotubular System

The muscle is supported by yet another system, which aids in the transmission of the electrical signal and provides an important activating substance for the muscle contractile mechanism. It consists of *tubules* that run transversely and longitudinally throughout the muscle fiber, known collectively as the *sarcotubular system*.

The sarcotubular system consists of two types of tubules, each apparently performing a somewhat separate function. The first is the *sarcoplasmic reticulum* (the endoplasmic reticulum of the muscle cell), which

11

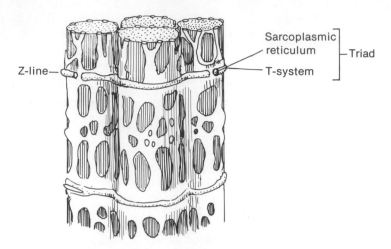

Figure 10. Relationship between Structures of the Sarcotubular System.
[K. R. Porter and M. A. Bonneville, *Fine Structure of Cells and Tissues.*
Philadelphia: Lea & Febiger (1968), p. 150.]

constitutes some 4 to 8 percent of the fiber volume, occupies the sarcoplasm
between myofibrils, and envelops each of the contractile elements of the
myofibrils, the sarcomeres. The structure of the muscle fiber will be explained in detail in Chapter 2. The second system is a transverse series of

Figure 11. The Sarcotubular System. [G. Hoyle, "How Is Muscle Turned
On and Off?" *Scientific American*, 222 (April 1970), p. 87.]

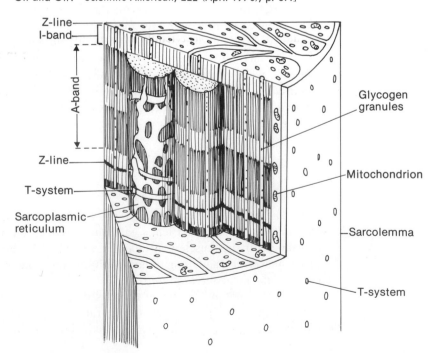

tubules, the *T-system*, which passes transversely through the fiber, forming almost a grid through which the myofibrils can pass. The relationship between these elements of the sarcotubular system is reflected in Figure 10. At one point (the Z-line of the sarcomere), two portions of the sarcoplasmic reticulum come together with a transverse tubule to form a *triad*. The T-system opens to the exterior of the fiber and provides an avenue down which the wave of depolarization can spread. The sarcoplasmic reticulum does not penetrate the cell membrane, nor does it connect with the T-system. Instead, its terminal cisternae bind the muscle activating substance (calcium) where it can be released upon arrival of the electrical excitation. The sarcotubular system is shown in Figure 11 in relationship to the contractile elements it supports.

SUMMARY

The nerve impulse is transmitted by the motor neuron, which for peripheral nerves is myelinated, is of varying lengths and diameters, and carries messages from the central nervous system to various receptor organs. The resting axon of a motor neuron is negative inside with respect to the outside, with relatively large amounts of sodium ions on the outer surface and potassium ions on the inner surface. Stimulation of the cell membrane causes a reversal of polarity, with sodium flowing inward during the rising portion of the spike potential. This is followed quickly by an outflow of potassium, restoring the resting state of the axon and propagating the action potential. At the myoneural junction the arrival of the nerve impulse causes release of acetylcholine, depolarizing the muscle cell membrane, setting up a muscle action potential, and resulting in a wave of excitation in the muscle fiber. This signals the release of calcium from the sarcoplasmic reticulum, which in turn activates the muscle contractile mechanism.

SELECTED REFERENCES

Aidley, D. J., *The Physiology of Excitable Cells*. Cambridge: Cambridge University Press, 1971.

Eccles, Sir John, "The Synapse," *Scientific American*, 212 (January 1965), 56.

Guyton, Arthur C., *Textbook of Medical Physiology*, 4th ed. Philadelphia: W. B. Saunders Company, 1971, chaps. 4–6.

Hoyle, Graham, "How Is Muscle Turned On and Off?" *Scientific American*, 222 (April 1970), 84.

Katz, Bernard, *Nerve, Muscle, and Synapse*. New York: McGraw-Hill Book Company, 1966.

Loofbourrow, G. N., "Neuromuscular Integration," in Warren R. Johnson, ed., *Science and Medicine of Exercise and Sports*. New York: Harper & Row, 1960, chap. 6.

Page, Sally, "Structure of the Sarcoplasmic Reticulum in Vertebrate Muscle," *British Medical Bulletin*, 24 (1968), 170.

Peachey, Lee D., "Transverse Tubules in Excitation-Contraction Coupling," *Federation Proceedings*, 24 (September–October 1965), 1124.

Porter, Keith R., and Mary A. Bonneville, *Fine Structure of Cells and Tissues*. Philadelphia: Lea & Febiger, 1968.

chapter 2

skeletal muscle

It has been argued that the single most important topic in the field of exercise physiology is the muscular system. While it is indeed true that muscles will fail to function normally if innervation is withheld or if the circulation is impaired, the fact remains that the total organism is put into motion and remains there because of the action of skeletal muscles. In a very real sense, then, it is essential that the structure and function of muscles be understood in some detail, so that an adequate explanation may be available concerning practical matters of exercise and training. This chapter will deal with factors surrounding the structure and function of skeletal muscle.

STRUCTURE OF MUSCLE

The student of kinesiology will immediately recognize that human skeletal muscles are arranged in a variety of configurations, depending upon the function for which they are intended. It is common to think of muscle as being composed of fibers that seem to run directly from tendon to tendon, such as in the biceps brachii, but in reality a large number of muscles in the human body are small, with their fibers arranged in a variety of ways. In one example, the *longitudinal type*, the fibers run approximately parallel to the long axis of the muscle, although they may not reach the entire distance covered by the muscle. In the longissimus muscle, for instance, the fibers need not be very long, running from the spinous processes of vertebrae to the transverse process and lateral surfaces of the ribs, a distance of only a few inches.

Several variations of the *penniform* type are illustrated in Figure 12. In the *unipennate* form, the fibers approach the tendon from only one side, as occurs with the tibialis posterior muscle, while the *bipennate* muscle has fibers converging on both sides of the tendon, as illustrated by the rectus femoris muscle. An example of the *multipennate* muscle is shown by the deltoid, where internal collagenous sheets divide the muscle into three parts, thus providing a mixture of the first two pennate forms. The advantage gained by these variations is easily seen, as there is provided a means for initiating movement, particularly for joints that may be involved with large masses, such as the trunk where the surface area is large, or in

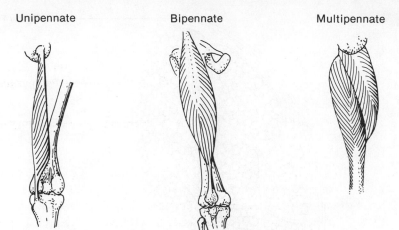

| Unipennate | Bipennate | Multipennate |

Figure 12. Variations of Fiber Arrangements. [D. L. Kelley, *Kinesiology: Fundamentals of Motion Description*. Englewood Cliffs, N.J.: Prentice-Hall, Inc. (1971), p. 147.]

other specialized areas of the body where range of motion may not be great. One can compare the function of the trapezius with that of the biceps to realize the great differences in joint function that are served. The fact that the fibers in penniform muscles shorten less than longitudinal muscles probably only attests to the types of functions they are intended to serve.

The contractile portion of the muscle gradually gives way to connective tissue, which is continuous with the tendons of origin and insertion, and forms a rigid adherence to bone so that it may bear the full tension of contraction. As the structure of the tendon interweaves with the muscle, the collagenous threads form a network that binds the muscle itself together without interfering either with contraction or the fiber arrangement. Figure 13 illustrates in cross-sectional form the gradually increasing size of the connective tissue. The individual fibers are surrounded by *endomysium*, and a group of as many as 150 individual fibers, called a *fasciculus*, is bound together by *perimysium*. The whole muscle is encased in a connective tissue sheath called the *epimysium*.

FIBER CHARACTERISTICS

In order to understand the complexities of total muscle contraction, it is first necessary to understand the detailed characteristics of the muscle fiber. Since the thrust of exercise physiology necessarily implies external work and usually movement, the discussion will be restricted to skeletal muscle, rather than smooth muscle or cardiac muscle, although the latter will receive special attention in Chapter 10.

As noted in Figure 13, skeletal muscles are composed of rather large

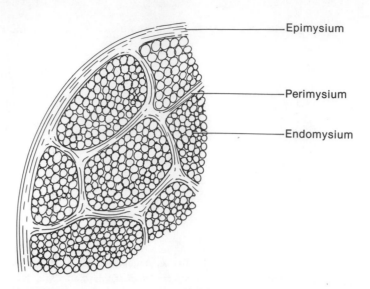

Figure 13. Cross-Section of a Small Portion of Muscle, Showing Relative Size of Connective Tissue. [J. R. Bendall, *Muscles, Molecules and Movement*. New York: American Elsevier Publishing Company Inc. (1971), p. xviii.]

numbers of fibers, amounting in large muscles to many thousands. In fact, individual fiber count of an older adult engaged in a lifetime of hard work revealed that the biceps contained over 316,000 fibers, arranged in more than 3,300 fascicles.[1] This would leave nearly 100 fibers to each fasciculus for that muscle. The fibers themselves range in size from 10 to 100 microns in diameter (.01 to .10 mm or 100,000 to 1,000,000 Å),[2] and are surrounded by the *sarcolemma*, the muscle cell membrane found just beneath the endomysium.

It is not the individual fiber *per se* that is crucial to understanding of the contraction characteristics of muscle so much as it is the constituency of the fiber. Figure 14 illustrates the progressively smaller subdivisions that can be dissected from an individual muscle (a). The fibers (b) have the striated appearance that characterizes skeletal muscle, and a single fiber (c) is composed of a number of *myofibrils*. The myofibril (d) can be further resolved into a series of repeating light and dark patterns known as *sarcomeres* (e). The sarcomere reveals that it consists of protein microfilaments, the thin filaments of *actin* and the thick filaments of *myosin* (f).

The sarcomere is further illustrated in Figure 15, an electron micrograph of the leg muscle of a frog. The persistent striations of the myofibrils result in a repeated pattern of light and dark areas. The less dense filaments

---

[1] A. A. Etemadi and F. Hosseini, "Frequency and Size of Muscle Fibers in Athletic Body Build," *Anatomical Record*, 162 (November 1968), 269.

[2] Note: Å = angstrom = 10^{-7} mm or one 10,000th micron.

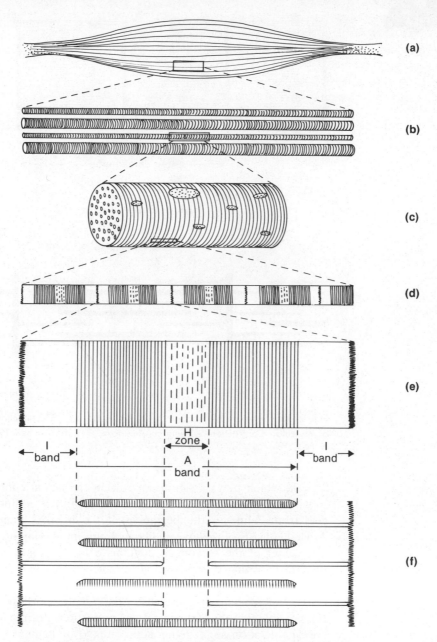

Figure 14. Ultrastructure of Skeletal Muscle. [H. E. Huxley, "The Contraction of Muscle," *Scientific American*, 199 (November 1958), p. 68.]

of actin form a light zone, called the *I-band*, and the thicker filaments of myosin, which includes some overlapping by actin, form the more dense *A-band*. The actin filaments themselves arise from a membrane called the *Z-line*, which clearly marks the boundary between adjacent sarcomeres. The Z-membrane, in addition to actin, contains another protein, *tropo-*

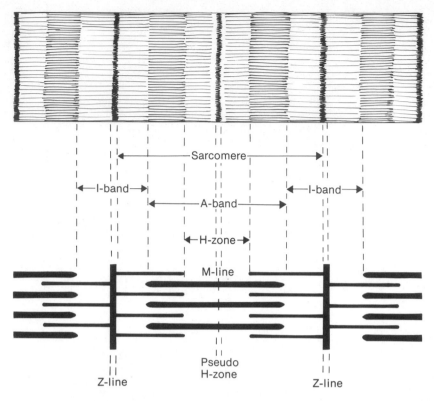

Figure 15. Structure of the Sarcomere. [H. E Huxley, "The Mechanism of Muscular Contraction," *Scientific American*, 213 (December 1965), p. 18.]

myosin, which plays a significant role in the actual contraction sequence, as will be seen subsequently. Thus, the I-band is composed of actin and goes from Z-line to the beginning of the myosin filament, whereas the A-band consists of the myosin filament plus an overlapping portion of actin. The center of the sarcomere contains a lighter zone, called the *H-zone*, the size of which depends upon muscle length, or the extent of overlap of thick and thin filaments. In the center of the H-zone is a region of low density, the *pseudo H-zone*, and a dark center portion called the *M-line*. It is possible that the M-line contains projections not made of myosin which are capable of linking together adjacent myosin filaments.[3]

While it is attractive to present the structure of muscle almost in two-dimensional array, it should be stressed that muscle fibers, and therefore their myofibrils, are packed in rather high density as bundles, and hence should be thought of as three-dimensional. In fact, the thick and

[3]Frank A. Pepe, "Some Aspects of the Structural Organization of the Myofibril as Revealed by Antibody-Staining Methods," *Journal of Cell Biology*, 28 (1966), 505.

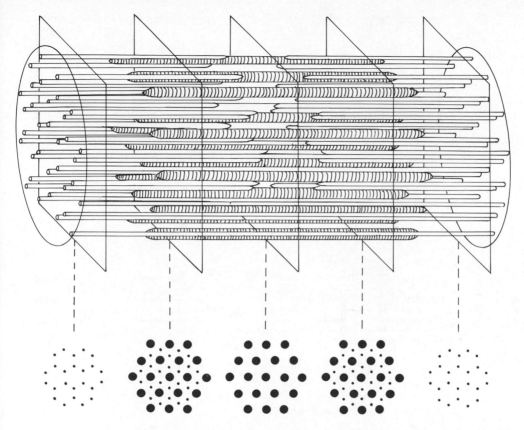

Figure 16. Relationship of Actin to Myosin. [H. E. Huxley, "The Contraction of Muscle," *Scientific American*, 199 (November 1958), p. 70.]

thin filaments are arranged in a six-sided (hexagonal) pattern, as shown in Figure 16. In the region of overlap, which occurs in the A-band, the actin filament lies between three myosin filaments. Stated in another way, it can be seen that myosin lies symmetrically between six actin filaments. The question, then, centers around what characteristics actin and myosin have that permit the sarcomere to shorten during contraction.

Evidence is quite conclusive that projections, called *cross-bridges*, exist on myosin at regular intervals. Figure 17 illustrates the recurring position of the cross-bridges which makes it feasible for myosin to contact the actin filaments on six sides. Thus, at a given level on myosin, two of the cross-bridges project directly opposite each other. Rotating 60 degrees, the next set of projections occurs 143 Å lower, continuing in this manner until finally the pattern repeats itself. This makes it possible for the myosin filament to interdigitate with the actin filament, which in turn is thought to have receptive "active sites." Actin, however, consists of beadlike molecules connected together in a double helical form, as shown in Fig-

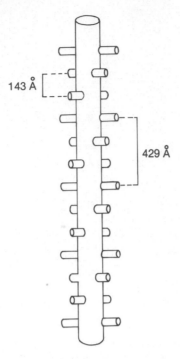

143 Å

429 Å

Figure 17. The Projections on the Myosin Filaments. [H. E. Huxley and W. Brown, "The Low-Angle X-Ray Diagram of Vertebrate Striated Muscle and its Behaviour during Contraction and Rigor," *Journal of Molecular Biology*, 30 (1967), p. 394.]

ure 18. Presumably, this arrangement would make it possible for actin to present the active sites to a variety of myosin filaments. The myosin molecule, on the other hand, consists of two parts, a head and a tail, as illustrated in Figure 19. The tails, more appropriately termed *light meromyosin* (LMM), become attached to each other to form a filament, and the heads, known as *heavy meromyosin* (HMM), project from the body of the filament. The HMM has the ability to interdigitate with actin, while LMM does not. Note that the heads on the two sides of the filament oppose each other, with a projection-free area in the center; this corresponds to the pseudo H-zone, a region of especially low density. It will soon become clear that the placement of HMM in this manner makes it possible for effective shortening of the sarcomere to take place.

THE SLIDING-FILAMENT MODEL OF CONTRACTION

The most widely accepted model to explain the contraction of muscle is embodied into the sliding-filament concept. The major occurrence is for the Z-lines of the sarcomere to be drawn in toward the A-band, gradually narrowing and finally even eliminating the I-band, but without

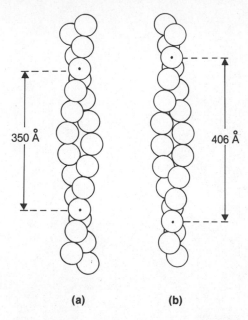

350 Å   406 Å

(a)   (b)

Figure 18. Arrangement of the Actin Filaments. Note two possible arrangements involving either thirteen (a) or fifteen (b) monomers per unit of the actin helix. [J. Hanson and J. Lowy, "The Structure of Actin Filaments and the Origin of the Axial Periodicity in the I-Substance of Vertebrate Striated Muscle," *Proceedings of the Royal Society* B, 160 (1964), p. 450.]

changing the length of the A-band. In this manner, the myosin filaments of the A-band retain a constant length, and the actin filaments are thought to slide over the myosin as the sarcomere approaches full shortening, perhaps even overlapping near the center of the sarcomere, as shown in Figure 20. Theoretically, this overlapping would place the actin filaments on the one side in the way of effective movement on the other, and has been suggested as a possible explanation for the loss in tension experienced by muscles contracting in a shortened position.[4] At any rate, the sliding is caused by a series of reactions between the HMM and the active sites on the actin filaments, so that the actin filament is pulled along, permitting the HMM to be released for reattachment at another site further along. It should be noted that the direction of pull is different on either side of the M-line, so that the movement of the actin filaments is always toward the center in each sarcomere. Thus, the tension produced becomes proportional to the number of cross-bridges that can be formed between the A- and I-filaments. Acting in concert, the entire isometric tension of the muscle will be determined by the total number of interdigitating elements that are brought into play.

[4]H. E. Huxley, "The Mechanism of Muscular Contraction," *Scientific American*, 213 (December 1965), 18.

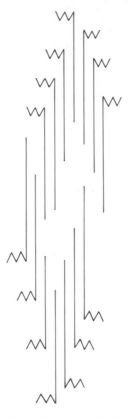

Figure 19. The Myosin Molecule. [H. E. Huxley, "Structural Arrangements and the Contraction Mechanism in Striated Muscle," *Proceedings of the Royal Society* B, 160 (1964), p. 444.]

A MOLECULAR THEORY OF CONTRACTION

In order to bring the known elements of contraction together to form an integrated theory that not only explains the mechanical aspects of contraction but accounts for the energization process as well is a difficult task, since all aspects of the mechanism are not presently known. However, an important theory has been proposed which attempts to account for the movement of myosin heads as they move actin toward the center of the A-band.[5] This model, when modified slightly,[6] helps us understand the contraction sequence.

The major premise upon which this theory rests is that an electrostatic bond is formed between the HMM of myosin and the actin filament, the latter of which contains, in addition to actin, *troponin* and *tropomyosin*.

[5] R. E. Davies, "A Molecular Theory of Muscle Contraction: Calcium-Dependent Contractions with Hydrogen Bond Formation Plus ATP-Dependent Extensions of Part of the Myosin-Actin Cross-Bridges," *Nature,* 199 (September 14, 1963), 1069.

[6] J. R. Bendall, *Muscles, Molecules and Movement* (New York: American Elsevier Publishing Company, Inc., 1971), pp. 193–200.

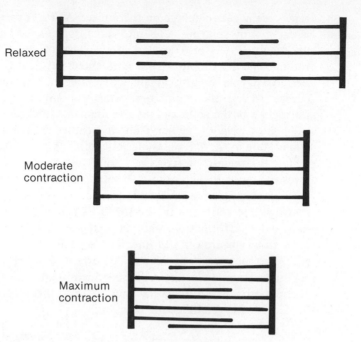

Relaxed

Moderate contraction

Maximum contraction

Figure 20. The Shortening of the Sarcomere.

In the presence of *calcium* (Ca^{++}), the HMM contracts, pulls the actin along one step, and then reextends for a second cycle. Schematically, this can be represented as in Figure 21. Ionized *adenosine triphosphate* (ATP), a high-energy compound, is present at the end of the HMM, bearing a negative charge. At the base of the HMM is a fixed negative charge, which

Figure 21. Schematic Arrangement of H-Meromyosin. [R. E. Davies, "A Molecular Theory of Muscle Contraction: Calcium-Dependent Contractions with Hydrogen Bond Formation Plus ATP-Dependent Extensions of Part of the Myosin-Actin Cross-Bridges," *Nature*, 199 (1963), p. 1069.]

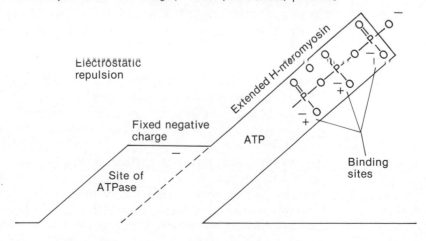

Electrostatic repulsion

Fixed negative charge

Extended H-meromyosin

ATP

Binding sites

Site of ATPase

L-meromyosin

repels the negative charge on the ionized ATP. The enzyme ATPase which is capable of splitting ATP into *adenosine diphosphate* (ADP) and free phosphate (Pi) is also located at the base of the HMM, so that in the resting state this mobile HMM is extented, repelled by the similar charges. Bound ADP is present at an active site on actin and bears a negative charge. At rest, the complex of actin, troponin, and tropomyosin prevents interaction of the actin and myosin filaments, and relaxation is maintained.

The arrival of the nerve impulse causes the release of Ca^{++} from its bound state in the sarcoplasmic reticulum, as explained in Chapter 1. This signals the release of free Ca^{++}, and by some reaction involving tropomyosin, troponin binds the Ca^{++} and removes the inhibition, permitting the liberated calcium ions to attach to the negative charge on the cross-bridge site of actin and the HMM. This forms an electrostatic depolarization and link formation, and the extended HMM contracts, moving the actin along towards the M-line. The sequences can be seen in Figure 22.

The contraction of the mobile portion of the HMM brings the ionized ATP into the range of the ATPase, which breaks the ATP down into ADP and a phosphate ion, releasing energy. Thus, the energization sequence can be visualized in the following reaction:

$$ATP \rightleftharpoons ADP + Pi + \text{free energy};\qquad (2\text{-}1)$$

the bond is then broken between actin and myosin filaments. The ATP is quickly replenished by a fresh molecule of cytoplasmic ATP and the negative charge to the end of the HMM is restored. This results in electrostatic repulsion with the fixed negative charge and causes the HMM to be extended. As long as calcium ions are still present, the cycle will repeat itself, but during relaxation, when calcium is withdrawn into the sarcoplasmic reticulum, the HMM remains extended, and no electrostatic attraction occurs. In fact, special changes occur in the myofibrils themselves, which involve not only troponin and tropomyosin, but magnesium (Mg^{++}) and ATP as well (MgATP). The role of magnesium seems to be that of binding ATP to myosin. The details of relaxation are not as clear as those of contraction, but the reader will find references in the literature to a *relaxing factor system* which accounts for the return of the sarcomere to resting length.

The amount of tension generated by each sarcomere is understandably small and will not be constant, because it will depend upon the amount of overlap of actin and myosin filaments. Increasing the number of myosin heads that can come into contact with actin will, up to a point, increase the amount of active tension that can be developed. The reactions described above occur at a rate of perhaps 100 cycles per second, so when it is realized that each myofibril contains a large number of sarcomeres, and each fiber contains a number of myofibrils, and, finally, the motor unit contains several muscle fibers, we see that, taken together, the maximum muscle tension must depend upon activating the largest number of sarcomeres through innervation of the greatest number of motor units. Whole-muscle tension development will be described in the next chapter.

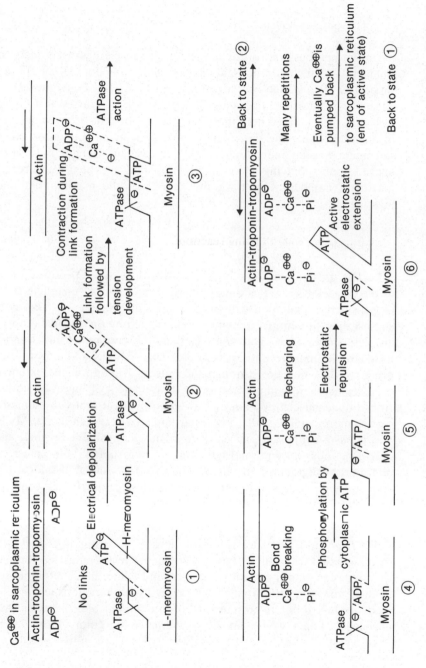

Figure 22. Sequence of Reactions of H-Meromyosin and Actin. [R. E. Davies, "A Molecular Theory of Muscle Contraction: Calcium-Dependent Contractions with Hydrogen Bond-Formation Plus ATP-Dependent Extensions of Part of the Myosin–Actin Cross-Bridges," *Nature,* 199 (1963), p. 1068.]

Nervous Regulation

The nervous control for activation of muscle has been dealt with in Chapter 1, so it should be clear that normally functioning muscle must be supported by adequate nerve supply. Some of the consequences of inadequate or interrupted action potentials will be discussed in Chapter 13. It should be reiterated here that since the motor unit behaves on the basis of an *all-or-none law*, no direct procedure can be found for increasing sarcomere tension individually. Any increase in strength must therefore depend upon supplying nerve impulses of sufficient intensity to recruit the maximum number of motor units, and thus, the maximum number of muscle fibers.

Circulation

The great importance of the circulation to the effective functioning of the muscular system cannot be ignored, and a more complete treatment of peripheral circulation will be presented in Chapter 11. This is not to suggest that the central circulation, represented by the cardiac output, is of any less importance. The point is that, for continuing functioning, the local muscles must receive appropriate oxygen supply and removal of waste products via blood flow through the muscle. Therefore, the extent of the *capillary network* is important to the development of muscular endurance. In addition, muscles contain *myoglobin*, a pigment that can combine with oxygen more readily, and at lower partial pressures, than blood. Myoglobin may act as a temporary oxygen store in muscle, available in small amounts during periods when normal flow may be interrupted. Some muscles contain more myoglobin than others, and therefore under histologic examination appear redder. It is felt that such muscles are better equipped for endurance activity than the paler muscles, whose function seems better suited for more rapid, hence anaerobic, action.

Fiber Types. The reader should be aware of terminology that is in use to designate various fiber types in human skeletal muscle. Rather than simply designating muscle fibers as red and white, it is preferable to refer to their *fast twitch* (FT) and *slow twitch* (ST) characteristics. While both types are mixed in human muscles,[7] a predominance of one over the other may exist, which would impart a characteristic color. More important, however, is the fact that the FT fibers (white) are more capable of high

[7]P. D. Gollnick *et al.*, "Enzyme Activity and Fiber Composition in Skeletal Muscle of Untrained and Trained Men," *Journal of Applied Physiology*, 33 (September 1972), 312.

speed activity of short duration, while the ST fibers (red) seem better able to sustain more long term endurance activity. The reason for this difference is that the FT fibers have high myosin ATPase activity and high glycolytic capacity, while the ST fibers have low myosin ATPase activity and low glycolytic capacity. Translated into functional terms, this means that the ST fibers are best suited for long term endurance activity, and the FT fibers for high speed or sudden muscular contraction. The role played by glycolytic activity will become more clear in Chapter 5.

Energization

The matter of energy supply, a central issue in the study of exercise physiology, will be dealt with more fully in Chapter 5. The primary energy source is various foodstuffs in the diet, and the energy released is converted to ATP. Thus, the ATP is an essential ingredient in the metabolism of cells and, of course, the contraction of sarcomeres. The release of energy and consequent production of ADP [equation (2-1)] stimulates the re-synthesis of ATP. This is accomplished by *creatine phosphate* (CP), according to the following reaction:

$$ADP + CP \rightleftharpoons ATP + \text{creatine.} \tag{2–2}$$

Since a major source of energy is carbohydrates in the diet, the presence of *glycogen* in muscle is of major importance. It will be seen in Figure 10 in Chapter 1 that glycogen granules are intimately associated with the myofibrils, hence are a primary source of energy. Since the major portion of ATP will eventually be extracted in the *mitochondria*, it is also interesting to note their ready supply in the cytoplasm of the cell supporting the myofibrils.

HEAT PRODUCTION IN MUSCLE

The contraction of muscle causes the production of heat to increase greatly beyond resting values. This increase of heat takes place in conjunction with the events that precede contraction, the rise in tension brought on during isometric contractions or the shortening phase of isotonic contractions, and finally the events associated with relaxation and recovery. Thus, there are four phases of heat production in muscle.

1. *Activation heat.* Activation heat is the heat production attributed to the dissociation of calcium from its bound state in the sarcoplasmic reticulum. It follows depolarization and precedes actual tension development, which means that it begins during the latent period.
2. *Shortening heat.* The heat generated during the shortening or contraction phase of an isotonic contraction is identified with bond formation of the H-meromyosin and actin filaments. This will continue during

the sliding of the actin along the myosin filaments as new links are formed. Shortening heat is independent of load but proportional to the distance of shortening. There may be additional *maintenance heat* produced during an isometric contraction, associated with ATP breakdown steadily, preventing the slipping of actin filaments.

3. *Relaxation heat.* In an isotonic contraction, relaxation heat occurs with lowering the load and lengthening of the muscle during the relaxation phase of an isotonic contraction. The need of the contractile filaments at this point is for a supply of ATP for the relaxing factor system. No heat of relaxation is found unless the muscle relaxes under load. Stated in another way, if the load cannot pull out the muscle after it has shortened, work done is not degraded into heat.

4. *Delayed heat.* The above phases of heat production correspond to Hill's[8] description of initial heat, and as such are associated with the contractile events themselves. Following this, however, the muscle liberates *delayed* or *recovery* heat once the mechanical events have been completed. Under aerobic conditions—that is, when oxygen is available in sufficient amounts during contraction—the oxidative delayed heat is approximately equal to initial heat and represents the oxidative processes of recovery, the resynthesis of high-energy phosphate compounds, thus restoring energy given off during the performance of work.

SUMMARY

Skeletal muscle fibers are arranged in the muscle longitudinally or in some variation of penniform types. The latter may be unipennate, bipennate, or multipennate. Individual fibers are surrounded by endomysium, a group of which is known as a fasciculus, and is bound together by perimysium. Finally, the entire muscle is encased in a connective tissue sheath, the epimysium. The muscle fiber is composed of a number of myofibrils which contain a series of contractile elements called sarcomeres. The sarcomeres in turn are made up of thin and thick filaments, known respectively as actin and myosin, and representing the repeated pattern of light and dark areas. The less dense filaments of actin make up the I-band, and the thick filaments of myosin form the A-band, the sarcomeres being separated from each other by a Z-line. Myosin lies between six actin filaments and contains projections of heavy meromyosin (HMM), which contact actin filaments at certain active sites. The sliding-filament theory proposes that during contraction myosin moves actin filaments toward the middle of the sarcomere, so that the Z-lines are drawn closer together and the I-band is eliminated. In molecular terms, an electrostatic bond is formed between the HMM and actin, the latter of which also contains troponin and tropomyosin, with bound ADP present at an active site. Ionized ATP is available at the end of the HMM, and ATPase is present at its base, so that no interaction takes place in the resting state

[8]A. V. Hill, "The Priority of the Heat Production in Muscle Twitch," *Proceedings of the Royal Society*, B 148 (1958), 397.

because actin, troponin, and tropomyosin prevent contraction. This is abolished with the release of calcium, and an electrostatic depolarization and link formation occurs, causing shortening of HMM and release of energy as the actin filament is moved along myosin. The contraction and relaxation process causes the production of heat, known as initial heat and recovery heat, corresponding to known molecular elements of the shortening process.

SELECTED REFERENCES

Aidley, D. J., *The Physiology of Excitable Cells*. Cambridge: Cambridge University Press, 1971.

Bendall, J. R., *Muscles, Molecules and Movement*. New York: American Elsevier Publishing Company, Inc., 1971.

Davies, R. E., "A Molecular Theory of Muscle Contraction: Calcium-Dependent Contractions with Hydrogen Bond Formation Plus ATP-Dependent Extensions of Part of the Myosin-Actin Cross-Bridges," *Nature*, 199 (September 14, 1963), 1068.

Hill, A. V., "The Priority of the Heat Production in a Muscle Twitch," *Proceedings of the Royal Society*, B 148 (1958), 397.

Huxley, H. E., "The Contraction of Muscle," *Scientific American* (November 1958), 67.

———, "The Mechanism of Muscular Contraction," *Science*, 164 (1969), 1356.

———, "The Mechanism of Muscular Contraction," *Scientific American*, 213 (December 1965), 18.

Hoyle, Graham, "How Is Muscle Turned On and Off?" *Scientific American*, 222 (April 1970), 84.

Kelley, David L., *Kinesiology: Fundamentals of Motion Description*. Englewood Cliffs, N.J.: Prentice-Hall, Inc., 1971.

chapter

3

mechanical
and
dynamic properties
of
muscle

A great deal is known about the various mechanical properties of muscle, as they have been favorite topics of physiologists for decades. Some of the characteristics to be described are so "classic" in nature that they have become suitable subjects for laboratory experiments in undergraduate physiology courses. These experiments are ordinarily conducted on isolated vertebrate muscle, such as that of the frog. Considerable progress has been made in learning about muscle tissue, but the crucial tests for human physiology will come when more complete information is available on muscle characteristics *in vivo*—that is, in the intact organism, not only with normal blood and nerve supply but with the muscle or group of muscles exerting tension through the usual muscle-tendon-joint complex. This chapter is devoted to such inquiry and will present a wide variety of topics, ending with a section on muscle training and hypertrophy.

LENGTH-TENSION CURVES

The amount of tension that a muscle can obtain depends upon its initial length. As shown in Figure 23, the maximum tension generated is not at resting length but when the muscle is slightly stretched beyond *equilibrium length*. A muscle that is foreshortened is at some disadvantage, as the amount of active tension produced becomes reduced. Even lengthening has its own built-in limitations, for excessive stretching can result in a decrement of active force. Considering the position of the actin and myosin filaments, one can understand how extreme stretching can place actin just out of reach of the myosin cross-bridges. The shortened sarcomere is also at a disadvantage, as discussed in Chapter 2. The lower curve in Figure 23 describes the tension produced when a resting muscle fiber is lengthened. The relationship between isometric tension and joint angle for the measurement of human elbow flexion is shown in Figure 24. Changing the joint angle effectively alters the muscle length, and for this particular test it reveals that 115 degrees is the most effective angle (most appropriate muscle length) for obtaining maximal tests of strength. Force drops off on either side of this value.

33

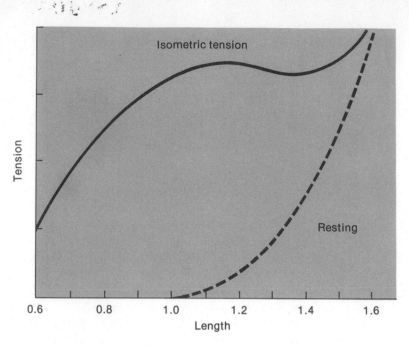

Figure 23. Length-Tension Curves.

FORCE-VELOCITY CURVE

The muscle has been examined for speed of shortening after being loaded. As shown in Figure 25, the relationship is curvilinear and has been found to be mathematically predictable.[1] The figure shows that when there is no load on the muscle, maximum velocity occurs. It also reveals that under essentially isometric conditions, where the velocity is zero, the force becomes maximal. It is difficult to load intact human muscles in quite the same way as the frog sartorius muscle, although the *force-time* curves of hand-gripping muscles have been examined when the muscles have adopted a preliminary tension varying from zero to 30 kg (66 lb). These curves are shown in Figure 26. There is a curvilinear (exponential) nature to these curves, also, the best force being obtained when the performer begins with very little or no preliminary tension. If he adopts some force to begin with, the velocity of contraction noticeably slows, and there is likely to be some reduction in the amount of maximum tension achieved.

ELASTICITY

For muscle to exert tension it must activate its contractile components, as discussed in Chapter 2. What may not be apparent is that the

[1]A. V. Hill, "The Heat of Shortening and the Dynamic Constants of Muscle," *Proceedings of the Royal Society*, B 126 (1938), 136.

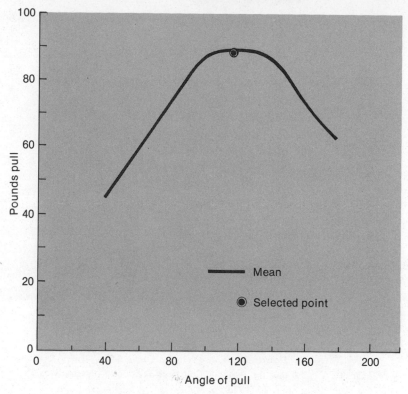

Figure 24. Elbow Flexion Strength Curve as a Function of Joint Angle.
[H. H. Clarke, *Muscular Strength and Endurance in Man.* Englewood
Cliffs, N.J.: Prentice-Hall, Inc. (1966), p. 47.]

effective force generated is dampened by viscoelastic properties of the muscle and tendon. These elements must first be overcome during the uptake of force. The result of their activity is a reduction in the force measured externally, as compared with actual forces created by the contractile elements themselves. These elastic components are arranged both in series and in parallel and represent the portions of the muscle that do not contract. These are shown in Figure 27, where their effects on tension can be seen.

The *series elastic component* is so named because the elastic elements occur directly in line with the contractile components; it is thought that these elastic elements are located in the tendons into which the muscle fibers are inserted, and are probably present at the Z-line region of the sarcomere. The *parallel elastic component* does not lie in series with the contractile mechanism, but in parallel, located specifically in the sarcolemma. Figure 27 illustrates the effect of this elasticity on effective tension. The contraction of the muscle imparts a given force, as illustrated in 35 (b), but this can be increased if, at the time of stimulation, the muscle is

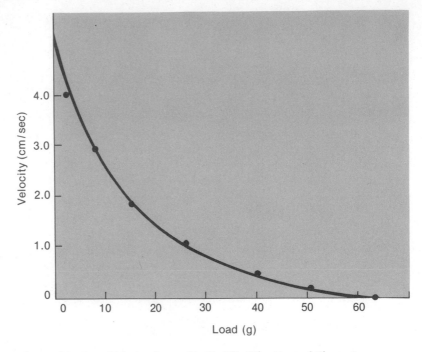

Figure 25. Force-Velocity Curve. [A. V. Hill, "The Heat of Shortening and the Dynamic Constants of Muscle," *Proceedings of the Royal Society* B, 126 (1938), p. 177.]

Figure 26. Force-Time Curves at Varying Preliminary Tensions. [D. H. Clarke, "Force-Time Curves of Voluntary Muscular Contraction at Varying Tensions," *Research Quarterly*, 39 (December 1968), p. 904.]

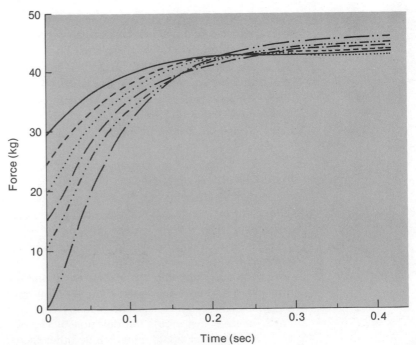

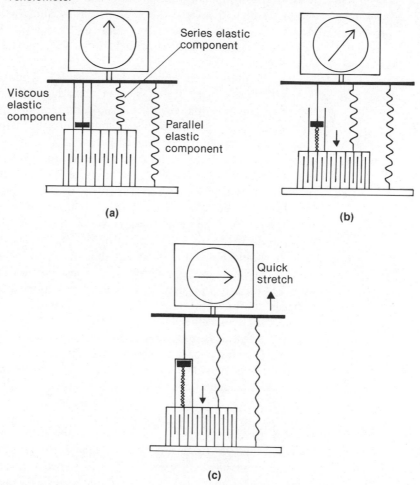

Tensiometer

Series elastic component

Viscous elastic component

Parallel elastic component

(a)

(b)

Quick stretch

(c)

Figure 27. Elastic Properties of Muscle. [G. Hoyle, "How Is Muscle Turned On and Off?" *Scientific American*, 222 (April 1970), p. 91.]

first given a quick stretch so as to pull out the elastic elements. The increase in measured tension, (c), results from the elimination of the elastic elements. These elements smooth out changes in tension, lessening to some degree the sudden force invoked by the act of contraction.

REACTION LATENCY

A term often employed in physical education and athletics is *reaction latency*, or *reaction time*. The latent period is the time elapsing between the onset of the stimulus and the initiation of response by the contractile mechanism. It represents the duration of the nerve impulse. The reaction time, on the other hand, may include other factors that makes its duration

37

somewhat longer than pure latency. The typical method of measuring re-action time is to present the subject with a stimulus, either auditory or visual, which starts a timer. As soon as the subject is able, he initiates some movement, which immediately stops the timer. The elapsed interval is reaction time (RT).

If the mass to be moved is large, the RT is longer than if the mass is small. Thus, finger RT is shorter than leg RT, because included in the measurement is time for the muscle contraction to move the mass of the limb involved. Since more motor units must be activated to move the heavier leg than the lighter finger, there will be a slight delay while this is being accomplished. This has led to use of the concept of premotor and motor reaction time,[2] in which we separate RT into two components, em-ploying an electromyograph to detect the instant that depolarization of the muscle cell membrane occurs. The *premotor time* is the time that elapses from the onset of the signal to initiation of the muscle action potential, and *motor time* is the time remaining for the actual response to be initiated.

It should also be pointed out that the onset of the signal is usually external, a sound or light stimulus, so some portion of the response time must be taken up with signal detection, to be followed by descending motor patterns to the appropriate body parts. Having the performer make a choice usually lengthens RT appreciably while he sorts out extraneous stimuli and decides upon the correct ones. Reaction time may be subject to some learning over a series of trials, the amount of this learning being greater if the individual must make a choice between alternatives in his response. The actual act of moving the body or its limbs is not a part of reaction time, since this is usually referred to as *movement time*. The time consumed by a ball carrier to the line of scrimmage is preceded by his reaction time; the time it takes for the action to be completed once it has been initiated is movement time. It may seem surprising, but a number of experiments indicate a low correlation between reaction time and move-ment time. In other words, an individual who has a fast reaction time does not necessarily have a fast movement time.

SUMMATION OF CONTRACTION

Strength of contraction can be increased in two different ways. Since the *motor unit* is the basic contractile entity, consisting of the motor nerve and all of the muscle fibers that it innervates, then it follows, first of all, that the force generated can be increased by bringing more motor units into play. However, a second factor involves the rate at which individual motor units are contracting. If a muscle stimulus is followed by a second one before the first is over, the total tension produced is increased. Thus,

[2]D. Lainé Santa Maria, "Pre-Motor and Motor Reaction Time Differences As-sociated with Stretching of the Hamstring Muscles," *Journal of Motor Behavior*, 2 (September 1970), 163.

increasing the rate of firing up to 60 per second successively increases the maximum tension, and is an example of *wave summation*. This principle is presented in Figure 28. However, at a firing rate of approximately 60 per second, the successive contractions fuse together—a state of tetanus; further increases in rate lead only to slight increases in maximal tension. The individual motor units that become active contract rhythmically, but it turns out that they are out of phase with each other and so contract *asynchronously*. This serves a useful purpose by making the overall contraction appear to be smooth, even during weak contractions.

STAIRCASE PHENOMENON (TREPPE)

When a series of maximal stimuli are delivered to a muscle below a frequency that would cause tetanus, an increase in the tension during successive stimuli occurs, resulting eventually in a uniform tension. This is known as the *staircase phenomenon*, or *treppe*, from the German word for *staircase*. Undoubtedly, some sort of activation facilitation within the sarcomere allows the actin and myosin filaments to interdigitate more effectively.

Figure 28. Wave Summation. [A. Guyton, *Textbook of Medical Physiology*, 4th ed. Philadelphia: W. B. Saunders Company (1971), p. 88.]

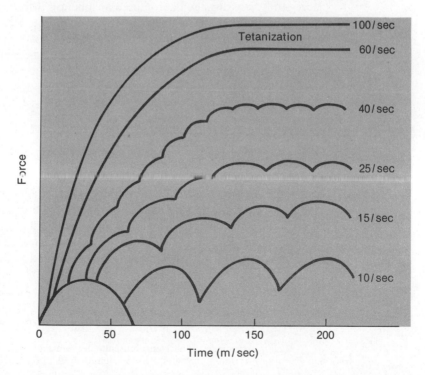

Repeated muscular exertion will soon lead to a fatigued state, greatly reducing the ability of the muscle to contract. There seem to be three potential sites where the focus of the fatigue process comes together: (1) the synapses of the central nervous system, (2) the neuromuscular junction, or (3) the muscle itself. It is difficult to imagine how the central nervous mechanisms could actually become fatigued during voluntary effort, although the following type of experiment would seem to indicate otherwise: voluntarily fatigue a muscle by a series of maximal contractions and then stimulate it directly by electrical means. It will be observed that the muscle seems to respond with renewed strength. Merton,[3] however, indicated that perhaps in humans some fibers are not under control of voluntary effort, and demonstrated that a muscle does not contract by electrical stimulation after it has fatigued by voluntary effort. Employing the adductor pollicis muscle of the hand, he compared voluntary strength with maximal tetani and found them equal. As strength declined during the exercise bout, electrical stimulation of the motor nerve did not restore the tension, thus suggesting that the site of fatigue was peripheral—that is, in the muscle itself.

Further support was given this position by the finding that muscle action potentials evoked by nerve stimulation were not significantly reduced even in extreme fatigue, meaning that the wave of depolarization was successfully crossing the neuromuscular junction. Moreover, recovery from fatigue did not take place if circulation to the muscle was occluded. Asmussen[4] has stressed that local muscular fatigue involves the many chemical reactions, both aerobic and anaerobic, that are responsible for delivering energy to the contractile mechanism of the myofibrils. The events associated with metabolism and energy transfer will be dealt with in Chapter 5.

FORM OF THE UPTAKE AND RELEASE OF FORCE

There have been very few efforts to study the characteristics of muscle contraction in the human with normal innervation and all other mechanical factors which produce maximal effort intact. The question involves how fast a maximal contraction can be made and what is the shape of the contraction curve. Figure 29 shows the contraction curve of the uptake of force of a single maximal contraction of the hand-gripping muscles. The force reaches half its maximum in approximately .08 sec, and three-fourths its maximum in .15 sec. By .4 sec the contraction is essentially complete.

[3]P. A. Merton, "Voluntary Strength and Fatigue," *Journal of Physiology*, 123 (1954), 553.

[4]Erling Asmussen, "The Neuromuscular System and Exercise," in Harold Falls, ed., *Exercise Physiology* (New York: Academic Press, 1968), p. 39.

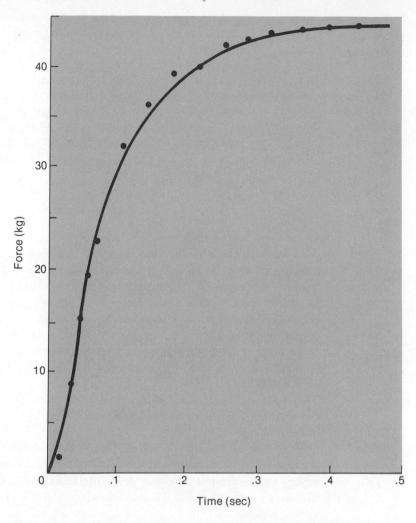

Figure 29. Form of the Contraction Curve. [D. H. Clarke and J. Royce, "Rate of Muscle Tension Development and Release under Extreme Temperature," *Int Z. angew. Physiol. einschl. Arbeitsphysiol.* 19 (1962), p. 331.]

This compares with the mechanical responses of mammalian skeletal muscle fiber to a single maximal stimulus of .04 sec for the gastrocnemius and .1 sec for the soleus.[5] Remember the earlier discussion (Chapter 1) of the slow twitch red and fast twitch white muscles reflecting different capacities, and the role of myoglobin in helping to make such a distinction. An interesting observation that can be made from Figure 29 is that the greatest speed occurs in the early portion of the effort, but any increase in force later comes much more slowly. The release of tension, on the other hand, is

[5]W. W. Tuttle and Byron A. Schottelius, *Textbook of Physiology*, 14th ed. (St. Louis: The C. V. Mosby Company, 1961), p. 74.

much more rapid. Half the drop occurs in only .04 sec, and by approximately .15 sec resting tension has been achieved once again. Thus, release can take place some four times faster than contraction. As might be expected, the ability to exert force is affected by such things as prior activity and temperature. It is not surprising to find that immersion in cold water will reduce tension and markedly slow the rate of contraction, since this is a common experience encountered in cold weather. Its effect is to cut the speed of contraction approximately in half. A passive warm-up effect is less pronounced; that is, immersing the muscles in hot water does not lead to a very large change in contraction speed or strength.[6] The release phase is lengthened by cold, but not by heat.

MUSCULAR FATIGUE

Since the turn of the century, there has been great interest in problems of muscular fatigue, and several experimental approaches have been tried. A complete understanding, however, has not been achieved. Such things as type of exercise and rate of work are crucial concepts. For example, is the exercise performed to be *isometric*, with no change in joint angle, or *isotonic*, employing a full range of motion? If the latter, is the resistance to be lifted a fixed amount, or some percentage of the person's maximum strength? Will he perform contractions according to some prescribed rhythm? If so, how much? If isometric, what is the criterion of fatigue? The topic is of practical significance to the teacher or coach, who should know something about the manner in which strength declines as a result of repeated effort.

Figure 30 shows the fatigue curve that results from an isometric contraction maintained maximally for two minutes. The decline in strength is very rapid, dropping halfway from the initial value to a *steady state* or plateau in approximately 38 seconds. Contrast this curve with that for a series of maximal isotonic contractions, given at a rate of 30 per minute for six minutes (Figure 31). The drop-off to half strength under these conditions is 89 seconds; that is, fatigue is delayed at least three times longer employing rhythmic exercise (at the specified rate of contraction) rather than nonrhythmic isometric exercise. Later on, the effect of isometric muscular contraction on the peripheral blood flow will be discussed (Chapter 11), but for the present it is clearly an advantage to have brief periods of rest, however small. Thus, the results of isotonic exercise are dependent upon the cadence used, so if the intercontraction rest interval is varied, the rate of fatigue and the level of steady state are both affected. This relationship can be seen in Figure 32. Reducing the rate of contraction from

---

[6]David H. Clarke and Joseph Royce, "Rate of Muscle Tension Development and Release under Extreme Temperatures," *Int. Z. angew. Physiol. einschl. Arbeitsphysiol.* 19 (1962), 330.

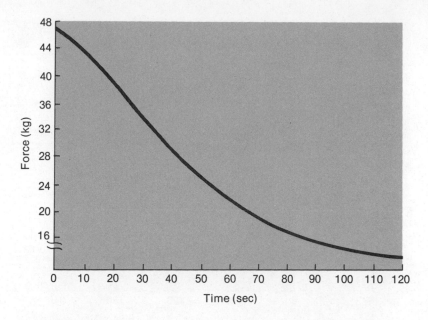

Figure 30. Isometric Fatigue Curve. [D. H. Clarke, "Strength Recovery from Static and Dynamic Muscular Fatigue," *Research Quarterly*, 33 (October 1962), p. 351.]

Figure 31. Isotonic Fatigue Curve. [D. H. Clarke, "Strength Recovery from Static and Dynamic Muscular Fatigue," *Research Quarterly*, 33 (October 1962), p. 351.]

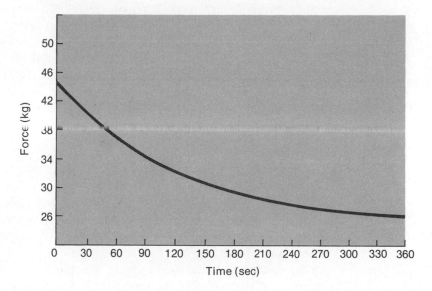

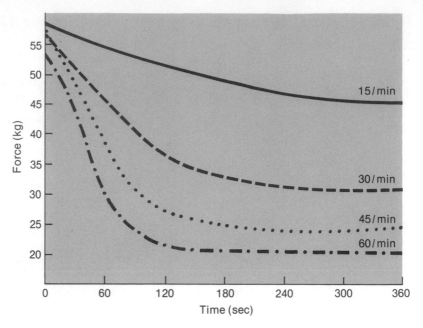

Figure 32. Effect of the Intercontraction Rest Interval on Muscular Strength. [D. H. Clarke, "The Influence on Muscular Fatigue Patterns of the Intercontraction Rest Interval," *Medicine and Science in Sports,* 3 (Summer 1971), p. 85.]

30/min, as in Figure 31, to 15/min raised the steady state appreciably—from approximately 31 kg to 45 kg. On the other hand, increasing the cadence to 60/min reduced the fatigue level even more, down to approximately 20 kg. Thus, as the intercontraction rest interval decreases, the steady state becomes lower, although the rate of this change is gradually becoming smaller. It is interesting to point out that so-called "complete fatigue" is absent when the subject is free to exert his maximum tension on each effort, rather than lifting a fixed weight. In the latter case, it would eventually develop that the individual could no longer move the load. This is the common experience in weight-lifting exercises.

Physiologically, strength is related to the energy supplies available at the beginning of any exercise task. The muscles contain high energy reserves and will use them in proportion to the rate at which work is done, assuming—as we have in the present examples—that a constant cadence alternating between contraction and relaxation is employed. Thus, as the rate of exercise increases there will be a steadily diminishing ability of the muscles to be supplied with oxygen and to remove metabolic waste products. Apparently even a small rest between contractions permits some recuperation, for even with a cadence of 60/min a steady state is established well above zero. Initial occlusion of the blood flow (by a mechanical pressure cuff) is probably the only practical method of guaranteeing that complete fatigue will occur from isotonic exercise.

After a bout of exercise, the resulting decrement must be paid back in the recovery period. This is payment of the *strength debt*, analogous to the oxygen debt that involves the oxidative processes of recovery from exercise. The strength debt, or recovery, from fatiguing work has not received the same attention as the exercise phase itself, even though a number of practical problems in dealing with training and adjustment to optimal working conditions are involved. In a study by H. H. Clarke *et al.*,[7] subjects isotonically exercised the elbow flexor muscles until fatigue occurred when lifting a load equal to three-eighths of their strength. The recovery curve showed an initial rise during the first two minutes, followed by a slower gain for the next ten, so that recovery was still not complete for most subjects two hours after the cessation of exercise. Lind[8] found fast and slow components in the ability of subjects to perform additional static contractions following fatigue.

The progress of recovery from isometric and isotonic exercise is difficult to compare, since the two exercise forms can easily result in quite different levels of fatigue. However, this can be controlled, so that the payoff of the strength debt can begin at about the same value. In Figure 33, recovery from exercise is quite rapid; in fact the gain in the first minute is appreciable, being 72 percent for the isotonic condition and 58 percent for isometric. After this first minute the recovery from isometric is about 35 percent faster than from isotonic. This points out the finding—typical of experiments of this sort—that the recovery process consists of two components, one operating during the very early time period, the other controlling events later. There is almost a spontaneous nature to the recovery from fatigue during the early seconds following exercise, and by three minutes a steady state has been achieved, resulting in no futher gains.

RESIDUAL MUSCULAR SORENESS

One of the handicaps associated with the resumption of exercise after an extended layoff is the usual experience of soreness in the exercised muscles. It ordinarily appears anywhere from 8 to 24 hours after activity and can be rather debilitating. This *residual muscular soreness* should be differentiated from the local discomfort that may be experienced during exercise. Residual soreness may last for several days, depending

[7] H. Harrison Clarke *et al.*, "Strength Decrement of Elbow Flexor Muscles Following Exhaustive Exercise," *Archives of Physical Medicine and Rehabilitation,* 35 (September 1954), 360.

[8] A. R. Lind, "Muscle Fatigue and Recovery from Fatigue Induced by Sustained Contractions," *Journal of Physiology,* 8 (1956), 608.

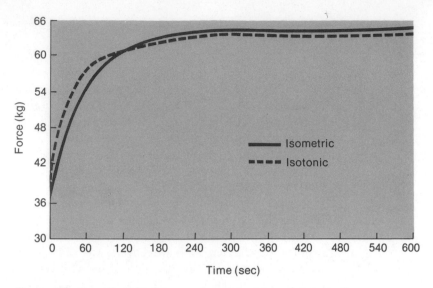

Figure 33. Strength Debt Recovery from Isometric and Isotonic Exercise. [D. H. Clarke and G. A. Stull, "Strength Recovery Patterns Following Isometric and Isotonic Exercise," *Journal of Motor Behavior*, 1 (1969), p. 240.]

upon the degree of exercise and the type of activity engaged in, and there is the assumption that no acute injury has occurred, since this would be reflected in immediate symptomatology.

The causative factors are not known, although minute tears in the muscle and connective tissue have been implicated, as well as an increase in extra or intracellular fluid,[9] and the existence of tonic muscle spasms.[10] Apparently not just any form of exercise leads to the same degree of residual soreness. Talag[11] found the eccentric phase of exercise to produce the most pain. As shown in Figure 34, when the shortening (concentric), lengthening (eccentric), and static (isometric) phases are compared in terms of subjective feelings of residual pain, the lengthening aspect is clearly predominant. Notice that the peak occurs around 48 hours after exercise.

MUSCULAR TRAINING

A great deal may be said about the many aspects of training for muscular strength and endurance, but there are limitations in a text of this

[9]Erling Asmussen, "Observations on Experimental Soreness," *Acta Rheumatologica Scandinavica*, 2 (1956), 109.

[10]Herbert A. deVries, "Electromyographic Observations of the Effects of Static Stretching upon Muscular Distress," *Research Quarterly*, 32 (December 1961), 468.

[11]Trinidad S. Talag, "Residual Muscular Soreness as Influenced by Concentric, Eccentric, and Static Contractions," *Research Quarterly*, 44 (December 1973), 458.

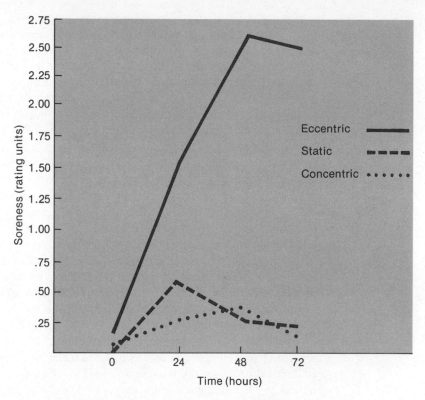

Figure 34. Effect of Concentric, Eccentric, and Static Contractions on Residual Muscular Soreness. [T. S. Talag, "Residual Muscular Soreness as Influenced by Concentric, Eccentric, and Static Contractions." *Research Quarterly*, 44 (December 1973), p. 458.]

scope. Therefore, we shall briefly consider training techniques and then the physiological effects of training. Changes in cardiovascular endurance will be dealt with in later chapters.

The individual will select his exercises from a system involving either *isotonic* or *isometric* forms. Isotonic exercises involve raising and lowering a load, whereas isometric require a static contraction to be held against a resistance. A number of factors can still be considered. For example, the isotonic exercises, usually known as *progressive resistance exercises*, are generally given in *sets*, or groups of *repetitions*, based on some criterion ranging from 6 to 15 repetitions maximum (RM). Since no really definitive standards have been established, a great deal of individual preference apparently exists, based on customs and convenience. There is reason to believe, though, that an optimal combination may be to train at 6 RM for three sets, three times a week.[12] Isometric exercise, popularized as an effective strength-improving procedure, has not proved as effective as at first supposed. The reader will find references to the early 1950's which

[12]Richard A. Berger, "Effect of Varied Weight Training Programs on Strength," *Research Quarterly,* 33 (May 1962), 168.

seemed to indicate that strength gains as much as 5 percent per week could be expected when isometric tractions of two-thirds maximum were held for 6 sec per day.[13] Confirmation of these findings has not been forthcoming, and it seems much more realistic to expect up to a 2 percent gain per week with these exercises, when the tension applied varies from 50 percent to maximum, and the duration of contraction lasts at least 5 sec.[14] When two forms of exercise have been compared, it is difficult to draw clear conclusions, particularly since it has been so difficult to equate the amount of effort involved. It may be a safe presumption that the isometric exercises are particularly helpful for individuals who are beginning training and have a long way to go to become conditioned, and also for those who have a limitation in range of motion. However, even in the former case it may be desirable to engage in typical resistance exercise of an isotonic nature, since the results seem to be clearly successful in increasing muscular strength and hypertrophy.

Still another form of exercise that has been inaugurated in recent years is what has come to be known as *isokinetic* exercise, or *accommodating resistance* exercise. It resembles the isotonic contraction, in that the joint moves through its range of motion, but the device that is used holds the speed of movement constant. Thus, the desired rate of limb motion may be preset, causing any effort to encounter an equal opposing force. An increase in exertion fails to increase the acceleration, but merely raises the resistance throughout the movement. This means that there is a high force applied at all times during the exercise. Typical weight lifting is subject to great fluctuations during the range of motion as the mechanical advantage changes. This means that the effort is often difficult at certain angles (called "sticking points"), and is relatively easy at others. The isokinetic exercise tends to equalize this factor.

We might raise the question of whether this form of exercise makes any difference in training. Thistle and colleagues[15] compared isokinetic training with isotonic and isometric procedures, and after eight weeks found that the isokinetic group gained approximately 35 percent in quadriceps strength, as compared with increments of 27.5 percent for the isotonic group and 9.2 percent for the isometric group. A control group decreased 9.4 percent over the same interval. A similar experiment was performed by Moffroid and co-workers[16] utilizing quadriceps and hamstring muscles. Significant increases in isometric strength of the quadriceps occurred at the end of four weeks in subjects who trained with isokinetic,

---

[13]T. Hettinger and E. A. Müller, "Muskelleistung und Muskeltraining," *Arbeitsphysiologie*, 15 (1953), 111.

[14]David H. Clarke, "Adaptations in Strength and Muscular Endurance Resulting from Exercise," in Jack H. Wilmore, ed., *Exercise and Sport Sciences Reviews*, Vol. 1 (New York: Academic Press, 1973), pp. 73–102.

[15]Howard G. Thistle *et al.*, "Isokinetic Contraction: A New Concept of Resistive Exercise," *Archives of Physical Medicine and Rehabilitation*, 48 (June 1966), 279.

[16]Mary Moffroid *et al.*, "A Study of Isokinetic Exercise," *Physical Therapy*, 49 (1969), 735.

isometric, and isotonic procedures, although the latter group failed to show a change when tested at a knee joint angle of 90 degrees. When the hamstring muscles were tested at this angle, only the isometric group gained significantly in isometric strength, although at 45 degrees both the isokinetic and isometric groups were significantly improved. When an isokinetic test was employed at the end of the training period, no improvement was noted for the quadriceps muscles, but the isokinetic group was significantly better than the other groups when the hamstrings were tested. Thus, it seems reasonable to conclude that isokinetic exercise provides a training stimulus that is comparable to or even better than isotonic exercise.

Strength vs. Endurance

It is often very confusing to the student to differentiate between strength and endurance, since they are often used interchangeably. Yet the differences should be pointed out. For example, a test of maximum effort against a dynamometer or tensiometer can be considered a test of strength, since it seeks to learn the outcome of a maximal voluntary innervation and subsequent contraction of the available motor units. It can be argued that employing a series of repetitions gradually introduces muscular endurance. The maximum numbers of sit-ups or push-ups, for example, are tests of muscular endurance.

No doubt each is important in its own way, but remember that different physiological events accompany the two forms. The endurance event must be supported by the circulation; the energy requirements will be very different than those for the single-effort test of strength. It is typical to develop strength by deemphasizing endurance—that is, by employing a weight training regimen involving high resistance but few repetitions. Endurance may be more satisfactorily developed in the opposite way: keep the resistance low and increase the number of repetitions. While this may be a satisfactory generalization to begin with, it may be inadequate when we examine their relative influence in delaying fatigue. This will be discussed later.

Maximum Strength

It is interesting to contemplate the actual amount of tension that can be developed within a muscle during its contraction. Since the usual tests are administered by attaching straps to limbs and connecting them to some measuring device, they then become estimates of external force, and not true measures at all. They are instead subject to the reduction associated with the mechanical application of resistance and force arms of a particular joint and muscle arrangement. A standardized system for strength testing of individual muscle groups is available,[17] however, and the reader may wish to consult these procedures before beginning an exercise program.

Though the true measure of muscle force is difficult to calculate, several attempts have been made. Such findings are generally expressed in kilograms per square centimeter (kg/cm^2), of cross section of muscle, and Ralston and his associates[18] point out the wide variability that exists from one muscle to another. In the cat quadriceps it may average 1.23 kg/cm^2, and in the cat gastrocnemius some 6.36 kg/cm^2. Their own data on human amputees with surgically prepared muscles (cineplastic tunnels) was 1.63 kg/cm^2 for pectoralis, 2.38 kg/cm^2 for biceps, and 1.31 kg/cm^2 for triceps. It may be useful to conclude that the maximum tension varies from 1.5 to 2.5 kg/cm^2 in vertebrate, nonhuman muscles, and perhaps slightly higher in the normal human. If one assumes a value of 3 kg/cm^2, and assuming that large muscles of the thigh may have 100 cm^2 of cross section, the resulting internal force that could be developed would be 300 kg, or 660 lb. This is a large force, as one can readily appreciate.

Hypertrophy

Muscular *hypertrophy*, an increase in the number or the size of individual fibers, is normally attributed to the long-term effects of heavy-resistance exercise. The prevailing view is that there is no formation of new muscle fibers (called hyperplasia), even though some rather bizarre changes can sometimes occur when muscles are placed under unusual stress. Goss[19] explains that it is the capacity of the so-called *functional unit* of an organism that grows in response to external demands. This functional unit is the smallest irreducible structure that can still carry out the basic physiological activities, and for the muscle this would refer to the myofibrils, or more specifically, the sarcomeres. One of the prime questions, then, would be whether the myofibrillar portion of muscle increases as a result of training.

Helander,[20] employing guinea pigs, found a 15 percent increase in the nitrogen component (actomyosin) of the myofilament as a result of training, when compared with control muscles in animals not exercised. Other investigators have also shown increases in the myofibrillar portion, which can be interpreted as enhancing the contractile ability of muscle fibers. Penman[21] worked with college students in a progressive-resistance

[17]H. Harrison Clarke and David H. Clarke, *Developmental and Adapted Physical Education* (Englewood Cliffs, N.J.: Prentice-Hall, Inc.), 1963, chap. 4

[18]H. J. Ralston *et al.*, "Dynamic Features of Human Isolated Voluntary Muscle in Isometric and Free Contractions," *Journal of Applied Physiology*, 1 (January 1949), 526.

[19]Richard J. Goss, "Hypertrophy versus Hyperplasia," *Science*, 153 (September 30, 1966), 1615.

[20]E. A. S. Helander, "Influence of Exercise and Restricted Activity on the Protein Composition of Skeletal Muscle," *Biochemistry Journal*, 78 (1961), 478.

[21]Kenneth A. Penman, "Human Striated Muscle Ultrastructural Changes Accompanying Increased Strength without Hypertrophy," *Research Quarterly*, 41 (October 1970), 418.

program aimed at developing the quadriceps muscle. Muscle biopsies revealed increased myosin filament concentration, a reduction in the distance between myosin filaments, and fewer actin filaments in orbit around a myosin filament. In other words, there would seem to be an increase in the packing density of the interdigitating filaments within a cell, plus a changing ratio of actin to myosin.

It is quite well established that eventually a change in the cross section of muscle will occur if heavy-resistance exercises are carried out systematically. These alterations are reflections of *ultrastructural* changes, which have been observed only with the use of biochemical or histochemical analysis. However, in practical terms, the use of limb circumference has proven to be helpful for reflecting changes in hypertrophy. Provided that a tape measure is employed carefully, with exactly the same tension on each occasion, changes in hypertrophy can usually be expected from isotonic exercise. Such changes do not always accompany isometric training.

Resistance to Fatigue

Recently the concept has been challenged that strength training and endurance training always lead to different results.[22, 23] When a fixed weight is used, one that can be handled readily, it is obvious that trained muscles can perform more work for each unit of time than can untrained muscles. However, when strain-gauge ergography is employed, where the individual exerts maximum tension rather than lifts a weight, the picture is somewhat different. It apparently doesn't matter whether the training involves low resistance and high repetition (characteristic of endurance training) or the opposite (thought to lead primarily to strength development). Both forms of training lead to increases in absolute muscular endurance, but also they result in approximately the same strength gains. In other words, the fatigue curves after training closely resemble those before training, except that they are simply displaced upwards. This leads to speculation that the main result of both strength and endurance training is an increase in strength. Endurance changes may be a secondary outgrowth.

Recovery

Training also improves the strength recovery rate after exhaustive exercise.[24] In an experiment utilizing an ergograph loaded with weight equal to three-eighths of each subject's elbow flexor strength, the recovery

[22]David H. Clarke and G. Alan Stull, "Endurance Training as a Determinant of Strength and Fatigability, "*Research Quarterly*, 41 (March 1970), 19.

[23]G. Alan Stull and David H. Clarke, "High Resistance, Low Repetition Training as a Determiner of Strength and Fatigability," *Research Quarterly*, 41 (May 1970), 189.

[24]H. Harrison Clarke *et al., op. cit.*

of trained muscles was much faster than that of untrained muscles. More-over, the strength recovery of trained muscles was more rapid when the subjects were permitted to move about and generally increase their circulation than when they were required to lie quietly during the recovery period.

Effect of Training on Connective Tissue

The changes that result from muscular training can also be seen in the connective tissue. Of particular interest has been the strength of ligaments supporting various joints. Specifically, a primary target has been the knee joint, partly because it can be isolated for study rather easily, and partly because leg action is so important in exercise and athletics. It is not surprising to learn that the subjects have often been experimental animals, such as the rat. In such a study involving male white rats, Zuckerman and Stull[25] examined the effect of a nine-week training program of swimming and running on the amount of force required to separate the medial and lateral collateral ligaments of the knee joint. Forced physical activity was found to increase this separation force, showing that training affects the strength of the ligaments as well as the muscles. With the prevalence of knee injuries so high in athletics, it serves as a further reminder of the importance of adequate physical conditioning. Ingelmark[26] summarizes the general area by indicating that exercise increases the thickness of ligaments, tendons, and other connective tissue in muscles; in fact, the hypertrophy of the tendon may be as great as that of the muscle. The hyaline cartilage, which covers the articulating surfaces of bones in joints, shows similar changes. Bones increase the amounts of calcium phosphate and calcium carbonate in response to training.

Effect of Training on Muscle Skill

One of the important questions to be asked relates to what changes can be expected to occur in the skill of movement, or the motor performance. It is one thing to demonstrate changes in strength, but quite another to translate these alterations into some form of coordination. It is not unusual for athletes and others to engage in weight training in the off-season, with the expressed belief that such activity will enhance their motor performance. In general terms, it seems clear that such activity is preferable to participating in no conditioning at all, and in fact, there may be some truth to the concept that *other things being equal*, the performer with the greatest muscular strength will probably have an advantage in athletic events. There are undoubtedly many situations in which

[25]Jerome Zuckerman and G. Alan Stull, "Effects of Exercise on Knee Ligament Separation Force in Rats," *Journal of Applied Physiology*, 26 (June 1969), 716.

[26]B. E. Ingelmark, "Morpho-Physiological Aspects of Gymnastic Exercises," *FIEP Bulletin*, 27 (1957), 37.

strength is a very important ingredient, so that enhancing the strength component establishes a foundation for the element of skill.

However, the question is whether or not increasing muscular strength will result in improvement in motor performance *per se*. Investigations reveal that prediction is really not possible, even though occasionally improvement in certain events has been found to occur.[27] Isotonic exercise is more beneficial than isometric, but the best method is clearly to practice the task itself, especially when the skill element is pronounced. In one investigation[28] where the two variables were isolated, the correlation between gain in arm strength and gain in arm speed was found to be quite low ($r = .405$). Apparently, changes in strength cannot very well predict changes in speed of movement.

SUMMARY

A number of mechanical and dynamic properties of muscle are applicable to the study of muscle function. Tension depends upon the initial length of the muscle, maximum force being greatest when the muscle is slightly lengthened and less when the muscle is foreshortened. The muscle will achieve maximum velocity of shortening when there is no load, and when the velocity is zero the force will be maximum. The curve of the development of maximum tension reveals an exponential function, and the tension development in the human will be greatest when there is very little preliminary load on the muscle. Various viscoelastic properties of muscles account for the reduction in force as measured by external recording devices. Both parallel and series elastic components must first be pulled out so that the development of tension may be smooth.

Reaction time is the lapse between the onset of a stimulus and the initiation of a response. It can be divided into premotor and motor time, the former involving depolarization of the muscle cell membrane, the latter being the remaining time for the movement to be initiated. Movement time, on the other hand, is the time that elapses during execution of the task. No correlation exists between reaction time and movement time.

Strength of a contraction can be increased by bringing into play additional motor units or by increasing their rate of firing. Wave summation can be brought about if one stimulus is followed by a second stimulus before the first is over. The successive contractions eventually fuse together, a state called tetanus. However, individual motor units contract asynchronously to smooth out the overall muscle contraction. Muscle fatigue occurs as a result of a repeated number of contractions, and it seems likely that

[27]David H. Clarke, "Adaptations in Strength and Muscular Endurance," *op. cit.*

[28]David H. Clarke and Franklin M. Henry, "Neuromotor Specificity and Increased Speed from Strength Development," *Research Quarterly*, 32 (October 1961), 315.

the site of muscular fatigue is in the muscles themselves. Muscular fatigue can be introduced both isometrically and isotonically, the decline in strength obeying mathematical laws. The pattern of recovery is known as the strength debt of exercise, is very rapid after fatiguing work, and consists of fast and slow components.

Strength training can be achieved through the use of progressive-resistance exercise or in some form of isometric contractions. The aim is to cause muscle hypertrophy, defined as the increase in size of the individual muscle fibers. Specifically, muscle may increase the nitrogen components of the myofilament, which enhances the muscle fibers' contractile ability. In addition, there seems to be an increase in the packing density of the interdigitating filaments within the cell, making the development of tension greater after training. Similar changes seem to occur in connective tissue. Ligaments respond by becoming stronger, and tendons and other components of connective tissue increase in thickness.

SELECTED REFERENCES

Asmussen, Erling, "The Neuromuscular System and Exercise," in Harold Falls, ed., *Exercise Physiology*. New York: Academic Press, 1968, chap. 1.

Clarke, David H., "Adaptations in Strength and Muscular Endurance Resulting from Exercise," in Jack H. Wilmore, ed., *Exercise and Sport Sciences Reviews*, Vol. 1. New York: Academic Press, 1973, pp. 73–102.

Clarke, H. Harrison, *Muscular Strength and Endurance in Man*. Englewood Cliffs, N.J.: Prentice-Hall, Inc., 1966.

————, and David H. Clarke, *Developmental and Adapted Physical Education*. Englewood Cliffs, N.J.: Prentice-Hall, Inc., 1963, chap. 4.

Close, R. I., "Dynamic Properties of Mammalian Skeletal Muscles," *Physiological Reviews*, 52 (January 1972), 129.

Edgerton, V. Reggie, "Exercise and the Growth and Development of Muscle Tissue," in G. Lawrence Rarick, ed., *Physical Activity, Human Growth and Development*. New York: Academic Press, 1973, chap. 1.

Goss, Richard J., "Hypertrophy versus Hyperplasia," *Science*, 153 (September 30, 1966), 1615.

Hill, A. V., "The Heat of Shortening and the Dynamic Constants of Muscle," *Proceedings of the Royal Society*, B 126 (1938), 136.

Merton, P. A., "Voluntary Strength and Fatigue," *Journal of Physiology*, 123 (1954), 553.

Ralston, H. J., *et al.*, "Dynamic Features of Human Isolated Voluntary Muscle," *Journal of Applied Physiology*, 1 (January 1949), 526.

Talag, Trinidad S., "Residual Muscular Soreness as Influenced by Concentric, Eccentric, and Static Contractions," *Research Quarterly*, 44 (December 1973), 458.

Wilkie, D. R., "The Relation between Force and Velocity in Human Muscle," *Journal of Physiology*, 110 (1950), 249.

chapter

4

proprioception

Knowledge of nervous excitation and of the characteristics of muscle contraction will not in itself allow us to understand the essentials of movement. It is true that the volitional act is basically one of motor-unit activation, and we know that without intact efferent pathways and sufficient innervation, normal function is impaired. So the task in learning complex skills is to direct effort along the most efficient lines, practicing the task, or a series of its parts, until such time as it is reasonably perfected. If it is a simple skill, the time involved may be short—a matter of a few trials. The more difficult the task, the longer the learning will take, until we come to events that require the utmost concentration and rehearsal, skills such that a lifetime of work is needed to achieve perfection. Endless examples in the realm of physical activities and athletics fit such a description. It would be a mistake, however, to conclude that the motor apparatus functions alone, unaided; it does not.

Assistance is provided by certain cues, called *feedback*, which provide essential information about external and internal conditions surrounding the task. The body is equipped with *receptors*, specialized sensory organs that can detect information and feed it back into the central nervous system, where it is sorted out and serves as a basis for modifying subsequent behavior. Accepting helpful stimuli and rejecting those that are detrimental make it possible for one to learn skills and to pattern movement. We call this *coordination*.

Actually, receptors may be divided into two categories. The *exteroceptors* respond to stimuli from outside the body, and consist of *distance receptors* (telereceptors), such as those situated in the visual, auditory, or olfactory sense organs, and *contact receptors*, such as those involved with touch and taste. The *interoceptors* are the second category and respond to stimuli originating inside the body. In this category are the numerous sensory organs that control such functions as arterial blood pressure (carotid sinus and aortic arch), partial pressure of oxygen (carotid and aortic bodies), inflation of lungs, and others. Also, *equilibrium receptors* monitor body position, and *proprioceptors* give information about the relative activity of muscles, tendons, and joints. The last category will be the subject of this chapter.

The three proprioceptors to be included are those of the skin and joints, of the muscles, and of the tendons. These are called, respectively, Pacinian corpuscles, muscle spindles, and Golgi tendon organs.

The Pacinian corpuscles are joint receptors embedded in subcutaneous tissues of the extremities and in tendons and joints. They are sensitive to quick movement and deep pressure. They must be thought of as different from so-called cutaneous receptors, which are sensitive to light touch on the skin, including *Meissner's corpuscles, Merkel's disks,* and nerve fibers surrounding the base of hair follicles. The cutaneous receptors are stimulated by light changes in pressure on the skin, while the Pacinian corpuscles respond to deep pressure. When located in ligaments they are very sensitive to quick movement or vibration.

Pacinian corpuscles are onionlike not only in shape but in their arrangement in thin layers, or lamellae. As shown in Figure 35, these lamellae surround a central non-myelinated nerve fiber. The axon acquires a myelin sheath and a node of Ranvier before leaving the capsule. Deformation or compression of this capsule exerts tension or pressure on the central core of the fiber; in this way a sensory stimulus is established. Thus, the Pacinian corpuscle is a single sensory neuron, whose peripheral end is adapted specifically to receive a stimulus and conduct it toward the central nervous system.

The deformation of the capsule causes the development of what is known as a *generator potential*—that is, a local nonpropagated depolarizing potential—and when it is of sufficient magnitude (about 10 mv), an action potential is generated in the sensory nerve. This is accomplished by increasing the permeability of the axon membrane to sodium ions, per-

Figure 35. The Pacinian Corpuscle.

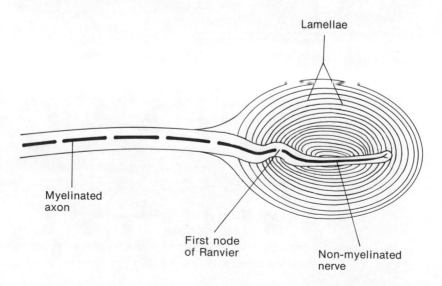

Lamellae

Myelinated axon

First node of Ranvier

Non-myelinated nerve

mitting the spread of depolarization in the terminal portion of the nerve. The current flow spreads to the myelinated portion and reaches the first node of Ranvier, where it initiates a propagated action potential as described in Chapter 1. The frequency of these action potentials increases when the magnitude of the applied stimuli is increased.

MUSCLE SPINDLE

Undoubtedly the most widely studied proprioceptors are the *muscle spindles*, or neuromuscular spindles, which are highly specialized sense organs located among the bundles of contractile fibers in the muscle (Figure 36). Each muscle spindle consists of from three to ten muscle fibers enclosed in a fibrous capsule. Smaller than the ordinary fibers of the muscle and having coarser striations, they are called *intrafusal fibers (extrafusal fibers* are the contractile elements of the muscle). Individual spindles are elongated, varying in length from .75 to 4 mm and in width from .1 to .2 mm. Their basic function is to respond to a stretch of a muscle and to produce, through reflex activity, contraction of the muscle in which they lie. Thus, they serve as monitors of muscle length.

Structure of the Spindle

The spindles are scattered through the belly of the muscle, and their structure is illustrated in Figure 37. In the central third, or *equatorial region*, of the spindle, the intrafusal fibers are surrounded by fluid contained in a *capsule*, which gives the spindle its characteristic fusiform shape. The intrafusal fibers lose the contractile material that is present at the *polar ends* when they enter the capsular region. Here two types of

Figure 36. The Muscle Spindle. [E. B. Gardner, "Proprioceptive Reflexes and their Participation in Motor Skills," *Quest*, XII (May 1969), p. 4.]

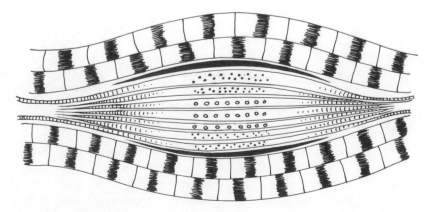

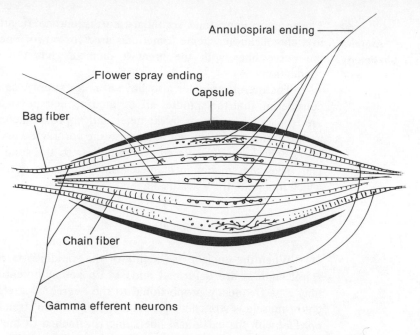

Figure 37. Structure of the Muscle Spindle. [E. B. Gardner, "Proprioceptive Reflexes and their Participation in Motor Skills," *Quest*, XII (May 1969), p. 5.]

fibers have been designated, differentiated by the arrangement of nuclei and also by length. The "percapsular" intrafusal fibers have nuclei arranged in aggregate form and are called *nuclear bag* fibers. The shorter "intracapsular" fibers have nuclei arranged in single file and are known as *nuclear chain* fibers. The muscle spindle typically contains two nuclear bag fibers, which are larger than the nuclear chain fibers and extend beyond the capsule to attach to the connective tissue and endomysium of the extrafusal fiber. On the other hand, the nuclear chain fibers, from three to five in number for each intrafusal fiber, are not only smaller than the nuclear bag fibers but do not extend beyond the capsule; instead, they terminate on the inside of the capsule itself.

Innervation of the Spindle

The key to spindle function as a sensory device lies in the distribution of sensory nerve terminals. The classification scheme employed to describe them is sometimes confusing, because several systems exist. However, there is a single primary sensory ending, called the *annulospiral ending* (Figure 37), which is entwined around the central portion of the intrafusal fibers. It averages 12 microns in diameter and passes from the spindle to the sensory roots of the spinal cord. A secondary ending 6 microns in diameter lies mainly in the *myotube region* of the nuclear chain fibers but sends a few connections to the bag fibers; these are the *flower spray endings*.

The terms primary and secondary correspond to Ia and II, respectively, in a classification scheme sometimes used for sensory neurons. In general, the nerve fiber with the greatest diameter has the greatest speed of conduction.

The muscle spindles also have a motor supply, as one would expect, considering that the spindles are striated at their polar ends. These nerves are from 3 to 7 microns in diameter and approximately 10 to 15 of them are distributed to motor end plates on the contractile ends of the intrafusal fibers. These *gamma efferent fibers* belong to the small motor nerve system. They are smaller in diameter than the *alpha efferents*, motor nerves which innervate the extrafusal fibers.

Stimulation of the Spindle

When the nuclear bag region of the spindle is stretched, the annulo-spiral endings are deformed and set up action potentials in the sensory fiber at a frequency proportional to the degree of stretching. Thus, if the entire muscle is stretched, the spindle will also be stretched, since it lies in *parallel* with the extrafusal fibers and is attached to the muscle connective tissue. This is followed very quickly by contraction of the muscle, and a lessening of the tension on the spindle as the muscle shortens. Following very quickly, a gamma efferent discharge increases to the polar ends. It should be kept in mind that this gamma efferent innervation does not contribute in any measurable way to muscle tension; however, contraction of the two ends of the spindle can cause the center portion to stretch and therefore become deformed, causing the annulospiral ending to increase its rate of sensory discharge. The role of the secondary flower spray endings is far less well defined, but they are also responsive to sudden stretching, although not as dynamically as the annulospiral ending. In addition, as we will learn below, their function is somewhat different.

Myotatic or Stretch Reflex

One of the simplest ways to understand the operation of the muscle spindle in responding to changes in muscle length is to describe its action in the *myotatic or stretch reflex*. This clinical example may not be a very functional one, but it does serve as a model for its action. For example, tapping the patellar tendon elicits a "knee jerk," brought about by a contraction of the quadriceps muscles that were briefly stretched. The mechanism is as follows: stretching the quadriceps by the tap on the tendon stretches the muscle spindles located in parallel with the muscle fibers. This in turn causes a deformation of the nuclear bag region and increases the firing of the annulospiral ending. The sensory message is transmitted to the spinal cord by way of the dorsal root, as shown in Figure 38, and synapses directly with an alpha efferent (motor) neuron.

The stretch reflex itself is *monosynaptic*; that is, afferent fibers from

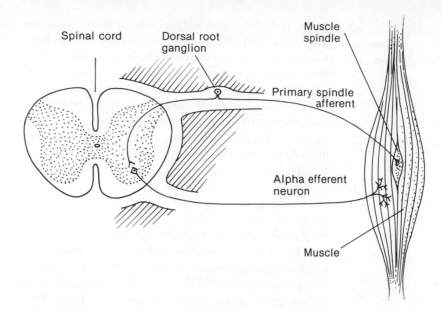

Figure 38. Sensory and Motor Pathways of the Stretch Reflex.

the muscle excite the dendrites of the motor neuron that supply the muscle, without employing any intervening neurons. Thus, the efferent impulse travels to the quadriceps and causes contraction. This shortens the muscle and takes the tension off the muscle spindle, causing it to slow its rate of firing, and at the same time abolishes the motor response so that the muscle relaxes once again. The additional support needed to make this an effective response is provided by activation of the *synergists* and inhibition of the *antagonists*. These responses, however, are not monosynaptic, but require the use of *interneurons*, whose function is to convey impulses within the central nervous system. They send facilitory impulses to the muscles that will assist in the response, and at the same time synapses with inhibitory neurons that inhibit the antagonists. This was dicussed in Chapter 1 as *reciprocal inhibition*. Both responses permit the effective response of the muscle to action.

The annulospiral endings have a lower threshold (3 g) than the flower spray endings (19 g), so they are the ones to respond to the stretch reflex. They respond by transmitting a large number of impulses even after only a slight stretch, and thus they monitor the *rate of change* of the spindle. The flower spray endings, on the other hand, function to monitor only the length of the spindle itself.

Postural Reflex

A great deal is known about posture as it relates to decerebrate animals, and on this basis we have gained understanding of the manner in which spinal reflexes function. In man, the maintenance of standing posture is controlled fundamentally by the stretch reflex. Comfortable standing is largely a matter of balancing the various body parts on each other in such a manner that very little muscular effort is required. In fact, electrical monitoring of the muscles supposedly involved in maintaining the erect position, using an electromyograph, reveals surprisingly little electrical activity. As the individual sways from a balanced position there is an immediate adjustment of the muscles antagonistic to the direction of movement. Since the body requires only a slight counteracting force, the contraction needs to be but slight, and relaxation ensues again once the readjustment has been made. The mechanism involves stretching of the counteracting muscles and eliciting an increased response from the annulospiral endings, and thus a reflex contraction of the muscles containing the spindles and righting of the imbalance.

The fact that posture can be maintained with only minor adjustments is also largely attributable to the eyes. Visual afferents are an important consideration in holding an upright posture; the amount of swaying and unsteadiness increases with the eyes closed. In fact, favorite tests of *kinesthesis* include items that involve steadiness and accuracy of muscular response, usually with the eyes blindfolded, to rule out the visual effect.

Movement Reflex

A more complex question in the realm of exercise is how the spindle functions in dynamically changing situations, rather than in the more static ones just described. After all, the spindles, to be effective, must be able to respond to new changes in muscle length even though the muscle is under tension or shorter than resting length. O'Connell and Gardner[1] describe the adjustment made to an added load. If the flexor muscles of the elbow joint are supporting a weight, and suddenly additional weight is added, at first the arm is depressed as the load puts a stretch on the muscles. After a brief interval (latent period), probably some 60 to 80 msec,[2] the muscles respond by adding a counteracting force. In fact, an exaggerated response occurs as the muscle contracts more strongly than needed in a slight overcompensation. The mechanism is this: the added stretch caused a lengthening of the primary spindle afferents (annulospiral endings), which caused a reflex contraction of the muscles. If the added load is abrupt, there is a greater overcompensation, which partially unloads the spindles and causes some uncertainty in response as the limb comes into equilibrium. This situation can be avoided if the load is added slowly; this finding reinforces a point made earlier—that the spindle has an important function in monitoring *rate* of change in muscle length.

[1]Alice L. O'Connell and Elizabeth B. Gardner, *Understanding the Scientific Bases of Human Movement* (Baltimore: The Williams & Wilkins Co., 1972), p. 201.

[2]P. H. Hammond, P. A. Merton, and G. G. Sutton, "Nervous Gradation of Muscular Contraction," *British Medical Bulletin*, 12 (1956), 214.

In order for the above reactions to occur satisfactorily, some mechanism must operate to keep the muscle spindle fully operative, even when the overall muscle length varies, as it surely must when it contracts or maintains other than a purely resting state. It is the function of the *gamma efferent* or *fusimotor* system to supply the motor control to the spindle and keep it operative no matter what the muscle length (and the spindle length) might be. Therefore, it is not surprising to find a persistently low level of firing over the gamma efferent neurons to the polar ends of the spindle. When stretching occurs and the muscle shortens in response to primary afferent innervation, there is increased discharge over the fusimotor neurons to cause contraction of the polar ends of the spindle, in effect *resetting* the spindle to new muscle length. The effect is to prepare the spindle for other lengthening reactions when the muscle may already be shortened. The amount of this change in spindle length by the gamma efferent neurons is known as *bias*. The pathway employed to bring about this response is presented in Figure 39. The whole system can be likened

Figure 39. Diagram of the Alpha and Gamma Pathways. Note the descending path to the gamma efferent neuron. [A. L. O'Connell and E. B. Gardner, *Understanding the Scientific Bases of Human Movement.* Baltimore: The Williams & Wilkins Co. (1972), p. 203.]

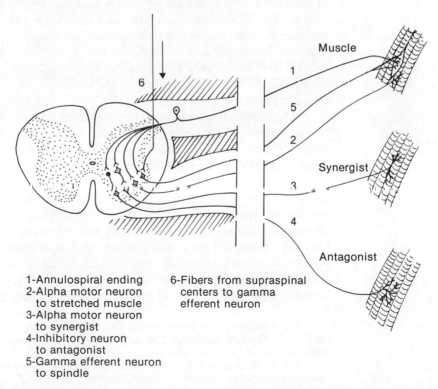

1-Annulospiral ending
2-Alpha motor neuron
   to stretched muscle
3-Alpha motor neuron
   to synergist
4-Inhibitory neuron
   to antagonist
5-Gamma efferent neuron
   to spindle

6-Fibers from supraspinal
   centers to gamma
   efferent neuron

to an automatic pilot equipped with a regulator that permits different speeds to be maintained.

Eldred[3] proposes a sequence of events which can occur in voluntary movement, involving gamma efferent activity. Immediately prior to a planned movement, impulses along pathways descending from supraspinal (brain) centers would synapse with the gamma efferent neuron and increase fusimotor activity to the polar ends of the spindle. This would stretch the primary spindle afferent, with the result that the muscle would be required to contract to a new length in response to this fusimotor lead. This is called a *servomechanism*, the muscle contracting without receiving a direct train of impulses from the brain to the motor neuron.

Such a mechanism raises further possibilities with respect to assuming various postures or positions. Often in athletic and physical activities a portion of the body must be stabilized by muscular contraction so that a firm foundation is established for the performance of some task. The weight lifter, for example, must have the body remain in a fixed position for the performance of a two-arm curl. It has been postulated that a servomechanism functions through the gamma efferent system to contract the appropriate hip and trunk muscles without intervention and constant readjustment from the brain.

Muscle Tone

One of the more controversial topics in exercise physiology is that of muscle tone. It is a state of muscle that can even be observed by the unaided eye. Physicians, therapists, and others can see differences in appearance between a muscle that is diseased and one that is normal. The loss of motor or sensory control abolishes tone in the muscle, and with it the fullness and appearance of normality. Clinically, tone may be tested by examining the resistance offered by the muscle to passive stretching and by direct palpation.

The classical definition of tonus accepted for so long has referred to the persistent bombardment of muscle by the alpha motor neuron by means of some rotational scheme established among the individual motor units. In light of more recent research evidence, however, the concept of tone must be modified. It has been known for quite some time, for example, that in a normal human subject at complete rest no action potentials are detectable in the corresponding skeletal muscles.[4] Thus, with the use of electromyography, electrical activity of the sort that should be found if the muscle were being bombarded with some low level action potentials cannot be detected. Yet, the muscle has not lost its tone at rest. It has been argued that some very low level of activity may actually be present, which does consist of muscle action potentials but is confounded

[3]Earl Eldred, "Functional Implications of Dynamic and Static Components of the Spindle Response to Stretch," *American Journal of Physical Medicine*, 46 (February 1967), 129.

[4]H. J. Ralston and B. Libet, "The Question of Tonus in Skeletal Muscle," *American Journal of Physical Medicine*, 32 (April 1953), 85.

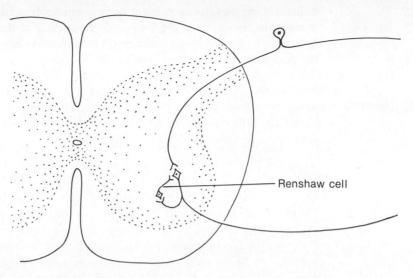

Figure 40. The Renshaw Cell.

by amplifier and thermal noise caused by difficulties in instrument sensitivity.[5] At any rate, Basmajian[6] suggests that muscle tone is determined by passive *elasticity* or *turgor* of both muscular and fibrous tissues and by contraction of muscle in response to some neural stimuli.

Whether muscles really remain at complete rest for any length of time is very speculative. The fact is, we are almost constantly changing position and moving about; sitting or standing perfectly still is a most difficult task. Thus, something operates to keep the muscles in a high state of readiness if not a state of partial contraction. The manner in which this can be accomplished is by means of the gamma efferent neuron, whose contraction of the polar ends sets the spindle so that the output via the sensory ending increases the alpha discharge, thereby preparing the muscles for the slightest stretch or increased bombardment of nervous stimuli.

Renshaw Cells

Present in the anterior horn of the spinal cord are recurrent loops that originate as collateral branches from the axons of alpha motor neurons. These collaterals make excitatory synaptic connections with a special category of interneuron, known as the *Renshaw cell*, the axons of which "loop back" and terminate on the original motor neuron and other neurons that go to synergistic muscles at the same segmental level. At this point, however, the Renshaw cell exerts an *inhibitory* effect. This feedback loop is illustrated in Figure 40. The overall effect is to smooth out reflex and

[5]Herbert A. deVries, "Muscle Tonus in Postural Muscles," *American Journal of Physical Medicine*, 44 (December 1965), 275.

[6]John V. Basmajian, "Electromyographic Analyses of Basic Movement Patterns," in Jack H. Wilmore, ed., *Exercise and Sport Sciences Reviews*, Vol. 1 (New York: Academic Press, 1973), pp. 261–262.

voluntary movement and prevent motor neurons from discharging impulses at rates that would exceed a frequency acceptable to the muscle fibers they innervate. Failure to do so could result in convulsive contractions and make fine coordination difficult or impossible.

GOLGI TENDON ORGAN

Another proprioceptor of significance to muscle control is the *Golgi tendon organ*, which consists of a netlike collection of nerve endings distributed among the fascicles of a tendon (Figure 41). The fibers from the Golgi tendon organs (afferent neurons), classified as belonging to the Ib group of myelinated, rapidly conducting fibers, cause reflex *inhibition* of the muscle to which they belong. Because these organs lie directly in line with the transmission of force from muscle to insertion on bone, they are said to be in *series* with the muscle, rather than in parallel as we found the spindles to be. Therefore, the Golgi tendon organs monitor muscle *tension*, rather than length, and instead of facilitating alpha neuron discharge, they inhibit it. In addition, they have a much higher threshold of response than the annulospiral endings (100 g), so they operate at higher tensions. In fact, tension to the tendon may be imparted by both active contraction of the muscle and by strong stretch.

The mode of operation for the Golgi tendon organ first involves tension on the tendon, which sets up activity in the afferent neuron and transmits it to the spinal cord, as illustrated in Figure 42. A synapse with an inhibitory interneuron in turn inhibits the alpha motor neuron, causing muscle relaxation. There is also evidence that at the same time there is facilitation of the antagonists. Relaxation in response to a strong stretch

Figure 41. Golgi Tendon Organ. [W. F. Ganong, *Review of Medical Physiology*, 2nd ed. Los Altos, Calif.: Lange Medical Publications, p. 72.]

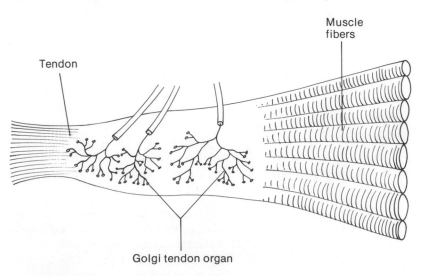

Muscle
fibers

Tendon

Golgi tendon organ

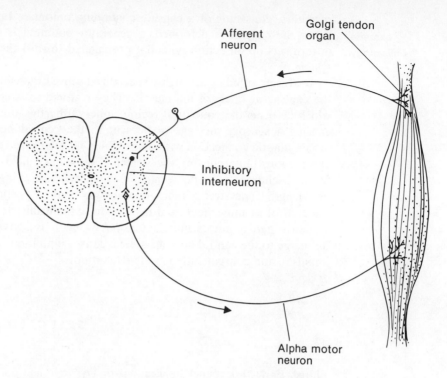

Figure 42. Diagram Representing Golgi Tendon Organ Pathways.

is called an *inverse myotatic reflex* or *autogenetic inhibition*; when operating in situations of high muscular contraction, it can be considered a safety device, protecting the muscle from dangerously high tensions.

The limits of physical strength may be determined in large measure by the control exerted by Golgi tendon organs. As tension mounts, the amount of sensory feedback increases, until finally the point is reached where further alpha discharge is dampened. It is interesting to speculate on what role training may play, if any, in modifying tendon organ response. Another example can be seen in arm wrestling. With two competitors struggling isometrically to gain supremacy, one may suddenly overcome the other when the limits of Golgi activity of the latter are reached. Similar examples are undoubtedly found in combative events, notably in competitive wrestling.

SUMMARY

Learning to perform motor acts is assisted by the feedback of certain cues from various receptors, some from outside the body (exteroceptors) and some from inside (interoceptors). Proprioceptors give information about muscles, tendons, and joints. The Pacinian corpuscles are joint receptors, consisting of a capsule containing onionlike layers or lamellae. When the capsule is deformed, a generator potential is developed which in turn sets up an action potential propagated toward the central nervous system.

Muscle spindles are highly specialized sense organs distributed among the contractile fibers of the muscle. They respond to stretch of the muscle which deforms the equatorial region, innervating the annulospiral ending, causing a sensory message to be sent to the central nervous system. A monosynaptic connection with an outgoing motor nerve results in a muscle contraction, thus relieving the stretch. Following quickly is a gamma efferent discharge to the polar ends of the spindle, resetting the spindle to a new length. The stretch reflex operates to control posture and assists in the control of movement, and it helps to explain muscle tone. The Golgi tendon organ monitors muscle tension; when it is activated, the sensory discharge to the central nervous system causes inhibition of outgoing motor impulses, and consequently muscle relaxation.

SELECTED REFERENCES

Eldred, Earl, "Functional Implications of Dynamic and Static Components of the Spindle Response to Stretch," *American Journal of Physical Medicine*, 46 (February 1967), 129.

————, "The Dual Sensory Role of Muscle Spindles," *Journal of the American Physical Therapy Association*, 45 (April 1965), 290.

Hammon, P. H., P. A. Merton, and G. G. Sutton, "Nervous Gradation of Muscular Contraction," *British Medical Bulletin*, 12 (1956), 214.

Hunt, C. C., and E. R. Perl, "Spinal Reflex Mechanisms Concerned with Skeletal Muscle," *Physiological Reviews*, 40 (July 1960), 538.

Matthews, P. B. C., "Muscle Spindles and Their Motor Control," *Physiological Reviews*, 44 (April 1964), 219.

O'Connell, Alice L., and Elizabeth B. Gardner, *Understanding the Scientific Bases of Human Movement*. Baltimore: The Williams & Wilkins Co., 1972, chap. 14.

chapter 5

metabolism
and
energy transfer

The contraction of muscles seems almost to be taken for granted, since about all that is required is proper excitation-contraction coupling and activation of the contractile machinery. Except for reference to ATP, very little has been said so far of the overall metabolic requirements for muscle activity. Given an individual free of neuromuscular disease, one can say that the act of contraction can take place with minimum involvement of the metabolism. In fact, oxygen is not required to initiate muscle activity, since it has long been known that muscle contraction is essentially an anaerobic process, able to occur in an atmosphere completely devoid of oxygen. However, for work to continue for any length of time, a number of adjustments must be made in order to keep supplying the necessary ingredients. After all, the supply of ATP is probably only good for 5 to 10 seconds or so of maximal effort; consequently, other mechanisms must be found if exercise is to be prolonged.

It is generally conceded that metabolic activities can be divided into anaerobic and aerobic phases, and that the ultimate goal is to provide energy for the cellular processes required of an individual. The minimum energy required to maintain life, called *basal metabolism*, is a rather carefully defined quiet state. In exercise physiology, however, there is less concern over basal metabolism than over what is known as *resting metabolism* (which is above basal level) and the metabolism of exercise. In this connection, this chapter will deal with anaerobic and aerobic metabolism, the concept of electron transfer and ATP production, aspects of carbohydrate and fat metabolism, and the changes that result from training.

ANAEROBIC METABOLISM

The process whereby ATP is produced in the muscle cell, and is therefore available as an immediate source of energy for metabolism, can be understood in terms of the manner in which fats and carbohydrates are disposed of or degraded in the various metabolic pathways. These initial processes do not require oxygen for their functioning, and so it is appropriate to speak of them as *anaerobic*. It should be clear, however, that their ability to continue functioning, and to supply energy, is dependent upon an adequate supply of oxygen, although for a while the muscle must wait for the necessary respiratory and circulatory adjustments to take place which are responsible for bringing oxygen to the cells.

Carbohydrate Metabolism: Glycolysis

The degradation of one molecule of glucose in the sarcoplasm of muscle results in the net gain of two molecules of ATP and the formation of two molecules of pyruvic acid. The detailed steps comprising this metabolic pathway are presented in Figure 43. Several of these steps are of major importance, since they result in the formation of ATP, ADP, or

Figure 43. Carbohydrate Metabolism-Glycolysis.

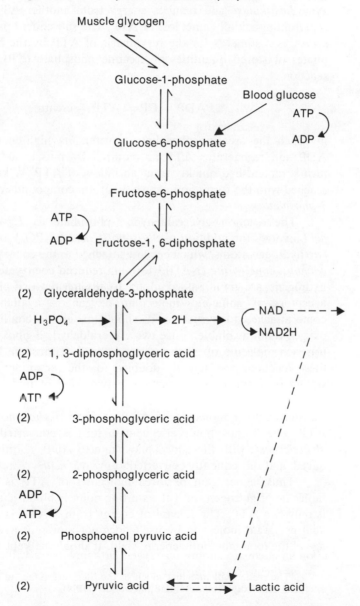

hydrogen atoms (2H), and are thus responsible directly or indirectly for energy production.

The glycogen is brought to the muscle by the blood as blood glucose and converted into glycogen, which in turn remains as a polymer of glucose. Thus, it becomes a storage form for carbohydrates, and when energy is needed for the muscle contractile process the glycogen is degraded by the enzyme *phosphorylase* into *glucose-1-phosphate*. The glucose-1-phosphate is metabolized further in a process called *glycolysis* in stages to *fructose-1, 6-diphosphate*, utilizing energy from the cleavage of ATP into ADP and inorganic phosphorus. When the starting point is blood glucose the conversion to *glucose-6-phosphate* is accomplished by the enzyme *hexokinase* and requires energy from another ATP, both reactions representing initially a net loss of ATP. The subsequent production of ADP serves as a stimulus for the resynthesis of ATP by the high-energy phosphates of stored quantities of creatine phosphate (CP) in the reversible reaction

$$ADP + CP \rightleftharpoons ATP + \text{creatine}, \qquad (5-1)$$

in which the creatine phosphate transfers its high-energy phosphate to ADP and regenerates ATP as required by muscle activity. The CP in turn is replenished quickly from an inflow of ATP. A key stage has been reached with the formation of two 3-carbon compounds of *glyceraldehyde-3-phosphate*.

The reaction glyceraldehyde-3-phosphate to *1,3-diphosphoglyceric acid* involves the addition of *phosphoric acid* (H_3PO_4) and the removal of two hydrogen atoms, which become attached to the coenzyme, *nicotinamide adenine dinucleotide* (NAD),[1] forming reduced coenzyme, NAD2H. These hydrogens are then passed along to the respiratory chain of hydrogen acceptors, if sufficient molecular oxygen is available, or they become attached to pyruvic acid, should anaerobic conditions prevail and oxygen is not available. Since two glyceraldehyde-3-phosphates are formed for each molecule of glycogen metabolized, it must be kept in mind that these reactions are actually doubled for the remainder of glycolysis, resulting from the present reaction in two *pairs* of hydrogens. In the next stage, the energy-rich phosphate group in 1,3-diphosphoglyceric acid is transferred to a molecule of ADP to form *3-phosphoglyceric acid* and ATP. The 3-phosphoglyceric acid in turn is converted into *2-phosphoglyceric acid*; with the added phosphate to ADP, additional ATP is produced, and subsequently converted to *pyruvic acid*.

Thus, a net gain of three molecules of ATP is made from each molecule of glycogen, or if the starting point is blood glucose the net yield is only two ATP. The release of energy from 3 ATP is approximately 36 kcal per gram mole and by itself does not represent a very high percentage of the total metabolic energy yield. It should be kept in mind, however,

---

[1]The reader will find that much of the literature refers to the coenzyme by an alternate name, diphosphopyridine nucleotide (DPN).

that the removal of hydrogen in the reaction NAD + 2H → NAD2H will result in additional ATP under aerobic conditions, as will the degradation of pyruvic acid. In the event that oxygen is not available in sufficient amounts to oxidize the NAD2H, as in heavy exercise when the muscles are using oxygen faster than the circulation can supply it, the NAD is no longer able to oxidize the glyceraldehyde-3-phosphate, and glycolysis is unable to continue. Pyruvic acid in this case acts as a temporary hydrogen store, and in the presence of the enzyme *lactic dehydrogenase* (LDH) the pyruvic acid is reduced to *lactic acid*, according to the equation

$$\text{pyruvic acid} + \text{NAD2H} \overset{\text{LDH}}{\rightleftharpoons} \text{lactic acid} + \text{NAD}. \qquad (5\text{--}2)$$

The reactions are reversible and temporary, since the accumulation of lactic acid is a self-limiting operation, dependent on factors associated with the prolonged performance of work beyond the steady state. Either the exercise rate must be reduced or it must be stopped completely before the lactic acid can be oxidized in payment of an *oxygen debt*, as will be discussed in Chapter 6. This very important chemical event serves as an essential anaerobic mechanism for the performance of prolonged and severe exercise. During the recovery period the lactic acid will be reconverted back into pyruvic acid and disposed of metabolically.

AEROBIC METABOLISM

The steps outlined above for glycolysis are clearly anaerobic, since they include no mention of oxygen. The point must be emphasized further, though, that the amount of work performed will be restricted if the intake of oxygen does not keep up with the demand. In the resting state and during submaximal exercise we would expect oxygen to be introduced into the cell in accordance with the metabolic requirement, where normal *aerobic* conditions prevail. The end product of glycolysis is pyruvic acid, and while the intensity of anaerobic metabolism can be gauged in large part by the production of lactic acid, a small amount of lactic acid may even be evident under aerobic conditions. However, this should be considered small and not particularly important. The reduction of pyruvic acid and the subsequent production of energy and disposal of metabolic byproducts, on the other hand, are of major concern to this discussion.

Krebs Cycle

Pyruvic acid is degraded to carbon dioxide and hydrogen atoms by passing into the *Krebs cycle* (also called the *citric acid cycle* or *tricarboxylic cycle*). This is accomplished initially by having a carbon dioxide (CO_2) molecule cleaved from pyruvic acid as it combines with *coenzyme A* to yield *acetyl coenzyme A*, as shown in Figure 44. The acetyl Co A com-

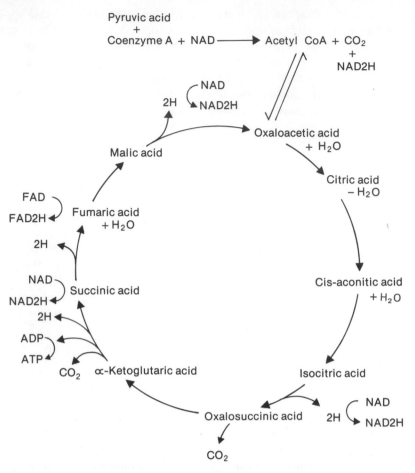

Figure 44. The Krebs Cycle.

bines with *oxaloacetic* acid to form *citric acid* in the first step of the Krebs cycle, thereby releasing hydrogen to NAD, reducing it to NAD2H. As usual, the hydrogens will be transported to the respiratory chain, the *cytochrome oxidase system*, where they will produce ATP and combine with oxygen. The Krebs cycle itself will be responsible for eliminating two additional CO_2 molecules, removing four pairs of hydrogen atoms, and producing one ATP molecule. Therefore, in order for pyruvic acid $(C_3H_4O_3)$ to be able to cause the elimination of 3 CO_2 molecules and a total of 5 H_2, there is the net addition of 3 H_2O molecules at various sites, including oxaloacetic acid, as shown in Figure 44.

The citric acid, by internal rearrangement and the removal and addition of water, becomes *isocitric acid*, which in turn is oxidized by the removal of 2H to NAD, forming NAD2H. This leaves *oxalosuccinic acid*, which loses CO_2 and adds water to form *α-ketoglutaric acid*. The *α-ketoglutaric* acid is metabolized in a series of reactions which results in the formation of *succinic acid*, at the same time releasing CO_2, transferring 2H to NAD, and creating a molecule of ATP in the reaction ADP + P ⇌ ATP. The succinic acid is oxidized by releasing 2H to the coenzyme *flavin adenine dinucleotide* (FAD), reducing it to FAD2H, resulting in the formation of *fumaric acid*; this in turn takes on a molecule of water and becomes *malic acid*. The removal of 2H in the oxidation of malic acid regenerates the oxaloacetic acid, and the cycle has come full turn, permitting oxaloacetic acid to combine once again with acetyl Co A from pyruvic acid in the initial step of the Krebs cycle.

Respiratory-Chain Oxidation

Thus, as long as the coenzyme can continue to oxidize the various stages of the cycle, oxaloacetic acid will continue to act to condense acetyl Co A. Should insufficient oxygen become available to satisfy the demand brought about by the formation of NAD2H, then the Krebs cycle would not be able to dispose of all of the pyruvic acid formed from glycolysis; as already demonstrated, this will result in the formation of lactic acid. The key to aerobic metabolism is the ability of the *flavoprotein-cytochrome oxidase* system to accept hydrogens and pass them along the respiratory chain to combine eventually with molecular oxygen from the atmosphere. In doing so, each pair of hydrogen atoms will produce 3 molecules of ATP for those attached to NAD, and 2 molecules if the coenzyme is FAD.

The two hydrogen atoms attached to NAD are transported from the outer surface of the mitochondrian to the inner surface where they react with the *flavoproteins*, metal-containing enzymes of a riboflavin derivative (FAD) that remove the hydrogens in a reaction that produces a molecule of ATP from ADP, and releases the NAD. These reactions are shown in Figure 45. The hydrogens are transferred to the *cytochrome system*, the

Figure 45. Respiratory Chain Oxidation.

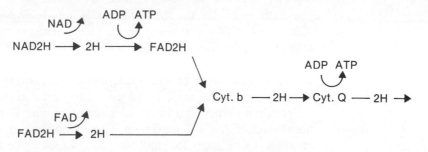

cytochromes being pigments that contain iron, bearing superficial re-
semblances to hemoglobin. The hydrogens are passed along to *cytochromes b* and *q*, where another ATP is formed, and to *cytochrome c*.
At cytochrome c the hydrogen undergoes *electron transfer*, and the electron
from each hydrogen atom is passed along to *cytochrome a* and cytochrome
oxidase, at the same time producing another ATP. Cytochrome oxidase has
the ability to transfer an electron to an oxygen atom and then combine
with two hydrogens to give water. In this manner, one molecule of oxygen
would combine with four molecules of hydrogen, and in the process each
pair of hydrogens introduced as NAD2H would produce three molecules
of ATP. In contrast, the introduction of FAD2H from succinic acid in the
Krebs cycle would only give 2 ATP, since it entered at a lower stage on
the respiratory chain.

Energy Yield

Oxygen serves the function of a hydrogen acceptor, and the amount
of hydrogen produced as a result of work performed will regulate the
oxygen uptake, and of course the extent of energy expended. When the
ATP produced as a result of glycolsis is compared with that of the Krebs
cycle, it should be clear that the majority comes from the latter. For every
molecule of pyruvic acid that is condensed, with the stepwise removal of
five pairs of hydrogen atoms, the respiratory chain will provide 14 molecules of ATP (12 from NAD2H, 2 from FAD2H), and an additional ATP
from the Krebs cycle itself, making a total of 15. Since the degradation of
glucose or glycogen results in two molecules of pyruvic acid, rather than
one, the totals are simply doubled, and the gain in ATP becomes 30. In
contrast, glycolysis produces two pairs of hydrogens in the reaction gly-
ceraldehyde-3-phosphate to 1,3-disphosphoglyceric acid and passes them
along to the respiratory chain, where they will produce 6 ATP. This,
together with the net gain of three ATP directly, gives a total of 9 for
glycolysis (provided the starting point is muscle glycogen; if it is glucose,
then only 8 ATP's are gained here). The conclusion must be not only that
more energy by far is produced under aerobic conditions than anaerobic,
but that the initiation of muscle activity must be essentially anaerobic.

The generation of hydrogen provides the stimulus for oxygen consumption, since the more hydrogen that is created the more oxygen will
be required. When the limits of circulation and oxygen transport have
been reached (termed maximum oxygen uptake), pyruvic acid does not
continue to be degraded and enter the Krebs cycle but is converted to
lactic acid, as described above, and diffuses into the blood. The oxidation
of lactic acid, which takes place in the recovery period after exercise, requires lactic acid to be converted back to pyruvic acid in the presence of
LDH; lactic acid cannot be converted directly into glucose or glycogen
but must involve a reversal of glycolysis, the reconversion occurring
primarily in the liver. Approximately 20 percent of this pyruvic acid is

utilized by the Krebs cycle, the energy from ATP employed to resynthesize the remaining 80 percent into glycogen.

The amount of energy that is produced by the complete oxidation of one gram-mole of glucose is 686,000 calories, 266,000 of which (39 percent) are stored in the form of ATP. The other 61 percent of the energy is lost as heat and can be considered a measure of the inefficiency of the metabolic process.

FAT METABOLISM

The great majority of the ATP produced metabolically comes from the breakdown of both fats and carbohydrates. While the fuel for exercise is thought to be composed primarily of carbohydrates, it is becoming increasingly evident that fat metabolism is important as an energy source, and that the fat that is used comes from *free fatty acids* (FFA) hydrolized from the *triglycerides* of the adipose tissue by the enzyme *lipase*, as follows:

$$\text{triglyceride} + 3 \text{ H}_2\text{O} \xrightarrow{\text{lipase}} 3 \text{ FFA} + \text{glycerol.} \tag{5-3}$$

The FFA diffuse into the blood and are transported to the muscles, where the fatty acid molecule undergoes *beta oxidation* to yield acetyl coenzyme A. The acetyl Co A enters the Krebs cycle by combining with oxaloacetic acid in the same way to yield ATP as the carbohydrates described above.

Since about 40 percent of the calories in the diet come from fats, an amount approximately equal to those provided from carbohydrates, their role as an energy source in normal metabolism becomes apparent. Moreover, it has been estimated[2] that 30 to 50 percent of the ingested carbohydrates are converted to triglycerides, which means that anywhere from two-thirds to three-fourths of all energy may be derived from fats rather than carbohydrates in the diet. Carbohydrates are probably used for short, strenuous bouts of activity, and fats in increasing amounts for light and moderate bouts which are maintained for prolonged periods. The efficiency of conversion is different for fats than for carbohydrates; fats require 2.01 liters of oxygen for their oxidation, and carbohydrates need only .75 liters. However, fats actually produce over twice as much energy per gram (9.5 kcal/g) as carbohydrates (4.3 kcal/g).

The fact remains, too, that fat, after absorption, may be stored in the body in large amounts by being taken up by the cells of adipose tissue. Not only may fat be employed in this manner, but carbohydrates may be converted to fat and stored in fat depots. The reverse does not seem to occur—that is, the conversion of fat to carbohydrate—and thus it is not a major source of blood glucose. Since body tissue, including muscle, is

[2]Arthur C. Guyton, *Textbook of Medical Physiology*, 4th ed. (Philadelphia: W. B. Saunders Company, 1971), p. 802.

unable to store glycogen in large amounts, fat synthesis is an important means by which energy can be stored in the body and called upon for later use. The fact that fat contains more than twice as many calories per gram as carbohydrates means that more energy is stored in fat than in carbohydrate.

AMINO ACID METABOLISM

Recent studies of protein metabolism have uncovered a previously unsuspected source of liver glucose, present in the amino acid *alanine*. It has been found to be released from working muscle in exercising man, and its presence in arterial blood roughly parallels arterial pyruvic acid concentration both at rest and during exercise.[3] Further, it is found that the uptake of alanine by the liver increases during exercise, and thus it may serve as an end-product of glycolysis and a source of liver glucose. In fact, the release of alanine may account for 12 to 18 percent of the total glucose extracted by muscle.

The manner in which these actions can be visualized is shown in the *glucose-alanine cycle* of Figure 46. Blood glucose is converted to pyruvic acid in the muscle. In a process called *transamination* of pyruvate, alanine is formed and released to the circulation. Alanine in turn is taken up by the liver where it is reconverted to glucose and released to the blood, thus completing the cycle.

ENERGY RELEASE

The object of metabolism is to break down the foodstuff molecules in such a way that energy can be liberated for cellular oxidations. As we have seen, the basal state simply means the lowest level of energy transfer consistent with the life processes, and since all cells need oxygen, the central feature of physiology could well be the mechanisms whereby oxygen is delivered to the cell. The previous descriptions serve to emphasize the manner in which oxygen can be utilized. In the final analysis, it turns out that molecular oxygen from the atmosphere serves as a hydrogen acceptor, and thus the production of hydrogens is the determining factor in metabolism.

Stress has been placed on the difference between aerobic and anaerobic phases of metabolism, and it should be clear at this point that a complete description of energy transfer must include both concepts. The important thing is to consider the sequence of events that occur with an

[3]Philip Felig and John Wahren, "Interrelationship Between Amino Acid and Carbohydrate Metabolism During Exercise: The Glucose Alanine-Cycle," in Bengt Pernow and Bengt Saltin, eds., *Muscle Metabolism During Exercise*. (New York: Plenum Press, 1971), pp. 205–214.

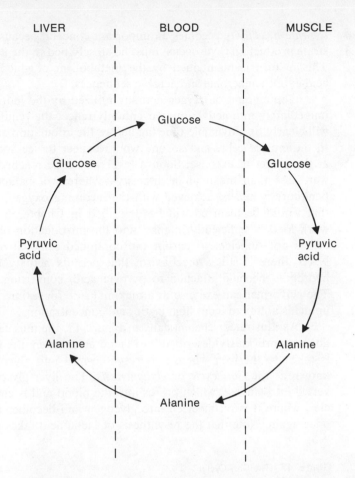

LIVER	BLOOD	MUSCLE

Glucose

Glucose

Glucose

Pyruvic acid

Pyruvic acid

Alanine

Alanine

Alanine

Figure 46. The Glucose-Alanine Cycle. [P. Felig and J. Wahren, "Interrelationship between Amino Acid and Carbohydrate Metabolism during Exercise: The Glucose Alanine-Cycle," in B. Penrow and B. Saltin, eds. *Muscle Metabolism During Exercise.* New York: Plenum Press (1971), p. 212.]

increase in activity, such as would accompany the start of exercise. Measurement of the resting metabolism would be essential so that the excess cost of work could be known. Physiologists would then subtract any values for rest from work-related values to arrive at the net cost of exercise.

The human organism has the capability of going from a condition of rest to one of high intensity without a moment's hesitation, and it can often hold this level for some time. Clearly, if we had to wait for the circulation and other factors to bring in a new supply of oxygen, some few minutes might be required. The amount of work done would be severely restricted, and the whole pattern of human behavior would be different. Fortunately, however, muscle contraction can be inaugurated fully just as soon as it receives the stimulus and can continue for a short time at maximum effort, or for a longer period at submaximal effort. Thus,

79

the *rate of activity* becomes an important concept, because the rate of substrate production (hydrogens) must be closely tied to the utilization of ATP. This in turn is maintained by the metabolism of glucose and free fatty acid in both anaerobic and aerobic sequences.

The amount of oxygen actually utilized by the individual in entering immediately into activity may eventually reflect the requirement, but there will clearly be a dynamic time lag before the circulation can deliver oxygen to the muscle cells, and so one would expect to see some sort of deficit at the outset of exercise. Soon a level would be reached—if the exercise were less than maximal in intensity—whereby a balance of energy expenditure would be achieved with the incoming oxygen. The *oxygen debt* that would be incurred will be described in Chapter 6. However, if the work load is sufficiently intense, and the introduction of oxygen into the cell is not sufficient to permit the continued removal of hydrogen from NAD, there is still a mechanism that permits activity to continue. The hydrogens become attached to pyruvic acid, converting it to lactic acid. The performer can exercise at a maximal rate for a time that is dependent upon his ability to incur high lactic acid concentrations.

As illustrated schematically in Figure 47, the muscle glycogen breaks down as previously described into lactic acid, enters the bloodstream, and is taken to the liver where it is resynthesized into glycogen in a process known as the *Cori cycle* or *glycogenesis*. The liver glycogen is then converted into glucose, which passes into the blood and is carried to the muscles, where it is reconverted into glycogen and becomes an energy source once again. Note that the resynthesis of lactic acid takes place in the liver

Figure 47. The Cori Cycle.

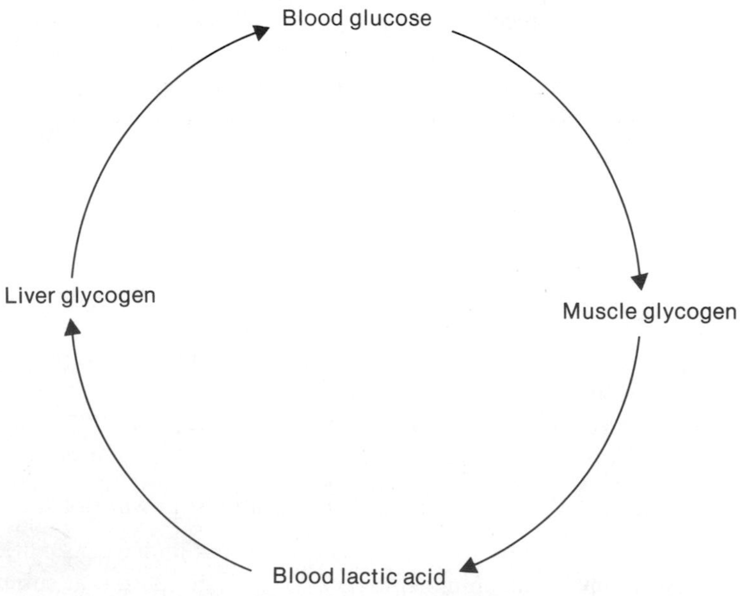

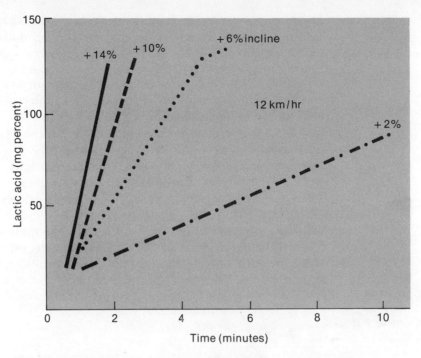

Figure 48. Lactic Acid as a Function of Time during Exhaustion Running. [R. Margaria *et al.*, "Kinetics and Mechanism of Oxygen Debt Contraction in Man," *Journal of Applied Physiology*, 18, (March 1963), p. 374.]

rather than the muscles that were involved in its production, so there is no specific recouping of the energy lost by the local tissues from this source. Muscles receive their energy from the general circulation.

Lactic acid determinations can be made from small blood samples when a subject has been run on a treadmill or exercised on a bicycle ergometer. For example, if the treadmill is set at 12 km per hour, the incline is varied from 2 to 14 percent, and lactic acid is measured in the blood at various time intervals during an exhausting run, the results appear as depicted in Figure 48. The increase in lactic acid concentration is a linear function of time during exercise.[4] In other words, during exhaustive running, there was a direct relationship between the length of running and the appearance of blood lactic acid. Since blood lactic acid is considered to be a satisfactory index of total lactic acid production, and hence an indication (but not a precise measure) of the extent of anaerobic work, it follows that as long as the rate of work in any of the designated conditions remains constant and sufficiently exhaustive, the lactic acid will continue to be produced in direct proportion to the expenditure of energy. The reader should bear in mind that this relationship will not hold true for low levels

[4]R. Margaria, "Energy Sources for Anaerobic Work," *Physiological Aspects of Sports and Physical Fitness* (Chicago: The Athletic Institute, 1968), p. 20.

of activity, as will be discussed in the next chapter. The maximum value for lactic acid was approximately 140 mg percent (140 mg per 100 ml of blood), achieved in three of the exercise conditions of Figure 48. The fourth condition, where the 2 percent grade was employed, was too mild to achieve exhaustion; hence the lactic acid production was reduced. It is generally felt that the maximum lactic acid increase in blood is approximately 150 mg percent.

Margaria[5] estimates that the energy production from glycolysis per gram of lactic acid formed is 230 calories. Further, he estimates that the maximum energy that can be obtained from the formation of lactic acid is about 260 calories per kilogram of body weight. The maximal rate of production of lactic acid is about 1.7 grams per kilogram of body weight per minute, which gives an energy yield of 390 calories per kilogram of body weight per minute. If one assumes that the maximum energy output from oxidation is some 220 calories per minute per kilogram of body weight, then it can be seen that the power available from glycolysis is approximately 50 percent higher than that from oxidation.

ENDOCRINE FUNCTION

The subject of endocrinology is an important one to the physiologist, because discharge from various endocrine glands affects cell behavior. This discharge consists of organic molecules known as *hormones*, and causes changes in cellular metabolism of other cells. The relationship of the secretion of *insulin* and the maintenance of blood glucose in the incidence of diabetes will be discussed later (Chapter 13). Insulin is secreted by the *beta* cells of the islets of Langerhans of the pancreas, and by increasing the permeability of cells to glucose makes glucose more readily available to be stored as glycogen (*glycogenesis*). The pool of glucose-6-phosphate is thus maintained by entrance of glucose into the cell.

Another hormone secreted by the pancreas, but by the *alpha* cells, rather than the beta cells, as is true with insulin, is *glucagon*. Glucagon also acts in a manner contrary to insulin. Its action in the liver is to stimulate the conversion of glycogen to glucose (*glycogenolysis*), which increases the concentration of blood glucose. Thus, glucagon helps to prevent blood hypoglycemia, a condition of reduced blood sugar.

TRAINING

The search for training effects within muscle occupies the attention of a number of investigators, who seek to uncover the adaptive changes that accompany the increase in strength and endurance known to occur.

[5]Rodolfo Margaria, "The Sources of Muscular Energy," *Scientific American,* 226 (March 1972), 84.

Most of the research has involved small animals that have been trained by swimming or running, and notable attention has been given to the enzyme systems that govern the metabolic activities of muscle. The reader will recognize some of the enzymes as having been mentioned earlier in this chapter. Others will be easily identified because they have been given the same names as the substance upon which they react. The main question is whether or not they change as a result of training, and whether this is an important change resulting in significant alterations in the capacity to perform exercise.

Very little change occurs in the basal concentration of ATP as a result of training,[6] and the change in ATPase activity is also very minimal, although Barnard and co-workers[7] found that the myosin and actomyosin ATPase activity may depend upon the type of muscle fibers involved. For example, muscle fibers which can be classified as slow-twitch (red in color) are found to have lowest, while those designated as fast-twitch (white in color) have highest ATPase activities (see Chapter 2). Gollnick *et al.*[8] found that fiber types themselves are not altered by physical training. Oscai and Holloszy[9] found mitochondrial ATPase to increase twofold in rat gastrocnemius muscle. Enzymes having an important bearing on the regeneration of ATP have also been studied, and Oscai and Holloszy found that the levels of CPase (creatine phosphokinase) did not change, reinforcing the idea that endurance exercise results in an increase in the capacity of the muscle to regenerate ATP aerobically, but not anaerobically.

Glycogen Loading

The glycogen content of working muscles, important as an indicator of the capacity to perform long-term endurance exercise, has been under rather intense study in recent years. The pattern of glycogen depletion of human subjects given exercise bouts of one-minute duration, and separated by a ten-minute rest period, of an intensity requiring an energy production equivalent to 150 percent of their aerobic power, is presented in Figure 49. The drop after the first one-minute bout was 20 percent; it then displayed a linear decline to a value more than 60 percent below resting levels after six bouts. One of the interesting developments has been the realization

[6]Julia W. Harris, "Effects of Exercise on the Basal Concentration of ATP in Muscle Tissue," *Research Quarterly*, 38 (December 1967), 598.

[7]R. James Barnard *et al.*, "Histochemical, Biochemical, and Contractile Properties of Red, White, and Intermediate Fibers," *American Journal of Physiology*, 220 (February 1971), 410.

[8]P. D. Gollnick *et al.*, "Effect of Training on Enzyme Activity and Fiber Composition of Human Skeletal Muscle," *Journal of Applied Physiology*, 34 (January 1973), 107.

[9]Lawrence B. Oscai and John O. Holloszy, "Biochemical Adaptations in Muscle. II. Response of Mitochondrial Adenosine Triphosphatase, Creatine Phosphokinase, and Adenylate Kinase Activities in Skeletal Muscle to Exercise," *Journal of Biological Chemistry*, 246 (November 25, 1971), 6968.

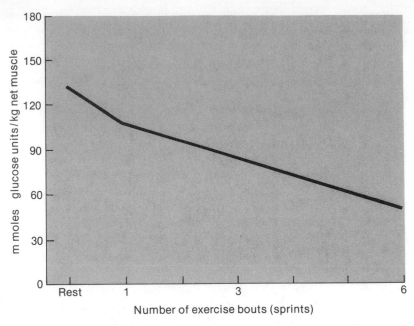

Figure 49. Muscle Glycogen Depletion Following Exercise. [P. D. Gollnick *et al.*, "Glycogen Depletion Pattern in Human Skeletal Muscle Fibers after Heavy Exercise," *Journal of Applied Physiology*, 34 (May 1973), p. 616.]

in man that exercise with glycogen depletion actually enhances the *resynthesis* of glycogen,[10] and that the factor controlling this resynthesis is a mechanism that operates locally in the exercised muscle. Moreover, the diet may play a role in causing elevated levels of muscle glycogen (called supercompensation) to occur. In one experiment of this sort, Bergström and colleagues[11] put subjects on a week's schedule as illustrated in Figure 50. The subjects were placed on a mixed diet and on Monday were measured for muscle glycogen content and work performance to exhaustion on a bicycle ergometer. They were then placed on a fat (1,300 kcal) plus protein (1,500 kcal) diet for three days and performed the work test again. For the next three days the subjects consumed a predominantly carbohydrate diet (2,300 kcal, plus 500 kcal protein), and were given a final work performance test. Glycogen determinations were made from muscle biopsy samples before each exercise and immediately after the subjects were exhausted. The increase in glycogen synthesis from the carbohydrate diet was nearly double the value achieved through a mixed diet, and five times more effective than the fat plus protein diet. As shown in Figure 51, there was also an increase in the work time of subjects given the high-

[10]Jonas Bergström and Eric Hultman, "Muscle Glycogen Synthesis after Exercise: An Enhancing Factor Localized to the Muscle Cells in Man," *Nature*, 210 (April 16, 1966), 309.

[11]Jonas Bergström *et al.*, "Diet, Muscle Glycogen and Physical Performance," *Acta Physiologica Scandinavica*, 71 (1967), 140.

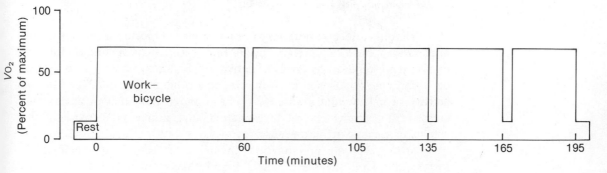

Mon		Tues	Wed	Thurs		Fri	Sat	Sun		Mon
Mixed	Work	Protein		1,500 kcal	Work	Carbo-hydrates		2,300 kcal	Work	
diet		Fat		1,300 kcal		Protein		500 kcal		

Figure 50. Schedule for Diet, Work, and Glycogen Determination. [J. Bergström *et al.*, "Diet, Muscle Glycogen and Physical Performance," *Acta Physiologica Scandinavica*, 71 (1967), p. 142.]

Figure 51. Relation between Initial Glycogen Content and Work Time. [J. Bergström *et al.*, "Diet, Muscle Glycogen and Physical Performance," *Acta Physiologica Scandinavica*, 71 (1967), p. 143.]

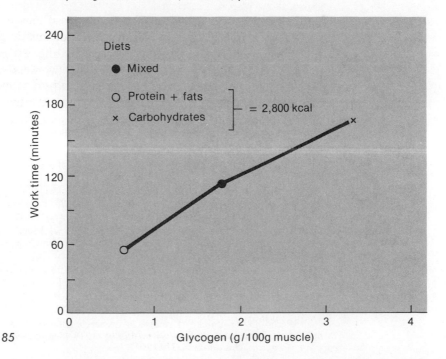

carbohydrate diet over those on a mixed or protein plus fat diet. In fact, the relationship between glycogen content and work time is approximately linear over the range of values studied. Thus, during one week, the muscles were able to synthesize greater concentrations of glycogen and consequently enhance work performance. Exercise depletes glycogen stores in heart and liver, also, but a supercompensation persists only in skeletal muscle.[12]

Respiratory Enzymes

Various mitochondrial enzymes have been subjected to analysis, and in particular those of the Krebs cycle. In a comprehensive study, Holloszy *et al.*[13] reported that the levels of activity of citrate synthase and isocitrate dehydrogenase doubled in rats subjected to a program of running, while the activity of α-ketoglutarate dehydrogenase and malate dehydrogenase increased 50 percent. Several investigators have noted an increase in the activity of succinic dehydrogenase.

In two separate investigations involving the respiratory chain, Holloszy[14] and Holloszy and Oscai[15] found that cytochrome oxidase and cytochrome c doubled as a result of training. According to Holloszy and co-workers,[16] evidence indicates that muscle mitochondria undergo an adaptive change in composition as a result of intense physical work, but unlike the constituents of the respiratory chain, the enzymes of the Krebs cycle do not increase to the same extent during response of skeletal muscle to a program of intense physical exercise.

Fat Metabolism

The degree to which skeletal muscle may alter fat mobilization after training has also been of interest to research workers in this field. For example, Gollnick[17] found that plasma and adipose tissue free fatty acid levels and FFA release from the fat pads of rats were elevated in both trained and untrained animals following exercise, although the mechanism

[12]David R. Lamb *et al.,* "Glycogen, Hexokinase, and Glycogen Synthetase Adaptations to Exercise," *American Journal of Physiology*, 217 (December 1969), 1628.

[13]J. O. Holloszy *et al.,* "Mitochondrial Citric Acid Cycle and Related Enzymes: Adaptive Response to Exercise," *Biochemical and Bio-Physical Research Communications*, 40 (1970), 1368.

[14]John O. Holloszy, "Biochemical Adaptations in Muscle. Effects of Exercise on Mitochondrial Oxygen Uptake and Respiratory Enzyme Activity in Skeletal Muscle," *Journal of Biological Chemistry*, 242 (1967), 2278.

[15]John O. Holloszy and Lawrence B. Oscai, "Effect of Exercise on α-Glycerophosphate Dehydrogenase Activity in Skeletal Muscle," *Archives of Biochemistry and Biophysics*, 130 (1969), 653.

[16]Holloszy *et al., op. cit.*

[17]Philip D. Gollnick, "Exercise, Adrenergic Blockage, and Free Fatty Acid Mobilization," *American Journal of Physiology*, 213 (September 1967), 734.

controlling FFA mobilization in untrained and trained rats appears to be different. Molé and Holloszy[18] found that exercised rats oxidized FFA (as calculated by the oxidation of palmitate) at rates significantly greater than sedentary controls; in fact, Molé et al.[19] found that the rate of palmitate oxidation was twice as great in the trained as in the sedentary. Apparently, one of the effects of physical training is to obtain a greater proportion of energy for submaximal effort from fat.

SUMMARY

Metabolism can be divided into anaerobic and aerobic phases, depending upon the role played by atmospheric oxygen. Glycolysis involves the degradation of the glucose molecule into pyruvic acid and is a reflection of carbohydrate metabolism. A number of intermediate products are involved, with the formation of some ATP and the transferrance of two hydrogen atoms to the coenzyme NAD, forming NAD2H. If oxygen is not present in sufficient quantities, the hydrogens are passed to pyruvic acid, converting it to lactic acid. The pyruvic acid is condensed aerobically in the Krebs cycle by first yielding acetyl Co A and combining with oxaloacetic acid. In the process three molecules of CO_2 are released, one ATP is produced, and five pairs of hydrogens are removed and passed by means of a coenzyme to the respiratory chain. Here they are accepted by flavoproteins and cytochromes, eventually undergoing electron transfer and combining with oxygen to form water. In this process the majority of ATP is produced; for every gram-mole of glucose, 686,000 calories are created, 39 percent of which are stored in the form of ATP.

Free fatty acids are hydrolized from the triglycerides of the adipose tissue, where they are transported by the blood to the muscles, entering the Krebs cycle to yield ATP. Carbohydrates are the preferred fuel for short, strenuous bouts of activity, and fats are used in longer endurance events. Another source of blood glucose may come from alanine, an amino acid released from working muscles.

The amount of energy utilized by the individual will reflect a dynamic time lag before the requisite circulatory factors can deliver sufficient oxygen. Moreover, if the exercise is severe, lactic acid will be formed. Both will result in an oxygen debt, which must be paid off in the recovery period. Training causes little change in basal concentrations of ATP, but mitochondrial ATPase can double. Glycogen content of working muscles

[18]Paul A. Molé and John O. Holloszy, "Exercise-Induced Increase in the Capacity of Skeletal Muscle to Oxidize Palmitate," *Proceedings of the Society for Experimental Biology and Medicine*, 134 (1970), 789.

[19]P. A. Molé, L. B. Oscai, and J. O. Holloszy, "Adaptation of Muscle to Exercise Increase in Levels of Palmityl Co A Synthetase, Carnitine Palmityltransferase and Palmityl Co A Dehydrogenase, and in the Capacity to Oxidize Fatty Acids," *Journal of Clinical Investigation*, 50 (November 1971), 2323.

can be enhanced if subjects first exercise to exhaust local glycogen stores, consume a diet of protein and fat for three days, undergo exhausting exercise again and go on a high-carbohydrate diet for three more days. This results in glycogen supercompensation and an increase in work time. Training also enhances plasma and adipose tissue free fatty acid levels, which results in a greater proportion of energy for submaximal exercise from fat.

SELECTED REFERENCES

Gollnick, Philip D., "Energy Production and Lactic Acid Formation," *Physiological Aspects of Sports and Physical Fitness*. Chicago: The Athletic Institute, 1968, p. 16.

————, and Lars Hermansen, "Biochemical Adaptations to Exercise: Anaerobic Metabolism," in Jack H. Wilmore, ed., *Exercise and Sport Sciences Reviews*, Vol. 1. New York: Academic Press, 1973, pp. 1–43.

————, and Douglas W. King, "Energy Release in the Muscle Cell," *Medicine and Science in Sports*, 1 (March 1969), 23.

Green, David E., "The Metabolism of Fats," *Scientific American*, 190 (January 1954), 32.

Guyton, Arthur C., *Textbook of Medical Physiology*, 4th ed. Philadelphia: W. B. Saunders Company, 1971, chaps. 67 and 68.

Holloszy, John O., "Biochemical Adaptations to Exercise: Aerobic Metabolism," in Jack H. Wilmore, ed., *Exercise and Sport Sciences Reviews*, Vol. 1. New York: Academic Press, 1973, pp. 45–71.

————, L. B. Oscai, P. A. Molé, and I. J. Don, "Biochemical Adaptations to Endurance Exercise in Skeletal Muscle," in Bengt Pernow and Bengt Saltin, eds., *Muscle Metabolism During Exercise*. New York: Plenum Press, 1971, p. 51.

Hultman, Eric, "Muscle Glycogen Stores and Prolonged Exercise," in Roy J. Shephard, ed., *Frontiers of Fitness*. Springfield, Ill.: Charles C. Thomas, 1971, chap. 2.

————, "Physiological Role of Muscle Glycogen in Man, with Special Reference to Exercise," *American Heart Association Monograph*, 20 (1967), p. 15.

Margaria, Rodolfo, "Biochemistry of Muscular Contraction and Recovery," *Journal of Sports Medicine and Physical Fitness*, 3 (1963), 145.

————, "The Sources of Muscular Energy," *Scientific American*, 226 (March 1972), 84.

chapter

6

work, oxygen debt, and aerobic capacity

The biochemical basis for the oxygen-debt mechanism was presented in Chapter 5, where it was brought out that the production of lactic acid reflects the need for energy which must be provided on an anaerobic basis. There seems little doubt that this is primarily the case, but whether it is sufficient alone to explain the presence of an oxygen debt is another matter. From what has been evident since the mid 1930's, there are actually two portions of the oxygen debt that appear to be consequences of anaerobic metabolic activity, and which together form the total debt. The purpose of the present chapter is to differentiate between these two types of debt and explain their relationship to work done and oxygen uptake.

WORK

The amount of energy expended by an individual engaged in muscular exercise depends upon how much *work* is accomplished in a given period of time. The term "exercise" has little scientific meaning because it cannot be *quantified*; we must turn elsewhere for some means of giving value to the amount of activity. The term work has been employed as a basis for the determination of energy expenditure. The formula for work is force times distance ($W = Fd$), and we can calculate it by knowing the weight of an object (which can be displaced by a muscular effort, or force) and the distance this object is moved. Thus, work results in *motion*. Should no movement occur, as in an isometric contraction, the product of force and distance would be zero, and it can be concluded that no work is done. Since it is clear that a considerable amount of energy expenditure is likely to have occurred, the physical definition is not always useful to the physiologist. Moreover, the calculation of total work does not take into consideration the time involved in its execution, so that what could amount to a very strenuous exercise when done in a short interval might turn out to be mild activity when spread out over a relatively long one. Yet, the calculation of total work would be the same, provided that the force and distance were the same.

This dilemma provides a rationale for the use of *power* as a substitute for work. Power is the rate of doing work, and it introduces the element of time: $P = W/t$, or $P = Fd/t$. While the term *horsepower* is familiar, it is not often employed in physiology. In fact, the term power is not used as much as it probably should be either. Time is accounted for by making the length of exercise a constant factor. This has the effect of cancelling out the variable of time, making the unit of work more acceptable in studies of the effects of exercise. Power is technically more valid, however, and it is being used more frequently in assessing the capacity of the individual to utilize oxygen. The *oxygen uptake* is being referred to as *aerobic power*, since the oxygen uptake is usually expressed in liters per minute or milliliters per kilogram of body weight per minute. This will be discussed in detail later.

A more realistic trend is to employ still another concept in expressing the extent of physiological stress during exercise. Rather than either work or power, which is sometimes extremely difficult to assess and is practically useless when the task is isometric,[1] a term of choice may be the *MET*. The metabolic cost at rest is one MET; two METS is two times the resting level, three METS is three times the value at rest, and so on. The resting energy cost (net oxygen requirement) is thus a standard for the relative assessment of the severity of further exercise loads, and theoretically can function in any type of activity. In actuality, though, the direct measurement of metabolic energy cost is time consuming and requires rather extensive equipment, so it is relatively inaccessible, except in the most well-equipped laboratories. Later we will see how approximations of the energy cost can be made from other predictive tests—relying on estimates from heart rate, for example, rather than actually measuring oxygen uptake and carbon dioxide elimination. Nevertheless, the MET will undoubtedly be in favor in future metabolic studies.

SUBMAXIMAL VS. MAXIMAL WORK

The human organism does not react in the same manner to all levels of muscular work. The reason is grounded in concepts expressed in the previous chapter. When the level of activity is light, normal disposal of metabolic byproducts takes place approximately as fast as they are produced. However, when the creation of these metabolites exceeds the ability of the circulation and other support mechanisms to bring in oxygen, the body makes use of the lactic acid mechanism as a means for sustaining activity. Exercise physiologists classify the former as *submaximal work*, the latter as *maximal work*.

Submaximal work, also known as *steady-state* performance, signifies theoretically that there is no limit to the length of time an individual can continue to exercise. It is a pay-as-you-go operation, with the rate of energy expenditure equal to the body's ability to supply oxygen. Most of the activities we undertake during the normal course of daily events are clearly of this nature, such as walking, light jogging, and of course more

---

[1]David H. Clarke, "Energy Cost of Isometric Exercise," *Research Quarterly,* 31 (March 1960), 3.

sedentary activities. When the steady state is exceeded, maximal exercise occurs, and now by definition the rate of energy expenditure exceeds the oxygen uptake, meaning that activity must be terminated because soon the body's capacity to tolerate the buildup of lactic acid will have reached its maximum. The individual actually has the ability to do considerable activity even when it is classified as maximal. Many athletic contests operate on this basis, as the performer strives to expend the greatest energy by the end of the contest or event. Later, there is a time of some considerable duration during which the performer remains in a state of heightened metabolic activity. As we have learned, this is the time when the oxygen debt is being repaid. The question that has been found intriguing, however, is whether an oxygen debt is associated only with maximal exercise, or whether it accompanies submaximal exercise as well.

ALACTIC VS. LACTIC OXYGEN DEBTS

The oxygen debt that accompanies exercise can be defined as the amount of oxygen required during recovery over and above the resting level. The most obvious causative factor is the oxidation of lactic acid that is known to accompany exercise beyond the steady state. This *lactic debt* is easily explained biochemically. After all, extensive exercise is known to result in a buildup of lactic acid; the hydrogen atoms become attached to pyruvic acid, which with the aid of the enzyme lactic dehydrogenase is converted into lactic acid. During subsequent recovery, the lactic acid is converted back to pyruvic acid, and as explained previously (Chapter 5), results in a resynthesis of glycogen. The fraction of pyruvic acid that enters the Krebs cycle eventually requires oxygen and thus forms an index of the reliance on this anaerobic mechanism. At the same time the requirement for oxygen in recovery can be measured and the oxygen debt calculated.

The difficulty with accepting the concept that the oxygen debt can be attributed solely to what has been called "excess lactate,"[2] which says that the blood lactic acid increases proportionately for all levels of work, is the persistent finding that there is more than one phase or component to the oxygen-debt mechanism. For example, Margaria and co-workers[3] in 1933 plotted the concentration of lactic acid in the blood against the oxygen debt with the results shown in Figure 52. For an oxygen debt of up to 3 or 4 liters there is no appreciable increase in blood lactic acid, but thereafter a linear increase occurs in the two functions. This means that for an oxygen debt beyond approximately 4 liters only the

[2]William E. Huckabee, "Relationships of Pyruvate and Lactate during Anaerobic Metabolism. II. Exercise and Formation of O_2-Debt," *Journal of Clinical Investigation*, 37 (1958), 255.

[3]R. Margaria, H. T. Edwards, and D. B. Dill, "The Possible Mechanisms of Contracting and Paying the Oxygen Debt and the Role of Lactic Acid in Muscular Contraction," *American Journal of Physiology*, 106 (1933), 689.

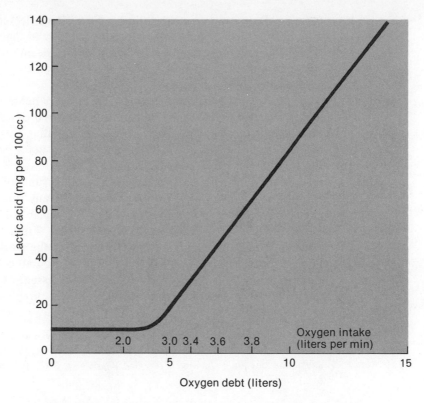

Figure 52. Relationship between Blood Lactic Acid and Oxygen Debt. [R. Margaria *et al.*, "The Possible Mechanisms of Contracting and Paying the Oxygen Debt and the Role of Lactic Acid in Muscular Contraction," *American Journal of Physiology*, 106 (1933), p. 694.]

lactic acid mechanism is involved. Moreover, the authors point out that it is not likely for an extra localized accumulation of lactic acid in the muscles to account for additional oxygen consumption after work. The question then is, to what do we attribute the early consumption of oxygen after exercise if it is not due to lactic acid?

The answer remains somewhat obscure, but research spanning many years makes it clear that there are two fractions to the oxygen-debt mechanism, one being lactic and the other, for want of a more specific term, *alactic* (sometimes called the *alactacid debt*). This says not so much what the debt is as what it is not; that is, it is not due to lactic acid. Exercise physiologists have long known that accompanying even rather mild levels of activity, a brief recovery period can be seen, involving such metabolic functions as heart rate, respiratory rate, and oxygen uptake. Ordinarily these functions have a short duration and, depending upon the severity of work load, return to normal quickly. Margaria and his co-workers found two mathematical constants in the data for recovery from exercise, a rapid one called alactic, and a slower one corresponding to the lactic acid function. Both are known to follow a logarithmic decrement; that is, they follow a curvilinear path, falling rapidly at first and then progressing more slowly toward the resting level. The half-time decline of the alactic debt is approximately 30 seconds, contrasting to a half-time of several minutes for the lactic debt.

The relationship of these two debt components can be seen from Figure 53. The total oxygen curve is the measured oxygen required during the recovery period, the starting point representing the steady-state value at the very end of exercise. The reader should note that the vertical axis shows the oxygen uptake plotted on a logarithmic scale. This is convenient for presenting the slope of the alactic and lactic functions, which would be curvilinear if plotted on a coordinate scale. At any rate, it reveals that an exercise of 680 kgm/min for 6 minutes resulted in a half-time decline of approximately 40 sec for the alactic curve and 4 min for the lactic component. The intriguing finding has been that as the work load increases, a greater proportion of the oxygen debt is attributable to lactic acid, but the rate of payoff of the alactic debt shows essentially no change. The lactic-debt recovery rate, in contrast, becomes progressively slower, thus

Figure 53. The Oxygen Debt Components. [F. M. Henry and J. C. De-Moor, "Lactic and Alactic Oxygen Consumption in Moderate Exercise of Graded Intensity," *Journal of Applied Physiology*, 8 (May 1956), p. 610.]

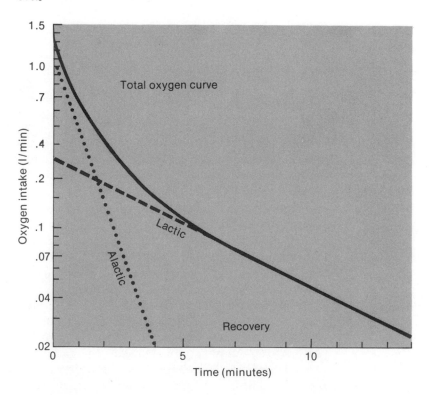

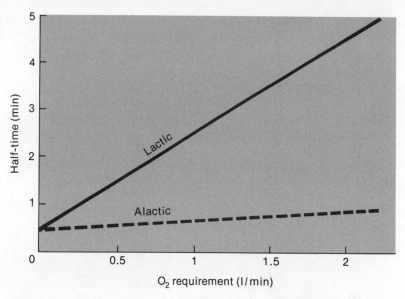

Figure 54. Changes in the Lactic and Alactic Parameters of the Oxygen Debt as Work Load Is Varied. [F. M. Henry and J. C. DeMoor, "Lactic and Alactic Oxygen Consumption in Moderate Exercise of Graded Intensity," *Journal of Applied Physiology*, 8 (May 1956), p. 613.]

taking longer to pay off as the work load becomes more severe.[4] This relationship is shown in Figure 54.

THE OXYGEN UPTAKE ($\dot{V}O_2$)

Turning our attention now to the *oxygen-uptake* side of the metabolic curve, we can see an interesting parallel between the initial uptake of oxygen and the repayment of the alactic debt in recovery. Current theory would indicate that the human organism is first activated by a biochemical scheme that does not require oxygen, but sets into motion a series of events that serves as a stimulus for the increased oxygen uptake ($\dot{V}O_2$).[5] In other words, as soon as exercise begins, and not before, the metabolic processes speed up and cause the increase in cellular use of oxygen. Some lag should be expected while this process is being completed, since time would be required for the respiratory and circulatory events responsible for increasing the oxygen uptake to actually exert their full influence. The tissues are unable to store large amounts of oxygen, so they must wait for the production of substrate materials associated with the new level of

[4]Franklin M. Henry and Janice C. DeMoor, "Lactic and Alactic Oxygen Consumption in Moderate Exercise of Graded Intensity," *Journal of Applied Physiology*, 8 (May 1956), 608.

[5]The dot over the V signifies rate, usually expressed in liters per minute (l/min).

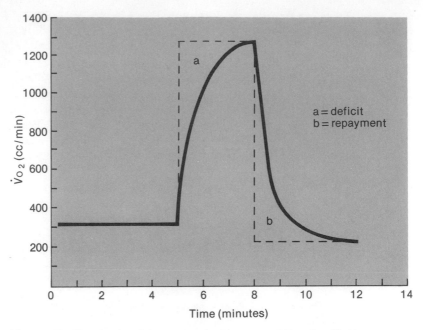

Figure 55. The Uptake of Oxygen at the Beginning of Exercise. [F. M. Henry, *Physiology of Work*. Berkeley: Associate Students' Store, University of California (1968), p. 48.]

activity before they can demand more oxygen. In a matter of a few minutes the O_2 intake has readjusted to this new level, which the individual has already assumed. If this is a submaximal load, then the steady state achieved will be a direct reflection of the metabolic requirement, since the $\dot{V}O_2$ will adjust to the demands created by the rate of work.

The pattern of increase in oxygen uptake from rest to the steady state is not linear, but curvilinear, bearing more than just a superficial resemblance to the alactic debt in recovery. Figure 55 reflects the intake curve during the first few minutes of a submaximal exercise, and it clearly shows a delay in the oxygen-uptake ability of the tissues. The difference between the observed oxygen intake and that which would have occurred if the rate of intake had instantly reached a steady state is termed the *oxygen deficit*. When compared with the corresponding debt after exercise, there appears to be a similarity in the rate of change. In fact, the half-time values for the uptake and repayment are quite close, being of the order of 30 seconds for both.[6] This means that approximately 30 seconds are required for the oxygen uptake at the outset of exercise to reach halfway to the steady state, or in the recovery period, for the alactic payoff to recede halfway to the resting level. In both cases an additional 30 seconds is required to take care of half of the remaining amount, and so forth, until the steady state has finally been reached.

[6]Franklin M. Henry, "Aerobic Oxygen Consumption and Alactic Debt in Muscular Work," *Journal of Applied Physiology*, 3 (January 1951), 427.

Whether the total amount of the deficit is equal to the repayment in submaximal exercise is somewhat uncertain, although Royce[7] found the deficit to be nearly the exact mirror image of the repayment. He also found them to be fairly highly correlated ($r = .79$). The interpretation that can be forwarded is that the alactic debt is a reflection of the oxidative delay that occurs in the early phase of exercise; after all, the increased oxygen uptake must first wait for an oxidizable substrate to be formed, and this must come as a result of the work itself. When values for oxygen debt are found to be greater than oxygen deficit, one possible explanantion is a disturbance in the resting metabolism, leading to increases in post-exercise oxygen uptake.[8]

In summary, while it would be attractive to attempt to ascribe the alactic debt to some single event, the likelihood is that a number of cellular processes not concerned with lactic acid removal contribute to the payoff of the alactic debt, as it is actually the combined effect that is seen. Wasserman, Burton, and Van Kessel[9] list the following "creditors" other than the conversion of lactate to pyruvate to which the oxygen debt is paid:

1. Regeneration of oxymyoglobin.
2. Renewal of ATP and other high-energy phosphate sources.
3. Replenishment of dissolved oxygen in tissue fluids.
4. Oxidation of reduced coenzymes.
5. Increase in the venous oxyhemoglobin concentration to its resting value.

Some of these factors will be discussed in later chapters, but the reader should note that each one represents a source of disposition of molecular oxygen. Theoretically, at least, each could serve as a basis for the alactic debt mechanism.

MAXIMAL OXYGEN UPTAKE ($\dot{V}O_2$ max)

Special attention should be directed to the concept of *maximal oxygen uptake* ($\dot{V}O_2$ max), or *maximal aerobic power*, currently so prominent in the exercise physiology literature. It involves an increase in the oxygen uptake to the highest level of severity, whereby the ability of the individual to utilize the greatest amount of oxygen is reached. This does not necessarily measure the individual physical work capacity, because that implies maximum performance. The $\dot{V}O_2$ max test does not need to reach the stage of exhaustion, because by definition it is the maximum aerobic capacity, not maximum anaerobic capacity. Once again we return

[7]Joseph Royce, "Oxygen Consumption during Submaximal Exercises of Equal Intensity and Different Duration," *Int. Z. angew. Physiol.* 19 (1962), 218.

[8]Howard G. Knuttgen and Bengt Saltin, "Muscle Metabolites and Oxygen Uptake in Short-Term Submaximal Exercise in Man," *Journal of Applied Physiology*, 32 (May 1972), 690.

[9]Karlman Wasserman, George G. Burton, and Antonius L. Van Kessel, "Excess Lactate Concept and Oxygen Debt of Exercise," *Journal of Applied Physiology*, 20 (November 1965), 1299.

to the biochemical scheme that suggests a direct relationship between the production of metabolites and the intake of oxygen; some point will be reached whereby the $\dot{V}O_2$ will fail to increase appreciably with an increase in work load. Quite clearly, it will involve the functional support of the respiratory and circulatory systems, as well as the metabolic pathways, and when the full contribution of each is realized, the $\dot{V}O_2$ stabilizes at its maximum value. Continued work is possible, of course, for reasons already explained, but this will be at the expense of the anaerobic mechanisms responsible for lactate build-up in the attainment of maximum work output.

The maximal oxygen uptake can be assessed by employing a test involving a treadmill, bicycle ergometer, or step-bench. The first two are the usual choices in research investigations, since they can be easily varied in adjusting work load or exercise severity. The technique is to monitor the $\dot{V}O_2$ during the progressive stages of work until the point is reached where it does not increase appreciably. This criterion value is usually 150 ml O_2, that is, if the next stage of work fails to increase the $\dot{V}O_2$ by this amount, the exercise is terminated, and this value is accepted as maximal. The details of testing are presented in Chapter 14, but the reader should bear in mind that the direct measure of $\dot{V}O_2$ max is a technical one, requiring great precision and skill. Moreover, the equipment that is required is expensive, and the whole procedure is not considered very useful as a field test for physical education classes in public schools. However, extensive efforts have been made to devise alternate forms of the test that reduce problems of measurement; consequently, we have procedures available which attempt to predict the $\dot{V}O_2$ max from submaximal tests employing a variable such as exercise heart rate. These will also be discussed later.

The fact remains that maximal oxygen uptake is regarded by an increasingly large number of exercise physiologists as the most appropriate measure of cardiorespiratory fitness, or perhaps even physical fitness. Caution should be exerted in accepting it as being synonymous with the broad concept of physical fitness, since it purports to measure only one element in total fitness, albeit an important one. Nevertheless, the cardiorespiratory system must be seen as a major element of fitness, and so the $\dot{V}O_2$ max test figures heavily in the total fitness scheme. A question of major importance to be answered, then, is how well $\dot{V}O_2$ max relates to the capacity of the individual for endurance performance. Wilmore[10] provided some information on this as a result of a bicycle ergometer task. The correlation between these two variables was found to be fairly high ($r =$ .84), and it was therefore concluded that considerable validity existed for using this test as a measure of performance capability and as an index of cardiorespiratory fitness.

[10]Jack H. Wilmore, "Maximal Oxygen Intake and its Relationship to Endurance Capacity on a Bicycle Ergometer," *Research Quarterly*, 40 (March 1969), 203.

Age and Sex

It would perhaps be appropriate to mention that the $\dot{V}O_2$ max undergoes alteration during a person's lifetime, increasing during the formative years to maturity, and then gradually declining throughout adulthood. This relationship with age is presented both in liters per minute (Figure 56a) and in ml O_2 per kg gross body weight (Figure 56b). Before puberty, no difference seems to exist in the $\dot{V}O_2$ max between boys and girls, when expressed in liters per minute, but the adult women appears to have a maximum aerobic capacity only about 75 percent of that of men, again expressed in liters per minute. However, since women generally increase in the amount of adipose tissue more than men, the difference is considerably modified when $\dot{V}O_2$ max is expressed in ml/kg body weight. In other words, sex differences are considerably modified when the oxygen intake is made relative to body size, as would be done by dividing $\dot{V}O_2$ by body weight. Some average values are given in Table 6–1 for men and women in various age-group categories, reflecting a range that would be expected to be found for each. Obviously, as average values, they do not represent the aerobic capacities of well-trained persons or of those who are extremely sedentary.

Figure 56a. Relationship between $\dot{V}O_2$ max and Age for Men ($\male$) and Women ($\female$), Expressed in l/min. [P. O. Åstrand and K. Rodahl, *Textbook of Work Physiology.* New York: McGraw-Hill Book Company (1970), p. 306.]

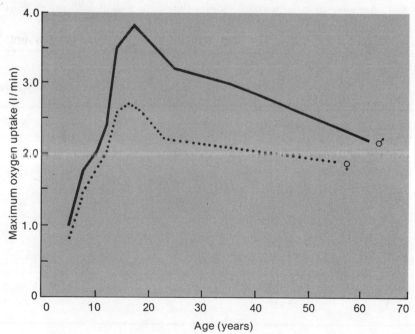

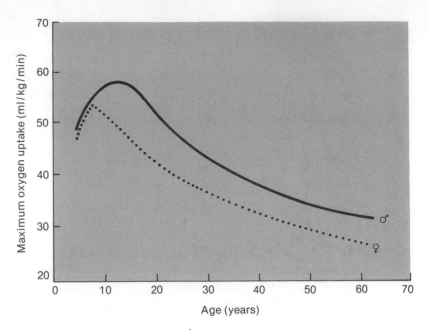

Figure 56b. Relationship between $\dot{V}O_2$ *max and Age for Men* (♂) *and Women* (♀), *Expressed in ml/kg/min.* [P. O. Åstrand and K. Rodahl, *Textbook of Work Physiology.* New York: McGraw-Hill Book Company (1970), p. 311.]

Table 6–1. Average Values for Maximal Oxygen Uptake for Men and Women at Various Ages

Men

	Age Group (Years)				
	20–29	30–39	40–49	50–59	60–69
$\dot{V}O_2$ (l/min)	3.10–3.69	2.80–3.39	2.50–3.09	2.20–2.79	1.90–2.49
$\dot{V}O_2$ (ml/kg/min)	44–51	40–47	36–43	32–39	27–35

Women

	Age Group (Years)			
	20–29	30–39	40–49	50–65
$\dot{V}O_2$ (l/min)	2.00–2.49	1.90–2.39	1.80–2.29	1.60–2.09
$\dot{V}O_2$ (ml/kg/min)	35–43	34–41	32–40	29–36

Adapted from I. Åstrand, "Aerobic Work Capacity of Men and Women with Special Reference to Age," *Acta Physiologica Scandinavica*, 49 Suppl. 169 (1960), 1.

Maximal Values

The interest in maximal oxygen uptake has extended to the recording of maximal values for $\dot{V}o_2$ max—partly, one would suppose, to know something of the extent of training, and partly out of curiosity. To the scientist such measures are similar to what world records are to the track coach; it is always interesting to know what limitations there are to human endurance. As will be explained later, the high values for aerobic capacity come from individuals engaged in activities such as cross-country skiing or orienteering (a cross-country running event guided by compass readings). Hanson[11] found the values for one skier to be as high as 88 ml/kg/min, which corresponded to 6.2 l/min. Compare this figure with the average values in Table 6–1.

Training

The changes that occur in maximal oxygen uptake as a result of training should be of considerable interest to the exercise physiologist. It is not surprising to learn that the amount of change to be anticipated depends to a large degree on the extent of fitness prior to the training period. The more sedentary and unconditioned one is, the greater will be the increase in $\dot{V}o_2$ max, whereas athletes in training can expect but a modest change. The greatest improvement, then, comes from those who have lost their usual level of fitness through inactivity such as that caused by bed rest. Age is also a factor, as older individuals seem unable to alter their maximal oxygen uptake appreciably. In fact, a moderately fit person can effect only about a 10 to 20 percent increment in $\dot{V}o_2$ max even after several months of strenuous training, while a low fit individual may achieve gains of 30 percent or more. How, then, are some athletes able to achieve the maximal values reported above? Perhaps this is a little like asking why some individuals are athletes, since the two questions seem to reflect the same thing. Endurance performance appeals to some because it seems to come naturally; the ability to achieve high performance was experienced perhaps early in life, and school athletic programs provided an opportunity for this capacity to develop fully. All of this may simply point out that an important determinant was perhaps the genetic inheritance of the performer—his natural endowment.

The mechanism for a change in aerobic capacity can be understood by considering the primary factors that are susceptible to change with training. The question here is not how the $\dot{V}o_2$ changes during exercise, but what causes a change in *maximum* values. Holloszy[12] suggests that the

[11]John S. Hanson, "Maximal Exercise Performance in Members of the U.S. Nordic Ski Team," *Journal of Applied Physiology*, 35 (November 1973), 592.

[12]John O. Holloszy, "Biochemical Adaptations to Exercise: Aerobic Metabolism," in Jack H. Wilmore, ed., *Exercise and Sport Sciences Reviews*, Vol. 1 (New York: Academic Press, 1973), p. 66.

primary factor for an increased utilization of oxygen comes about as a result of the extraction of a greater percentage of oxygen from the blood, brought about by a reduction in the oxygen tension in the muscle cells. In Chapter 8 we will gain a better understanding of the laws governing gas exchange, but what it means is that there would be a greater and probably more rapid uptake of oxygen from the blood by the muscle cells. This is enhanced by the increase in muscle mitochondria, which occurs as an individual adapts to prolonged endurance exercise.

SUMMARY

Work is the product of force and distance, and it results in motion. When divided by time it becomes a measure of power; oxygen uptake is often referred to as aerobic power, since it is usually calculated on the basis of time. The MET, the metabolic cost at rest, is the standard for assessment of relative severity of exercise intensity.

Submaximal exercise, known as steady-state performance, can be continued for long periods since the rate of energy expenditure is equivalent to the intake of oxygen. Exceeding the steady state leads to maximal exercise because the rate of energy expenditure is greater than the oxygen uptake capability; the result is a buildup of lactic acid. The early portion of the oxygen debt, which is not concerned primarily with lactic acid removal, is called the alactic debt. The portion involved with the oxidation of lactic acid is the lactic debt. The lag in oxygen delivery at the beginning of steady-state exercise is termed the deficit, and the corresponding debt in recovery is called the repayment.

The maximal oxygen uptake is the maximum aerobic capacity; it implies the stage where the greatest amount of oxygen can be used in cellular reactions. Many consider it the most representative measure of cardiorespiratory fitness, and it correlates fairly well with an individual's endurance performance. Maximal oxygen uptake increases with age during the formative years to maturity and gradually declines during adulthood. Women have lower absolute values, but when allowance is made for differences in body weight and adipose tissue, the difference is modified. The amount that can be changed with training depends on the initial state of fitness; the average increase may be no more than 10 to 20 percent, even after an extended period of strenuous training.

SELECTED REFERENCES

Andersen, K. Lange, "The Cardiovascular System in Exercise," in Harold B. Falls, ed., *Exercise Physiology*. New York: Academic Press, 1968, pp. 114–116.

Åstrand, Per-Olof, and Kaare Rodahl, *Textbook of Work Physiology*. New York: McGraw-Hill Book Company, 1970, chap. 9.

Henry, Franklin M., "Aerobic Oxygen Consumption and Alactic Debt in Muscular Work," *Journal of Applied Physiology*, 3 (January 1951), 427.

————, and Janice C. DeMoor, "Lactic and Alactic Oxygen Consumption in Moderate Exercise of Graded Intensity," *Journal of Applied Physiology*, 8 (May 1956), 608.

Holloszy, John O., "Biochemical Adaptations to Exercise: Aerobic Metabolism," in Jack H. Wilmore, ed., *Exercise and Sport Sciences Reviews*, Vol. 1. New York: Academic Press, 1973, pp. 45–71.

Margaria, R., H. T. Edwards, and D. B. Dill, "The Possible Mechanisms of Contracting and Paying the Oxygen Debt and the Role of Lactic Acid in Muscular Contraction," *American Journal of Physiology*, 106 (1933), 689.

Nagle, Francis J., "Physiological Assessment of Maximal Performance," in Jack H. Wilmore, ed., *Exercise and Sport Sciences Reviews*, Vol. 1. New York: Academic Press, 1973, pp. 313–338.

Tipton, Charles M., and R. J. Barnard, "Alactacid Debt," *Physiological Aspects of Sports and Physical Fitness*. Chicago: The Athletic Institute, 1968, p. 26.

Wasserman, Karlman, George G. Burton, and Antonius L. Van Kessel, "Excess Lactate Concept and Oxygen Debt of Exercise," *Journal of Applied Physiology*, 20 (November 1965), 1299.

chapter 7

nutrition and performance

The study of metabolism and production of energy and its use would not be complete without considering the broad topic of nutrition. After all, muscles receive their fuel from energy sources that consist of combinations of carbohydrates and fats in varying amounts, depending upon the type of exercise and duration of activity. As pointed out in Chapter 5, the short, fast bouts of activity are thought to rely more on carbohydrates, and the longer endurance events more on fats. Since the individual is likely to be on a mixed diet that contains a combination of nutrients, not just limited to carbohydrates and fats, but sufficient in water, proteins, minerals, and vitamins as well, the body should have little difficulty in performing large amounts of activity. This chapter will discuss the various factors associated with nutrition, including the respiratory exchange ratio, exercise and weight control, nutrition and athletic performance, energy equivalents, and the important topic of body composition.

GENERAL DIETARY CONSIDERATIONS

The three major constituents of the diet, classed as energy nutrients, are carbohydrates, fats, and proteins, and they are usually very abundant in foods. *Carbohydrates*, the chief source of energy, contain carbon, hydrogen, and oxygen, with the atoms of hydrogen and oxygen attached to the chain of six carbon atoms in a two-to-one ratio, the same as in water. Compounds with one carbohydrate unit are known as *monosaccharides*, such as glucose, fructose, and galactose; those with two sugar compounds, *disaccharides*, include sucrose, maltose, and lactose, and those with more than two carbohydrates in their chemical structure are *polysaccharides:* these include starch, dextrin, glycogen, and cellulose. The reader will recognize glucose and glycogen from earlier discussions of carbohydrate metabolism (Chapter 5). The process of conversion of a dietary monosaccharide (glucose) to a polysaccharide (glycogen) is called *glycogenesis*, and the glycogen thus formed is stored in the liver and muscles.

Fats are composed of carbon, hydrogen, and oxygen, just as are carbohydrates, but the ratio of hydrogen to oxygen in the fat molecule is much greater, and fats also contain more carbon than carbohydrates. Fats, or at least their form as *lipids*, include the neutral fat (triglycerides), the phospholipids, and cholesterol. The triglycerides, made up of three *fatty acids* bound to glycerol, function mainly to provide energy for metabolic processes. Some fatty acids contain as many hydrogen atoms as the carbon atoms can hold (*saturated fatty acids*), or a few hydrogen atoms may be missing in their carbon chains (*unsaturated fatty acids*).

In contrast with carbohydrates and fats, which are made up of carbon, hydrogen, and oxygen, *proteins* are the only class of nutrients that contain nitrogen. Proteins are abundant in the body, the major portion being located in muscle tissue. Proteins are composed of *amino acids* formed into chains by peptide linkages. When two amino acids are united by a peptide linkage, the resulting compound is called a *dipeptide*, and when three are joined together, a *tripeptide*. When many amino acids are linked together, the compound is known as a *polypeptide*. Each protein is a unique sequence of amino acids joined by such peptide bonds. Some twenty-two different amino acids are known and must be present for the building of new tissue and the maintenance of the tissue already formed. However, eight of the amino acids cannot be synthesized in the human body and must be supplied in the diet; they are called *essential* amino acids. The others can be synthesized by the body if insufficient quantities are available in food.

The need for energy is provided by the carbohydrate and fat content of the diet, as explained earlier, but when these substances are in insufficient supply, protein can be used for this purpose. However, the loss of stored fats and subsequent *deamination* of the amino acids of the blood cannot be considered a useful process in providing energy for athletic activity. The source of liver glucose from the amino acid alanine will be remembered from Chapter 5. Increased protein synthesis, on the other hand, accompanies hypertrophy.

A number of *minerals* also are required in the daily diet for the maintenance of health. These, including calcium, phosphorus, potassium, chlorine, sodium, magnesium, iron, and such important trace elements as manganese, copper, iodine, cobalt, zinc, fluorine, and others, make up less than 5 percent of the body weight. Although they are present in small amounts, the mineral elements are nevertheless indispensable to body functioning. In general, they serve as constituents in building and give rigidity to the hard tissues of the body, enter as components of soft tissue, and also serve in compounds essential to body functioning. For example, *sodium* and *chlorine* are contained in large amounts in the extracellular fluid, *potassium* is contained in the intracellular fluids, and together they play important roles in maintaining the normal osmotic pressure of the body, thus aiding in the movement of water in and out of tissues. Their role in nerve conduction was discussed in Chapter 1. Sodium bicarbonate ($NaHCO_3$) plays an important role in transportation of carbon dioxide from the cells to the lungs. Potassium is present in the muscles in so nearly a constant proportion that a method of determining the amount of lean tissue is based on counting the amount of radioactive potassium in the living body. The chloride ion also assists in the regulation of the acid-base balance of the body, a function shared by other mineral elements.

More *calcium* is contained in the body than any of the other minerals

(Table 7–1), amounting to approximately 2 percent of the body weight. Together with *phosphorus*, calcium is necessary for the formation of bones and teeth and, as we have seen, is required for musclar contraction. It is also necessary for blood-clot formation. Phorphorus provides energy in forming the high-energy phosphate bond in ATP and creatine phosphate; thus it is indispensable in metabolism. *Magnesium* serves to activate various intracellular enzymes, particularly those in carbohydrate metabolism that link phosphate groups to glucose in the formation and breakdown of glycogen. It is also necessary in the regulation of body temperature.

The remaining elements are required by the body in such small quantities that they are called *trace elements*, and although some fourteen are essential, only a few will be mentioned here. *Iron* is widely distributed about the body, and anywhere from 60 to 70 percent is present in the blood. Iron-containing hemoglobin serves as a carrier in the transport of oxygen to the tissues, and iron is also a component of myoglobin in muscles. It readily accepts and gives up electrons and is thus a necessary ingredient in the electron transport and respiratory enzyme systems. In short, it is essential both for the transport of oxygen to the tissue cells and for maintenance of oxidative systems within the cells. *Iodine* is taken up by the thyroid gland, where it forms an integral part of the hormone *thyroxine*, whose primary function is to influence the rate of oxidation in the cells; thus iodine is essential in the maintenance of basal metabolism. *Copper* plays an important role as a catalyst for the formation of hemoglobin and for the metabolism of glucose and release of energy. *Manganese* has a variety of metabolic functions; in particular it is a component of many enzymes of the body. *Zinc* is a constituent of the hormone *insulin,* which is secreted by the pancreas and thus is concerned with carbohydrate

Table 7–1. Elementary Composition of the Human Body

Element	Percent	Approx. Amount (grams) in a 70-kg man
Oxygen	65.0	45,500
Carbon	18.0	12,600
Hydrogen	10.0	7,000
Nitrogen	3.0	2,100
Calcium	1.5	1,050
Phosphorus	1.0	700
Potassium	0.35	245
Sulfur	0.25	175
Sodium	0.15	105
Chlorine	0.15	105
Magnesium	0.05	35
Iron	0.004	3
Manganese	0.0003	0.2
Copper	0.00015	0.1
Iodine	0.00004	0.03

metabolism. It is also an important part of the enzyme *carbonic anhydrase*, which makes possible the rapid combination of carbon dioxide with water to form carbonic acid in the red blood cells. Zinc is also present in *lactic dehydrogenase*, the enzyme involved in the interconversion of pyruvic acid and lactic acid.

Vitamins were discovered when it was found that individuals on diets adequate in calories, essential amino acids, fats, and minerals failed to remain healthy. Vitamins are organic compounds (in contrast to minerals which are inorganic) that are essential to human life and must be provided in the diet. The body is unable to synthesize them in quantities sufficient to maintain normal growth, maintenance of health, and reproduction. Vitamins may be classified as either fat-soluble or water-soluble. The *fat-soluble* vitamins include vitamins A, D, E, and K; the *water-soluble* vitamins include thiamine (B₁), riboflavin (B₂), nicotinic acid (niacin), pyridoxine (B₆), pantothenic acid, inositol, biotin, folic acid, ascorbic acid (C), choline, and cyanocobalamin (B₁₂).

Vitamin A promotes growth and aids in maintaining different types of epithelial cells, in particular those of the mucous membranes of the eyes, skin, mouth, gastrointestinal tract, respiratory tract, and genitourinary system. It protects the body against infection and the drying up and hardening of the mucous membrane, a condition called *keratinization*. Vitamin A is a constituent of the pigment in the retina, and lack of it is one of the causes of night blindness. *Vitamin D* is required for the proper absorption of calcium and phosphorus from the intestinal tract and their deposition in the bones and teeth. Deficiency of the vitamin produces rickets in children and osteomalacia in adults. *Vitamin E* has been found essential for normal reproduction in various species of animals; it is known as the *antisterility vitamin*. However, its role in this regard for man is questionable, and in fact vitamin E deficiency is believed to be extremely rare. The primary role of *vitamin K* is in the formation of *prothrombin* in the liver, one of the substances necessary in the process of blood coagulation. A deficiency prolongs bleeding and delays blood clotting.

All of the water-soluble vitamins with the exception of vitamin C are members of the vitamin B complex, which as noted above represents a rather large number of individual vitamins. *Thiamine* (B₁), widely distributed throughout the body, is particularly active in the coenzyme *thiamine pyrophosphate*, required in the decarboxylation of pyruvic acid—that is, the splitting off of carbon dioxide from pyruvic acid as a function of carbohydrate metabolism. Deficiency of thiamine results in beriberi, characterized by polyneuritis, disturbance of heart function, and various gastrointestinal disorders. The chief function of *riboflavin* (B₂) centers around its presence in two coenzymes, *flavin mononucleotide* (FMN) and *flavin adenine dinucleotide* (FAD), important in the oxidation-reduction reactions of the respiratory chain, described in Chapter 5. *Niacin*, or *nicotinic acid*, is an essential ingredient of two important coenzymes, *nicotinamide adenine dinucleotide* (NAD) and *nicotinamide adenine dinucleotide phosphate* (NADP). As such, niacin plays an essential role in hydrogen transport, and thus tissue oxidations.

Pyridoxine (B$_6$) in the body is converted to *pyridoxal phosphate* in the cells and functions as a coenzyme, playing an important role in protein and amino acid metabolism. Two of these reactions are known as *transamination* and *decarboxylation*. *Pantothenic* acid is a constituent of coenzyme A, and it is therefore involved in the intermediate metabolism of carbohydrates, fats and proteins. *Biotin* acts as a coenzyme in reactions involving the splitting off of carbon dioxide, as in the synthesis of fatty acids, and in the production of energy from glucose. *Ascorbic acid* (vitamin C) has as one of its chief functions the formation and maintenance of intercellular substances throughout the body that make up cartilage, dentine of teeth, matrices of bone, and collagen of connective tissue. Vitamin C deficiency in the diet results in scurvy. *Vitamin B$_{12}$* (cyanocobalamin) promotes growth and stimulates red blood cell formation. It is used in the treatment of pernicious anemia.

CALORIC VALUES

In order to maintain optimum body weight, the individual must make the caloric value of the dietary intake balance the daily expenditure of energy. When there is an imbalance, the individual may change his body weight, either up or down, depending upon the direction the imbalance takes. For example, when the caloric intake is not sufficient, the body draws upon its stores of fat, and perhaps even protein, and when it is excessive there is a synthesis of fat. The average daily requirement of kilocalories (kcal) for the average individual is 2,000 for basal needs plus an additional 500 to 2,000 for activity. This latter value is dependent upon the extent of physical activity during the day; it can be rather high in some individuals engaged in exercise. It is not beyond the realm of possibility that football players could consume over 5,500 kcal and still not gain weight during the season. Compare this with a sedentary clerk or secretary who might require but 2,300 kcal during a normal working day.

The average individual receives approximately 45 percent of his energy from carbohydrates, 40 percent from fat, and the remaining 15 percent from proteins. Fats contain the most available physiological energy, since they supply 9.3 kcal/gm, as compared with 4.1 for carbohydrates and 4.1 for protein. On the other hand, fats are also the most expensive; as pointed out in Chapter 5, fats require 2.01 liters of oxygen for oxidation, but carbohydrates need only .75 liters. In calculating the dietary needs of the body, Ganong[1] suggests that the protein requirement be met first to supply the essential amino acids, and that the calories remaining be divided between fat and carbohydrate. Thus, a man weighing 70 kg might require 3,000 kcal per day if moderately active, and he should eat 70 gm of protein per day, supplying 287 kcal. The total is calculated by multiplying body weight (70 kg) by the energy per gram for protein

[1]William F. Ganong, *Review of Medical Physiology,* 2d ed. (Los Altos, Calif.: Lange Medical Publications, 1965), p. 245.

(4.1). Fat intake could reasonably be 60 gm, resulting in the essential fatty acids and 558 kcal (60 × 9.3). The remaining caloric requirement, 2,155 kcal, can be met by supplying 526 gm of carbohydrate. The recommended dietary daily allowances of various food constituents for individuals of varying ages are presented in Table 7–2.

RESPIRATORY EXCHANGE RATIO

The concept has been advanced repeatedly that the fuel for exercise is provided by carbohydrate and fat. It has been well documented that protein is not involved where the supply of calories is adequate, which takes in the realm of normal activity. The result of the metabolism of protein in the body is excretion of the nitrogen, and so we can accurately gauge the quantity of protein metabolized by analyzing the nitrogen excretion during a given period. The fact that nitrogen excretion does not rise during muscular activity indicates that protein is not involved.

The method of determining the relative contribution made by the various constituents of the diet is to calculate the *respiratory exchange ratio* (R), given as the ratio of carbon dioxide produced by the body to the oxygen utilization. Thus,

$$R = CO_2/O_2$$

and for carbohydrates it is 1.00, as shown in Table 7–3. This means that during the oxidation of a molecule of glucose the number of oxygen molecules required for the oxidation processes is equal to the number of carbon dioxide molecules liberated. Fats, on the other hand, result in a respiratory exchange ratio of .70, as shown in Table 7–3 for the oxidation of stearin. Contrast these with the R for protein (.83), as indicated for alanine. Since most individuals consume a mixed diet of various combinations of the three foods, the resting R averages approximately .83. The ratio of CO_2 to O_2 is highest when carbohydrates are used as fuel; thus these are a more efficient source of energy. The R goes down with the use of fats, revealing (as already mentioned) that more oxygen is required for fat

Table 7–3. Respiratory Exchange Ratios (R) for the Oxidation of Carbohydrate, Fat, and Protein

	R
Carbohydrate (Glucose): $C_6H_{12}O_6 + 6O_2 \longrightarrow 6CO_2 + 6H_2O$	$\dfrac{6CO_2}{6O_2} = 1.00$
Fat (Stearin): $2C_{57}H_{110}O_6 + 163O_2 \longrightarrow 114CO_2 + 110H_2O$	$\dfrac{114CO_2}{163O_2} = .70$
Protein (Alanine): $2C_3H_7O_2N + 6O_2 \longrightarrow (NH_2)_2 CO + 5CO_2 + 5H_2O$	$\dfrac{5CO_2}{6O_2} = .83$

Table 7–2. Recommended Daily Dietary Allowances, Food and Nutrition Board, National Research Council, Revised 1974

	Age (yrs)	Wt. (lbs)	Ht. (in)	Energy (kcal)	Protein (g)	Fat-Soluble Vitamins			Water-Soluble Vitamins							Minerals					
						A Activity (IU)	D (IU)	E Activity (IU)	Ascorbic acid (mg)	Folacin (µg)	Niacin (mg)	Riboflavin (mg)	Thiamin (mg)	B-6 (mg)	B-12 (µg)	Calcium (mg)	Phosphorus (mg)	Iodine (µg)	Iron (mg)	Magnesium (mg)	Zinc (mg)
Children	1–3	28	34	1300	23	2000	400	7	40	100	9	0.8	0.7	0.6	1.0	800	800	60	15	150	10
	4–6	44	44	1800	30	2500	400	9	40	200	12	1.1	0.9	0.9	1.5	800	800	80	10	200	10
	7–10	66	54	2400	36	3300	400	10	40	300	16	1.2	1.2	1.2	2.0	800	800	110	10	250	10
Men	11–14	97	63	2800	44	5000	400	12	45	400	18	1.5	1.4	1.6	3.0	1200	1200	130	18	350	15
	15–18	134	69	3000	54	5000	400	15	45	400	20	1.8	1.5	2.0	3.0	1200	1200	150	18	400	15
	19–22	147	69	3000	54	5000	400	15	45	400	20	1.8	1.5	2.0	3.0	800	800	140	10	350	15
	23–50	154	69	2700	56	5000	—	15	45	400	18	1.6	1.4	2.0	3.0	800	800	130	10	350	15
	51+	154	69	2400	56	5000	—	15	45	400	16	1.5	1.2	2.0	3.0	800	800	110	10	350	15
Women	11–15	97	62	2400	44	4000	400	12	45	400	16	1.3	1.2	1.6	3.0	1200	1200	115	18	300	15
	15–18	119	65	2100	48	4000	400	12	45	400	14	1.4	1.1	2.0	3.0	1200	1200	115	18	300	15
	19–22	128	65	2100	46	4000	400	12	45	400	14	1.4	1.1	2.0	3.0	800	800	100	18	300	15
	23–50	128	65	2000	46	4000	—	12	45	400	13	1.2	1.0	2.0	3.0	800	800	100	18	300	15
	51+	128	65	1800	46	4000	—	12	45	400	12	1.1	1.0	2.0	3.0	800	800	80	10	300	15

Adapted from National Research Council, Food and Nutrition Board, *Recommended Daily Dietary Allowances*, 8th ed. Washington, D.C.: National Academy of Sciences, 1974.

oxidation. One liter of oxygen will release 5.05 kcal of energy from carbohydrate, 4.54 kcal from fat. The mixed diet will result in an energy equivalent of 4.83 kcal.

Exercise

If the protein content of the diet plays little or no role in providing the fuel for exercise, then calculation of the respiratory exchange ratio is useful in providing information concerning the relative reliance upon fats and carbohydrates. In this manner, the proper caloric value for a given exercise can be calculated, as shown in Table 7–4. It is actually more correct technically to refer to the *nonprotein R*, but at any rate, the *R* is calculated from the oxygen used and carbon dioxide produced. During steady-state exercise, the *R* generally approaches 1.0, revealing the dependence upon carbohydrates for muscular work. During prolonged periods of exhaustive work, the *R* goes steadily down toward .70, indicating the increased reliance upon fat. However, these values depend upon circumstances within the individual that are sometimes difficult to achieve during exercise; that is, certain consequences of severe exercise that affect *R* are not involved in the oxidation of food. In fact, the *R* during the period of exertion may rise considerably above 1.0, even to 1.5 or higher—values that cannot be justified on dietary considerations. It is not uncommon for the *R* to peak shortly after the end of exercise and during the subsequent recovery period to fall below normal, perhaps to as low as .5.

The explanation for this phenomenon can readily be found in consideration of the oxygen debt mechanism, where lactic acid is formed. The

Table 7–4. Caloric Values for Various Nonprotein Respiratory Exchange Ratios

R	kcal/liter O_2	R	kcal/liter O_2
0.707	4.686	0.85	4.862
0.71	4.690	0.86	4.875
0.72	4.702	0.87	4.887
0.73	4.714	0.88	4.899
0.74	4.727	0.89	4.911
0.75	4.739	0.90	4.924
0.76	4.751	0.91	4.936
0.77	4.764	0.92	4.948
0.78	4.776	0.93	4.961
0.79	4.788	0.94	4.973
0.80	4.801	0.95	4.985
0.81	4.813	0.96	4.998
0.82	4.825	0.97	5.010
0.83	4.838	0.98	5.022
0.84	4.850	0.99	5.035
		1.00	5.047

lactic acid accumulates in the blood and is buffered by sodium bicarbonate in a reaction that yields *sodium lactate*, often called simply *lactate*, and carbonic acid. Thus,

$$\underset{\substack{\text{Lactic} \\ \text{acid}}}{\text{HL}} + \underset{\substack{\text{Sodium} \\ \text{bicarbonate}}}{\text{NaHCO}_3} \longrightarrow \underset{\substack{\text{Sodium} \\ \text{lactate}}}{\text{NaL}} + \underset{\substack{\text{Carbonic} \\ \text{acid}}}{\text{H}_2\text{CO}_3}. \qquad (7\text{--}1)$$

The result of this reaction has been to replace a strong acid (lactic acid) with a weak one (carbonic acid); perhaps more important, the carbonic acid is more volatile and can be eliminated from the body via the lungs, as follows:

$$\text{H}_2\text{CO}_3 \longrightarrow \text{CO}_2 + \text{H}_2\text{O}. \qquad (7\text{--}2)$$

The resultant liberation of large amounts of CO_2 is not accompanied by a corresponding increase in the utilization of oxygen, so the respiratory exchange ratio rises. During the recovery period the R may continue to rise, as the lactic acid produced in the late portion of exercise is being buffered and the full effect of CO_2 formation is being experienced. Subsequently, the lactate must be oxidized, yielding CO_2, which enters the blood and is retained there to a considerable extent, rather than being blown off in the lungs. This retention of CO_2 is to reform the bicarbonate which was depleted during the exercise, and it causes the R to fall. It may take several minutes, even an hour or more, for the R to return to preexercise resting values. This is illustrated in Figure 57.

Figure 57. The Effect of Exercise on the Respiratory Exchange Ratio (R) during the Recovery Period. [C. H. Best and N. B. Taylor, *The Physiological Basis of Medical Practice*, 7th ed. Baltimore: The Williams & Wilkins Company (1961), p. 881.]

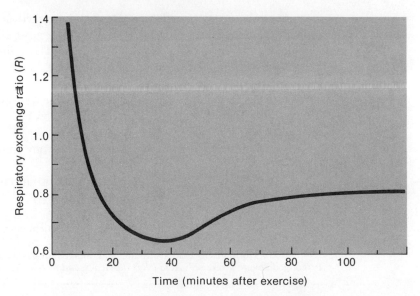

Since the respiratory exchange ratio can reflect the reliance upon the lactic acid mechanism during anaerobic exercise, the possibility arises that it can indicate the involvement of lactic acid. Further, if the exercise is sufficiently stressful, it would appear feasible that monitoring "excess CO_2" could be useful in determining the extent of this participation. Issekutz and Rodahl[2] calculated the excess CO_2 as

$$\text{total } CO_2 - .75 \times O_2,$$

the value .75 being the average metabolic R. The correlation between the change in blood lactate and excess CO_2 ($r = .92$) confirms the practicality of this procedure, and it has the added benefit of bypassing the analysis of blood lactate samples. The determinations of $\dot{V}O_2$ and $\dot{V}CO_2$ are more routine laboratory procedures.

Training

It has been found[3] that endurance-trained individuals have lower respiratory exchange ratio values than untrained at comparable percentages of their $\dot{V}O_2$ max—that is, during submaximal exercise. Apparently, trained persons derive a greater percentage of their energy from fatty acids and less from the carbohydrate portion than do sedentary individuals. This would help account for the finding that training results in decreased glycogen utilization and lower values for blood lactate, together with the increase in fatty acid oxidation. Both are reflected in lower values for R during submaximal exercise. This is revealed in Figure 58.

MECHANICAL EFFICIENCY

A fundamental consideration to those engaged in physical performance is efficiency—the ability to accomplish the most with the least effort. For the automobile, the mileage per gallon of gasoline is an important factor in assessing its general acceptability. The same may be said for the human: how much work can be accomplished for a given expenditure of energy? Does it matter what food provides the energy? Are some ways of exercising more efficient than others? How can the efficiency be increased?

Mechanical efficiency may be calculated from the following formula:

$$\text{Percent M.E.} = \frac{\text{kcal external work produced}}{\text{kcal energy used}} \times 100. \quad (7\text{--}3)$$

[2]B. Issekutz and K. Rodahl, "Respiratory Quotient during Exercise," *Journal of Applied Physiology*, 16 (July 1961), 606.

[3]Lars Hermansen, Eric Hultman, and Bengt Saltin, "Muscle Glycogen during Prolonged Severe Exercise," *Acta Physiologica Scandinavica*, 17 (1967), 129.

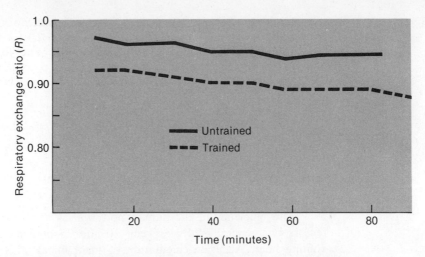

Figure 58. The Effects of Training on the Respiratory Exchange Ratio during Prolonged Exercise to Exhaustion. [L. Hermansen *et al.,* "Muscle Glycogen during Prolonged Severe Exercise," *Acta Physiologica Scandinavica,* 71 (1967), p .134.]

Two variables must be available in completing this problem—the physical work done and the oxygen requirement. Both are typical laboratory procedures, but the value for work is generally in units of ft-lb or more likely kgm (or kpm[4]), and the net O_2 requirement ($\dot{V}O_2$) is in liters per minute. The task is to convert them both to similar units, generally kcal, as the formula suggests. Thus, 3,087 ft-lb = 427 kgm = 1 kcal; 1 ft-lb = .13825 kgm = 0.000324 kcal; 1 liter of oxygen = 5.05 kcal = 15,575 ft-lb = 2,153 kgm (for carbohydrates); 1 liter of oxygen = 4.54 kcal = 14,108 ft-lb = 1,950 kgm (for fats).

It should be made clear in determining efficiency whether it is *net* efficiency or *gross* efficiency that is being considered. For net efficiency, the energy cost during rest is substracted from the total energy requirement—that is, the period of rest corresponding in time to the duration of the work period. Gross efficiency, on the other hand, includes the value of energy expenditure for rest; thus it is equivalent to the *total* metabolic rate for the exercise. In the calculation of both net and gross efficiency from the same problem involving the same amount of external work, the inclusion of values for the rest will inflate the denominator of the basic equation and will consequently cause gross efficiency to be lower than net efficiency. This is illustrated in the following example:

A weight lifter raising a 120-lb weight 3 ft 20 times in 2 minutes has a net oxygen consumption of 2.10 liters, taking into consideration both the oxygen intake during exercise and the oxygen debt. The rate at rest is .35

[4]The unit of kpm (kilopond meters) is often employed. One kp is the force acting on the mass of 1 kg at normal acceleration of gravity.

l/min. The caloric equivalent of 7,200 ft-lb $= 7,200 \times .000324 = 2.3328$ kcal, and the caloric equivalent of 2.10 liters $= 2.10 \times 5.05 = 10.605$ kcal. (The value of 5.05 kcal as the caloric equivalent per liter of oxygen intake is conventional practice in metabolic work, a practice which assumes that the calories resulted from carbohydrate oxidation.) Thus:

$$\text{Net M.E.} = \frac{2.3328 \text{ kcal}}{10.6050 \text{ kcal}} \times 100 = 22.0 \text{ percent,} \quad (7\text{–}4)$$

$$\text{Gross M.E.} = \frac{2.3328 \text{ kcal}}{14.1400 \text{ kcal}} \times 100 = 16.5 \text{ percent.} \quad (7\text{–}5)$$

The efficiency of the human body varies according to a number of factors but generally falls between 20 and 25 percent, the remainder becoming heat. Accurate calculation of mechanical efficiency is sometimes very difficult, owing to the problems involved in determining external work accomplished. Treadmill running, bicycle ergometry, and step tests are standardized procedures that can lead to reasonably accurate estimates of work, although not without some careful attention to detail. For example, work output in treadmill running is equal to the weight of the subject times the vertical distance he raised himself while exercising on an inclined surface. For the bicycle ergometer it is equal to the amount of resistance to the flywheel times the product of the circumference of the flywheel by the number of revolutions. Compare these determinations with those that might evolve from an individual's swimming, playing handball, or running in soccer.

Improvement in efficiency may be brought about in several ways. Given the problem above, anything that would increase the amount of weight lifted (work done) while keeping the energy cost the same would result in an increase in net mechanical efficiency. Conversely, lowering the energy cost for the same bout of work would have the same effect. Thus, it may be said that if the work load is standardized, the individual with the lowest $\dot{V}o_2$ is the most efficient. Improving physical fitness is another method of improving efficiency, since it has the desired effect of permitting more work to be accomplished at less cost. One could reasonably expect fairly wide individual differences in the performance of tasks even when the work load is held constant; it is not unusual to find the variability to range between 5 and 8 percent even in standardized exercise tasks.

A method of exercising designed to improve efficiency is to adjust the rate to an optimum level. In practical circumstances this may not always be possible, since athletic contests are often dictated by strategies other than physiological ones. Nevertheless, Henry[5] calculated for running that it is more efficient to employ a steady pace rather than to run all-out

[5]Franklin M. Henry, "Time-Velocity Equations and Oxygen Requirements of 'All-Out' and 'Steady-Pace' Running," *Research Quarterly* 25 (May 1954), 164.

or to use some variable-pace procedure. He suggested that the inefficiency of running at fast speeds is due to the increasing use of anaerobic metabolism. Walking, too, can be inefficient if the proper pace is not established. Very slow gaits increase isometric portions of muscle activity, as an individual must support his weight for longer than optimal times. Rapid walking seems to be wasteful of energy, as the individual develops increasing tension in the antigravity muscles which control the acceleration and deceleration of body segments. Cavagna *et al.*[6] found the most economical rate of walking to be 2.4 mph (4 km/hr). Above 5 mph the energy cost rises even above that of running.

A reat deal more is known about the relative efficiency of certain laboratory exercise procedures, such as the optimum pedal frequency for the bicycle ergometer. When performing submaximal exercise a frequency of from 40 to 50 pedal revolutions per minute results in the greatest mechanical efficiency, as indicated by lowest $\dot{V}_{O_2}$, whereas for maximal work the pedal frequency should change to 60 rpm.[7] In a study dealing with treadmill running, Knuttgen[8] found that with increased stride frequency the oxygen consumption increased more rapidly than with increased stride length for a comparable range of speeds. The latter would indicate improved efficiency.

The rate of contracting muscles seems to be an important factor in providing optimum work output. When performing maximal effort, experience has shown that approximately one second is the most efficient contraction time. Exceeding this rate may leave insufficient time to develop maximal force, dissipating energy in overcoming viscous resistance. Very slow contraction rates result in the production of large amounts of maintenance heat, thus decreasing efficiency.

If the reliance upon the lactate mechanism is less efficient than aerobic means, then it must be possible to examine whether or not differences in efficiency seem to parallel the increased reliance on the lactic oxygen debt portion of recovery from exercise. DeMoor[9] divided subjects into two groups, the more efficient men and women, and the less efficient men and women, and found a significant relationship between the lactate debt and efficiency ($r = -.694$). Moreover, the inefficient subjects increased the size of the lactate debt component by 56 percent over that of the efficient group. No differences occurred between the two groups in alactic debt. The relative contributions to the oxygen debt components for the efficient and nonefficient subjects are given in Figure 59.

[6]G. A. Cavagna, F. P. Saibene, and R. Margaria, "External Work in Walking," *Journal of Applied Physiology*, 18 (January 1963), 1.

[7]Per-Olof Åstrand and Kaare Rodahl, *Textbook of Work Physiology* (New York: McGraw-Hill Book Company, 1970), pp. 362–63.

[8]Howard G. Knuttgen, "Oxygen Uptake and Pulse Rate While Running with Undetermined and Determined Stride Lengths at Different Speeds," *Acta Physiologica Scandinavica*, 52 (1961), 366.

[9]Janice C. DeMoor, "Individual Differences in Oxygen Debt Curves Related to Mechanical Efficiency and Sex," *Journal of Applied Physiology*, 6 (1954), 460.

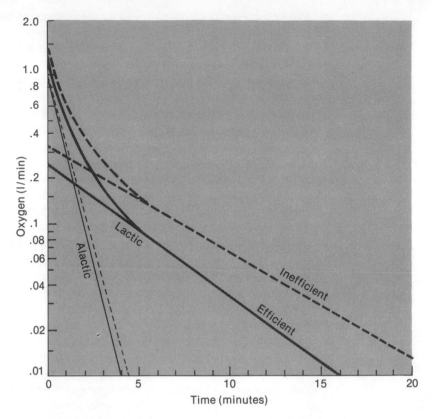

Figure 59. Oxygen Debt Components for Two Groups Differing in Mechanical Efficiency. [J. DeMoor, "Individual Differences in Oxygen Debt Curves Related to Mechanical Efficiency and Sex," *Journal of Applied Physiology,* 6 (1954), p. 462]

Training

Whether training improves efficiency may depend upon how one looks at it. For example, if Olympic cyclists and untrained individuals are compared at *submaximal* work loads on a bicycle ergometer, no differences in mechanical efficiency seem to exist. On the other hand, Knehr, Dill, and Neufeld[10] reported approximately a 10 percent increase in efficiency over a six-month training period involving graded treadmill walking. Other investigators have shown that efficiency can increase through training, although it must be cautioned that the changes may be somewhat modest.

An ancillary consideration in this regard, however, is the acquisition of *skill.* One could easily translate the learning of an activity into the improvement of efficiency. After all, one of the aims of skill instruction is the reduction of extraneous movement and perfection of technique, which can undoubtedly result in the use of less energy for the same

---

[10]C. A. Knehr, D. B. Dill, and William Neufeld, "Training and its Effects on Man at Rest and at Work," *American Journal of Physiology,* 136 (1942), 148.

amount of work or, conversely, improvement in the work done with a given amount of energy. The teacher of physical activities strives conscientiously to impart to the learner those elements of the skill which will conserve energy so that wasted motions are eliminated and purposeful activity ensues.

Diet

A number of studies have been conducted to evaluate the effect of a previous diet on efficiency. Once again, we go back to the idea that fats require more oxygen for their oxidation than do carbohydrates, and it is not surprising that the mechanical efficiency increases as much as 10 percent or even more when individuals are placed on carbohydrate diets as when the prior diet is predominantly fat. Thus, it would appear that in endurance events requiring sustained muscular activity the eventual drain on carbohydrate stores and subsequent increase in the proportion of fat metabolized would lower the mechanical efficiency.

ENERGY EQUIVALENTS FOR PHYSICAL ACTIVITIES

The relative severity of various physical activities has been a subject of interest to physiologists, physical educators, and physicians, but the search for a definitive taxonomy has been hampered somewhat by the development of adequate data-gathering procedures, particularly for those sports that do not lend themselves readily to laboratory examination. Since the caloric cost can be determined at least indirectly by the energy expenditure (net oxygen requirement), a number of activities can be simulated or measured in a laboratory, or even in a swimming pool. But team sports seem to offer the most difficulty, and even though we might categorize some as strenuous, exact determinations have been elusive. The advances in technology, such as the development of the portable respirometer (Kofranyi-Michaelis meter), have permitted the monitoring of some activities (such as handball, squash, tennis) that would be especially difficult to assess in any simulated manner.

Even then, it must be clear that no single value for caloric cost can be absolutely definitive; it is common experience that the level of competition, the skill of the performers, and other factors control the pace of play, and thus dictate the actual energy expenditure. Body size also may play a role, so in activities in which the individual moves about, as in running, a larger person will be doing more work than a smaller person, and consequently the expenditure of energy will be greater. This need not be the case when one is doing external work such as weight lifting or cycling; in these instances body size is not a factor in determination of work done. However, one would expect large individual differences in response to such tasks. The larger person could be expected to have more reserve capacity for the exercise.

Typical caloric values that might result from various physical activities are shown in Table 7–5. The number of kilocalories expended in any situation varies from individual to individual, and so these are what may be termed "representative" values for average subjects. They serve a useful purpose in illuminating the relative cost of some commonly en-

Table 7–5. Energy Expenditure for Various Physical Activities

Activity	Energy Cost (kcal/min)
1. Lying at ease	1.5
2. Sitting at ease	1.6
3. Standing at ease	1.7
4. Canoeing, 2.5 mph	3.0
5. Canoeing, 4.0 mph	7.0
6. Cycling, 5.5 mph	4.5
7. Cycling, 9.4 mph	7.0
8. Cycling, 13.1 mph	11.1
9. Volleyball	3.5
10. Baseball	4.2
11. Golf	5.0
12. Tennis	7.1
13. Handball	10.9
14. Swimming crawl stroke, 2.2 ft/sec	12.0
15. Swimming crawl stroke, 4.2 ft/sec	40.0
16. Swimming crawl stroke, 5.2 ft/sec	80.0
17. Swimming crawl stroke, 5.8 ft/sec	125.0
18. Swimming back stroke, 2.0 ft/sec	10.0
19. Swimming back stroke, 3.9 ft/sec	38.0
20. Swimming back stroke, 4.7 ft/sec	75.0
21. Swimming back stroke, 5.0 ft/sec	135.0
22. Swimming breast stroke, 2.5 ft/sec	18.0
23. Swimming breast stroke, 3.5 ft/sec	50.0
24. Swimming breast stroke, 4.0 ft/sec	78.0
25. Skiing, 8.1 mph	20.9
26. Long distance running	14.9
27. Running, 11 mph	23.6
28. Running, 14.5 mph	43.9
29. Running, 16.2 mph	62.1
30. Running, 18.6 mph	124.0
31. Running, 20.0 mph	186.0

Compiled from F.M. Henry, *Physiology of Work: The Physiological Basis of Muscular Exercise.* Berkeley: Associated Students' Store, University of California, 1968; P.V. Karpovich and N. Millman, "Energy Expenditure in Swimming," *American Journal of Physiology*, 142 (1944), 140; and R. Passmore and J.V.G.A. Durnin, "Human Energy Expenditure," *Physiological Reviews*, 35 (October 1955), 801.

countered activities. In the sports of baseball, volleyball, golf, tennis, and handball, the actual caloric expenditure is determined by the severity of play, as already discussed, and obviously there will be periods where maximum work will be performed, which will increase any average value for that interval, just as more quiet intervals can be less costly. In the case of handball, for example, simply playing against an opponent of superior ability raises the caloric cost to 12.2 kcal/min.[11]

Some of the values for swimming and running may seem exceptionally large, especially at the high speeds, but it must be kept in mind that the kcal/min are projected from the work rate established for the brief interval during which such speeds are established. In some cases (such as running at top speed) this may be but for a few seconds. Henry[12] estimates that running at 20 mph (9.8 yd/sec) would require approximately 37 liters of oxygen per minute. No wonder such speeds can be maintained for only a short time.

It may be noticed that the caloric values for swimming do not increase in increments directly comparable to increases in speed. In fact, the curve for each stroke becomes quite steep where the speed is greatest. This means that any increase in speed is accompanied by rather large expenditures of energy.[13] Also, a poor swimmer expends more energy than a good swimmer, pointing out the shift in mechanical efficiency brought about by training.

BODY COMPOSITION

Stress has been placed on the importance of various components of the diet and their caloric values. If more kilocalories are ingested than are utilized in energy metabolism, the excess will be converted and stored as adipose tissue, and of course the reverse will stimulate the reduction of fat stores. So it is possible to see the change that can come about through dieting or extended training. For example, dieting can lead to reduction of adipose tissue and can be sensed subjectively by noting the slimming effect that can be crudely measured by the differences in the way clothing fits. Weight training, on the other hand, may lead to muscular hypertrophy and a sense of feeling stronger, with larger and more noticeable muscle definition. Both regimens can be monitored by scale weight, which is the usual objective measuring device available to the average person. Simply obtaining body weight may be better than nothing and may provide a very general indication of changing nutritional status; however, it does not reveal much about the relative contribution of lean and fat tissue to total

[11]E. W. Banister *et al.*, "The Caloric Cost of Playing Handball," *Research Quarterly*, 35 (October 1964), 236.

[12]Franklin M. Henry, *Physiology of Work: The Physiological Basis of Muscular Exercise* (Berkeley: Associated Students' Store, University of California, 1968), p. 57.

[13]Peter V. Karpovich and Nathan Millman, "Energy Expenditure in Swimming," *American Journal of Physiology*, 142 (1944), 140.

weight. In fact, it can even be misleading. Take, for example, a 220-lb male. What does the weight alone tell us? Add the fact that he is 6 feet tall; does that provide much more information? Actually, this individual could be extremely lean, play professional football, and be in excellent physical condition, or he could be sedentary, poorly conditioned, and considered obese. Without additional information weight alone provides very little insight into the actual body composition.

The metabolically active tissue, such as muscle and bone, can be differentiated from the metabolically inactive tissue, such as fat, by careful measurement and calculation. Determining lean body weight (LBW) is important in assessing the nutritional status of individuals, as is fat content, and for these purposes several techniques have been developed. Some are readily accessible to the physical education teacher or clinician, while others are more usually found in research applications. Some are extremely technical, and beyond ordinary use in the laboratory. The reader will find reviews of various techniques helpful in providing additional background study.[14] The more commonly employed methods of determining body composition will be discussed briefly here.

Body Density by Underwater Weighing

A rather precise estimate of body composition can be obtained by applying Archimedes' principle of *body density*: when a body is immersed in water it is acted upon by a buoyant force, such that the loss of weight is equal to the weight of the displaced fluid. In actual practice this requires an individual to be weighed under water, having fully exhaled, to find the loss of weight in water. Certain corrections must be made, one for the density of water at that particular water temperature, another for the residual volume of air left in the lungs at the time the underwater weight was taken. This latter correction is important, because air left in the lungs exerts a buoyant effect upon the body when it is submerged, and it would readily distort the estimates of body fat unless taken into account. Moreover, a certain amount of gas remains trapped in the gastrointestinal tract, and it is necessary to take this amount (usually estimated to be 100 ml) into consideration. The pulmonary residual volume can actually be measured, and it is when body density is used for accurate determination. Sometimes, standard corrections are also used for men (1,300 ml) and women (1,200 ml), but this introduces some error in the measurement. The following formula may be used in determining body density (D):

$$D = \frac{W_A}{\dfrac{(W_A - W_w)}{D_w} - (RV + 100 \text{ ml})}, \qquad (7\text{--}6)$$

[14]Josef Brožek, ed., "Body Composition," parts I and II, *Annals of the New York Academy of Sciences*, 110 (September 26, 1963), pp. 1–1018.

where W_A = weight in air, W_w = weight in water, D_w = density of water at water temperature, and RV = residual volume. From these calculations, a low value would indicate a relatively large proportion of body fat; conversely, a high value would signify a lower porportion of fat. In order to calculate the percent of fat from knowledge of the body density, the following formula has been shown to be satisfactory:

$$\text{Percent fat} = 100\,\frac{4.570}{\text{body density}} - 4.142. \tag{7-7}$$

The *percent* of body weight that is fat can thus be used to determine the actual amount of fat weight; the remainder is *lean body weight* (weight in air less total fat).

Lean Body Weight by Anthropometric Measurement

Another method of estimating lean body weight that may be substituted for the underwater weighing procedure involves the measurement of the diameters of various body segments. This relieves one from immersing the body in water and requires instead that the width of the body be measured at selected sites employing sliding calipers.[15] The measurements must be taken with great care and precision, since the introduction of small errors will lead to an inaccurate estimation of LBW. The formula to be used is

$$\text{LBW} = D^2 \times h, \tag{7-8}$$

where D = sum of d divided by 8, and h is the individual's height (measured in decimeters), as shown in Table 7–6. The values for d are obtained by dividing the body diameters (measured in centimeters) by the appropriate constants for men and women. It will be found generally that D will fall between 1.80 and 2.10, and this will result in LBW's being expressed in kilograms. Multiplying by 2.2 will convert kilograms to pounds. Wilmore and Behnke[16] have found that employing only four of the diameters will yield essentially comparable results; they recommend that if this is done, the biacromial, bitrochanteric, wrist, and ankle diameters be used, primarily because the bony landmarks that must be employed are quite readily accessible.

[15]Albert R. Behnke, "Quantitative Assessment of Body Build," *Journal of Applied Physiology*, 16 (November 1961), 960.

[16]Jack H. Wilmore and Albert R. Behnke, "Predictability of Lean Body Weight through Anthropometric Assessment in College Men," *Journal of Applied Physiology*, 25 (October 1968), 349.

Table 7–6. Calculation of Lean Body Weight from Body Diameters

	(c) Measured Values	(d) Calculated Values (c/k)	(k) Constants Men	Women
1. Chest width	_____	_____	15.9	14.8
2. Bi-iliac diameter	_____	_____	15.6	16.7
3. Knee widths (R + L)	_____	_____	9.8	10.3
4. Elbow widths (R + L)	_____	_____	7.4	6.9
5. Biacromial diameter	_____	_____	21.6	20.4
6. Bitrochanteric diameter	_____	_____	17.4	18.6
7. Ankle diameters (R + L)	_____	_____	7.4	7.4
8. Wrist diameters (R + L)	_____	_____	5.9	5.6

Sum of d = _____

$$D = \frac{\text{Sum of } d}{8} = \underline{\hspace{1cm}}$$

Calculations:

$$\text{LBW} = D^2 \times h$$

$$\text{Percent fat} = 100 \times \frac{\text{Body weight} - \text{LBW}}{\text{Body weight}}$$

Body Density by Skinfold

By far the most popular and most widely used technique for body-density determination is the one that involves skinfold measures. It is obviously based on the proposition that the extent of adiposity can be estimated by measuring the thickness of the double layer of skinfold at various sites on the body. Not all of the adipose tissue resides in the subcutaneous areas; in fact, as much as half is located within the body itself. However, it is usually accepted that the skinfold may be used as an index of total body fat, and several equations have been advanced which involved two or three "representative" sites. One of these[17] involves the following formula, applicable to men:

$$\text{Density} = 1.1017 - .000282(A) - .000736(B) - .000883(C), \qquad (7\text{–}9)$$

where A is the abdominal skinfold, B is the chest skinfold, and C is the arm skinfold. Specially designed *calipers*[18] are employed which give con-

[17]J. Brožek and A. Keys, "The Evaluation of Leanness-Fatness in Man: Norms and Interrelations," *British Journal of Nutrition*, 5 (1951), 194.

[18]See Lange Skinfold Caliper, Cambridge Scientific Industries, Inc., 527 Poplar Street, Cambridge, Md. 21613.

stant spring tension, the measures are all obtained in millimeters, and the right side is used in each instance. The *abdominal skinfold* is measured at the midaxillary line at waist level, the *chest skinfold* at the level of the xiphoid in the midaxillary line, and the *arm skinfold* at the midposterior, midway between the tip of the acromion and the tip of the olecranon process with the elbow in 90 degrees of flexion and the arm hanging at the side. Once again, percent fat can be determined by use of formula (7–7).

The following formula is applicable to women:[19]

$$\text{Density} = 1.0764 - .00081(A) - .00088(C). \qquad (7\text{–}10)$$

Athletic Performance

Both body composition and body build play an important role in athletic performance. In fact, such factors seem to dictate the particular sport an individual will be best suited for. The tall basketball player, the stocky football player, and the well-proportioned gymnast are examples, but obviously much more than just structure is involved. One attribute that seems to be quite important is the amount of lean tissue. Put another way, it is seldom that a relatively high proportion of body fat is advantageous, although the reader can probably name successful athletes who appeared to have considerable adipose tissue. Nevertheless, if high body weight is desirable (even necessary, as in heavyweight boxing and wrestling), it is better that the bulk be composed of muscle tissue rather than fat tissue. Yet, this might mean that the individual could be 25 or even 30 percent or more above the average weight for normal individuals of the same height. It should be clear that partitioning body weight into its lean and fat components is essential to a proper understanding of nutrition as it relates to athletic performance. Keep in mind, too, that the precise balance between lean and fat tissue is apt to change during a season of competition depending upon the factors of diet and activity. Clearly, failure to continue intense early preseason conditioning right on through a competitive season that lasts for several months can actually cause the percentage of fat to increase, especially if the pattern of caloric intake remains high.

The amount of muscle tissue, however, is not the determining factor in athletic success, even though (as pointed out in Chapter 3) *if other things are equal*, in many activities the individual with the greatest strength may have an advantage. But the ability to use the strength—that is, the neuromotor coordination—is more important than strength alone, and repeated studies indicate that static muscular strength is essentially unrelated to what is sometimes called "strength in action."[20] Lean tissue, then, is not

---

[19]A. W. Sloan, J. J. Burt, and C. S. Blyth, "Estimation of Body Fat in Young Women," *Journal of Applied Physiology*, 17 (November 1962), 967.

[20]F. M. Henry and J. D. Whitley, "Relationships between Individual Differences in Strength, Speed and Mass in an Arm Movement," *Research Quarterly*, 31 (March 1960), 24.

likely to be a sole determiner of athletic ability. The coach must still appraise the ability of the individual in revelant physical activities before deciding on his or her probable contribution to the total team effort. If a change in body composition can be seen as detrimental, then efforts should be taken to obtain a more favorable balance. The scale weight is not adequately diagnostic for this purpose.

EXERCISE AND WEIGHT CONTROL

Teachers in health and physical education are frequently called upon to counsel students about nutrition and weight control. It is important to keep a few things in mind when doing so. First, it is probably best to take a long-term approach to weight reduction and avoid crash caloric restriction programs. Second, it is usually in the best interests of the individual to plan a program of systematic and progressive exercise to complement the diet. If there is any doubt about one's ability to undertake either, it is standard procedure to consult a physician. Sometimes the school nurse can offer information that might bear on the student's health; in particular she may know if there are any contraindications. The obese adult participant should also have a complete physical examination by a physician before beginning an exercise program.

There is occasional debate about the effectiveness of exercise in the control of body weight, and for good reasons. Barring complications, it still remains essentially a matter of counting calories, and it doesn't take long for one to realize just how much time would be required to lose a pound of body fat. Since it takes 4,222 kcal to metabolize one pound of fat, and since 1 kcal is equal to 3,087 ft.-lb, it is clear that the reduction of fat weight is not easily accomplished. What this can amount to is some 36 hours of walking, 11 hours of playing volleyball, or some other prodigious feat of exercise. The point is, weight reduction on a short-term basis by the use of exercise alone is not very successful, because so much work is required to mobilize body fat. However, if the diet is held constant, then over a period of time weight reduction can occur as a result of exercise. Simply apportion the hours required for the needed amount of work over intervals of days and weeks. In other words, the long-term approach is eminently more successful.

The control of weight through exercise can be confounded very easily if the individual simply replaces the expended calories by increasing the caloric intake. In this instance, the diet is not held constant, and the desired loss of fat weight may not actually take place. This serves to emphasize that effective weight reduction depends on achieving a *negative caloric balance*—that is, expending more calories than taken in. Obviously, the process can be hastened by reducing the intake of calories in the form of food while at the same time engaging in an exercise program. The speed with which weight will be lost will depend upon the vigor with which both aspects are pursued, but perhaps even more important is the fact that dieting alone is known to result not only in reduction of fat weight but in the loss of lean body weight as well. This can be prevented by systematic exercise.

Effect of Exercise on Food Intake

One concern is what happens to a person's appetite during his active period. We know that the athlete in training is consuming an enormous number of calories at the training table. But is it necessarily true that exercise itself stimulates the appetite? The answer depends upon whether the exercise is long-term or short-term. A classical study was carried out on an industrial population in West Bengal, India,[21] in which the diet was quite uniform, but the physical activity of the inhabitants ranged from sedentary to very heavy. Subjects in the latter category habitually carried twice their body weight on their heads and shoulders for nine hours a day. Figure 60 reveals that as the exercise increased from sedentary to light there was actually a decrease in caloric intake, a trend which was reversed through the categories of medium, heavy, and very heavy work. Body weight, on the other hand, decreased beyond the sedentary range, and stabilized throughout the heavy work categories. Apparently the increased caloric intake is essential for performance of the long hours of daily activity. On the other hand, short-term exercise, such as one hour a day, does not seem to stimulate the appetite.[22]

Effect of Exercise on Obesity

The classification of obesity is based on the amount of fat that is contained in the body. Standards vary from one authority to another, but it is generally felt that men should not exceed 15 to 20 percent body fat, and women 25 to 30 percent. It is becoming clear also that human obesity results in a marked increase in the *number* of adipose cells, as well as an increase in cell size. Figure 61 reflects the comparison in adipose cellularity of obese and nonobese subjects. Cell size increased by 40 percent, but cell number increased almost 190 percent.[23] A disturbing note is the finding that obesity in childhood (in fact as early as the first year) leads to a greater increase in cell number than obesity beginning later in life.[24]

[21]Jean Mayer, Purnima Roy, and K. P. Mitra, "Relation between Caloric Intake, Body Weight, and Physical Work: Studies in an Industrial Male Population in West Bengal," *American Journal of Clinical Nutrition*, 4 (1956), 169.

[22]Jerry A. Dempsey, "Anthropometrical Observations on Obese and Nonobese Young Men Undergoing a Program of Vigorous Physical Exercise," *Research Quarterly*, 35 (October 1964), 275.

[23]Jules Hirsch and Jerome L. Knittle, "Cellularity of Obese and Nonobese Human Adipose Tissue," *Federation Proceedings*, 29 (July–August 1970), 1516.

[24]C. G. D. Brook, June K. Lloyd, and O. H. Wolf, "Relation between Age of Onset of Obesity and Size and Number of Adipose Cells," *British Medical Journal*, 2 (April 1, 1972), 25.

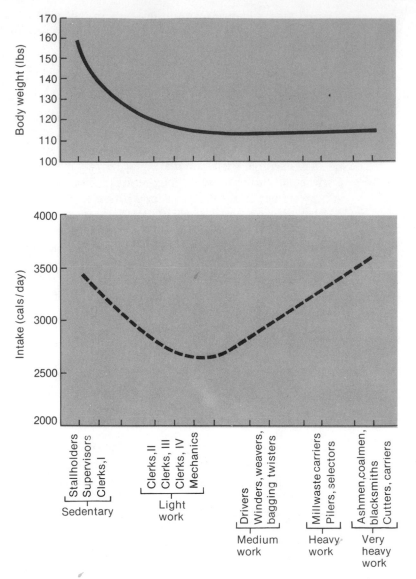

Figure 60. Effect of Exercise on Caloric Intake and Body Weight. [J. Mayer *et al.*, "Relation between Caloric Intake, Body Weight, and Physical Work: Studies in an Industrial Male Population in West Bengal," *American Journal of Clinical Nutrition*, 4 (1956), p. 172.]

Effect of Exercise on Body Composition

One of the aims of exercise and training is to cause changes in body composition. The individual may employ weight-lifting exercise to become stronger, in which case he is seeking to enhance muscle hypertrophy,

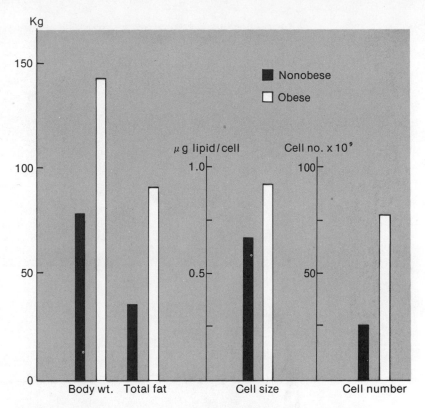

Figure 61. A Comparison of the Cell Size and Cell Number of Obese and Nonobese Subjects. [J. Hirsch and J. L. Knittle "Cellularity of Obese and Nonobese Human Adipose Tissue," *Federation Proceedings*, 29 (July-August 1970), p. 1518.]

which seeks to increase the quantity of lean tissue. Whether or not the fat content is reduced depends on the combination of energy expenditure and caloric restriction, as already explained. It is entirely conceivable that a balance could be effected between the gain in lean weight through hypertrophy and the loss of fat weight through mobilization of the adipose tissue. Thus the exercise regimen could actually result in no change in total body weight, once again pointing out the need to carefully evaluate body composition. Much the same can be said of the person who claims he weighs the same as he did when he competed in athletics many years ago. The body weight may be the same, but the chances are good that the ratio of fat to lean content may have altered considerably.

Most of the research literature substantiates the notion that regular physical exercise has a favorable effect on body composition for individuals of all ages. Athletes are known to have greater amounts of lean tissue, as reflected in higher body densities, and less body fat than the average person of comparable age. In fact, marathon runners, who are known for their lean appearance, possess approximately 9 percent less fat than men of

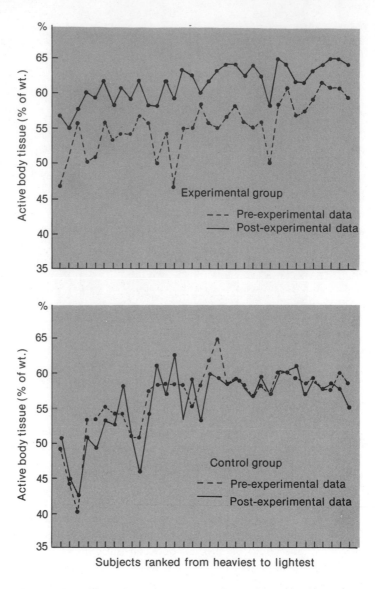

Figure 62a. Effect of Exercise on Lean Tissue. [E. Jokl, "Physical Activity and Body Composition: Fitness and Fatness," *Annals of the New York Academy of Sciences*, 110 (1963), p. 780.]

their age (26 years), and 5 percent less than younger, college-age men (20 years).[25] Clearly, the most efficient way to reduce body fat by means of exercise is to employ the longer-duration endurance activities where a more favorable opportunity exists to develop a negative caloric balance. This may even occur with vigorous walking, as Pollock *et al.* found when

---

[25]D. L. Costill, R. Bowers, and W. F. Kammer, "Skinfold Estimates of Body Fat Among Marathon Runners," *Medicine and Science in Sports*, 2 (Summer 1970), 93.

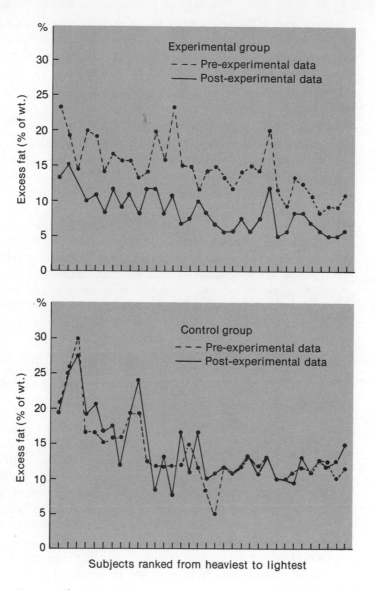

%

Figure 62b. Effect of Exercise on Excess Fat. [E. Jokl, "Physical Activity and Body Composition: Fitness and Fatness," *Annals of the New York Academy of Sciences*, 110 (1963), p. 781.]

middle-aged men trained for several months.[26] Similar results may be attained with young people, as Jokl[27] found when he studied adolescent boys and girls in a five-month daily physical training program. The change in body composition is shown in Figures 62a and 62b, where there is a

[26]Michael L. Pollock *et al.*, "Effects of Walking on Body Composition and Cardiovascular Function of Middle-Aged Men," *Journal of Applied Physiology*, 30 (January 1971), 126.

[27]Ernst Jokl, "Physical Activity and Body Composition: Fitness and Fatness," *Annals of the New York Academy of Sciences*, 110 (1963), 778.

significant increase in active tissue and decrease in excess fat at the conclusion of the training program. Note that the control group, made up of subjects not given the exercise program, did not experience such changes.

NUTRITION AND ATHLETIC PERFORMANCE

Almost no other topic in physiology of exercise involves more fad and fancy than that of the nutrition for athletes. In the more affluent athletic circumstances, training tables abound, stimulated in part, one would suspect, by the desire to provide an environment and the appropriate nutrition to foster winning performances. The additional use of supplements in the form of sugar-based foods and drinks and other substances attests to a somewhat mystical view of food with respect to the athlete and his performance. It is assumed that efforts to provide more energy in the diet are well-meaning. No one will argue that a proper diet is important, even essential, to proper functioning of the human organism, but from a physiological point of view some practices must be questioned in light of what is known about the source of energy for muscular contraction. These concepts have been sufficiently reviewed in previous chapters. Aside from the potential benefits of properly administering a carbohydrate-rich diet after first exhausting local glycogen stores (see Chapter 5), little advantage can be seen in providing special diets for athletes.

The Fuel for Athletic Performances

It would be a mistake to speak of athletic performance as if it were a single entity, always involving the same energy. Obviously, this is not true; some events involve rather isolated and single-effort activities, such as putting the shot, lifting weights, high jumping, and other field events. A second category consists of the short dash or hurdle events, as well as certain aspects of football and other sports that involve a relatively short period of high activity. Beyond these are the middle-distance running events, lasting, say, from a minute to several minutes, such as those contests up to the mile run. Finally, the relatively long endurance contests, leading up to the marathon, involve prolonged efforts where the energy expenditure may be moderate, but the duration may be an hour or even longer (in the case of the marathon, perhaps well over two hours).

To summarize previous discussions, it should be clear how the energy is supplied for the actual performance of these various athletic activities. First of all, we can conclude that the category involving a single burst of effort derives its energy from ATP and CP, which are eventually replenished from the breakdown of glycogen, a process that is essentially anaerobic. In the second category, the short-dash events, again we are dealing largely with an anaerobic situation during the running of the race, even though ultimately the energy requirement may be fairly substantial. The breakdown of glycogen to lactic acid permits the expenditure of energy, which is replenished in recovery. The subsequent payoff of the oxygen debt reflects the fact that little oxygen was actually taken in during the event. For longer contests, the slower pace reflects the combination of aerobic and anaerobic sources of energy. Considerably more time is available to utilize aerobic mechanisms while establishing the maximum oxygen debt. As Van Itallie, Sinisterra, and Stare[28] point out, the actual fuel supply is of minor concern, since the amounts of energy expended are relatively small. This is not necessarily true, however, for very long endurance efforts, where the fuel supply may be more important. It is here that the performer probably will be assisted if carbohydrate stores are plentiful. Even this is subject to some skepticism, for the infusion of large amounts of glucose during exercise apparently does not inhibit glycogen breakdown appreciably, pointing out that energy release from glycogen breakdown for heavy muscular work is indispensable.[29]

The Diet

The best advice still seems to be that the most appropriate diet for athletes is a well-balanced one, where all types of foods are available in quantities sufficient to meet the body's needs. This can be said for nonathletes as well, but the amount of food may be the differentiating factor, the individual in training requiring more calories to maintain a balance between energy expenditure and caloric intake. Special foods, given at special times, do not seem to enhance performance, except where glycogen loading is desired. In such cases, long-distance runners have noted improvement when the two or three pre-event days permit ingestion of large amounts of carbohydrate. When the local glycogen stores are first depleted by exhausting exercise and then held down for two or three days, an increase in endurance can be expected.

The practice of eating meat as an essential part of training derives from an ancient custom, supposedly to replenish muscle that was thought to be lost during severe muscular work.[30] Today, many still feel that steak is helpful to the athlete, even though it is clearly not an important fuel for physical work. Some protein is essential, of course, not only for normal dietary purposes, but also because protein is needed for rebuilding of muscle tissue. But normal dietary practices can provide sufficient pro-

[28]Theodore B. Van Itallie, Leonardo Sinisterra, and Fredrick J. Stare, "Nutrition and Athletic Performance," *Journal of the American Medical Association*, 162 (November 17, 1956), 1120.

[29]Eric Hultman, "Physiological Role of Muscle Glycogen in Man, with Special Reference to Exercise," in Carlton B. Chapman, ed., *Physiology of Muscular Exercise*, American Heart Association Monograph No. 15, 1967, p. 99.

[30]Jean Mayer and Beverly Bullen, "Nutrition and Athletic Performance," *Physiological Reviews*, 40 (July 1960), 369.

tein without resort to protein supplementation, and well-balanced meals during training are ordinarily sufficient. Again, additional protein than normal may be required during muscle training and during periods of growth, but even at these times the increased demand is likely to be met normally through the ingestion of larger portions of food at each meal.

The distribution of meals during the day is not critical, and the practice of three meals seems satisfactory. It is usually best to eat 2 to 2½ hours before a contest, and the meal should consist of light, easily digested foods, so that they may clear the stomach by game time. The difficulty otherwise may be the diversion of significant blood flow to the splanchnic region in response to the demand for digestion. When exercise starts, the blood flow to this region will be decreased and shunted to the working muscles. This may leave significant quantities of partially digested food in the stomach, which, if large enough, can impair full motion of the diaphragm, making breathing difficult and engendering an uncomfortable feeling of fullness. The ultimate effect is likely to depend upon the nature of the activity that follows.

A curious factor that cannot be ignored is the possibility of a psychological effect. If the athlete thinks there is a chance of improving through some special type of food, his belief itself may yield an improvement. This "proof" may reinforce his belief in the value of the dietary regimen. Unfortunately for exercise physiologists, some of these performers never really understand energy requirements and become coaches themselves, passing along misinformation and perpetuating fads rather than facts. The criticism here is less of the diet per se than of the misrepresentation.

DRUGS AND PERFORMANCE

A number of supplements and stimulants have been employed over the years by athletes and others in an effort to enhance performance. Indications from the popular press and elsewhere attest to their use, even though it is considered improper and even illegal in athletic competition. Ethical questions aside for the moment, it is rather important to know from a scientific point of view what can be expected when certain drugs are taken to improve performance. The knowledgeable coach or physical educator must be able to differentiate between the real effects of drugs and their psychological effects. Individual testimonials are seldom reliable indicators of physiological changes; indeed, athletes can be convinced that a superior effort had been due to some alteration in the training regimen. Therefore, controlled studies are needed to help decide if performance can indeed be improved through the administration of drugs. The discussion to follow will be limited to amphetamines, anabolic steroids, and caffeine.

Amphetamines

Amphetamines exert a direct effect on the central nervous system, stimulating activity of the post-ganglionic sympathetic nerves,[31] and are known to help overcome mental fatigue, boredom, and inattentiveness. Reports involving physical performance are not entirely unanimous in their results, due in part to differences in methodology, the amount of the dose, and absorption time. For example, Smith and Beecher[32] employed weight-throwers and shot-putters who were given either 14 mg of amphetamine per 70 kg of body weight, or a placebo. It was found that the amphetamine improved performance significantly, amounting to some 3 or 4 percent. Whether such an improvement is really better than taking a placebo has been questioned,[33] although Lovingood *et al.*[34] found that grip strength was significantly improved after administration of 15 mg of d-amphetamine sulfate. Ikai and Steinhaus[35] found that 30 mg of amphetamine sulfate improved by 13.5 percent the isometric strength of subjects. Other physiological effects of amphetamines seem to be nonsignificant, so apparently some minimal improvement may be experienced in muscular strength, but not in aerobic capacity or endurance. Much of the effect seems to be psychological rather than physiological.

Anabolic Steroids

The action of *anabolic steroids* is to cause the synthesis of protein tissue, thus leading to the increased retention of nitrogen in skeletal muscles, and a reduced nitrogen loss in the urine. Proponents for the use of anabolic steroids attest to an increased development of muscular strength and body weight, but there are potential hazards of side effects from their prolonged use. Among these hazards are a reduction in growth, a decrease in testicular size, and liver damage. Early puberty could be induced in young boys, so any use of steroids should be under control of a physician.

The research on anabolic steroids is in conflict, as we found with am-

[31]Melvin H. Williams, *Drugs and Athletic Performance*. Springfield, Ill.: Charles C. Thomas, 1974, p. 23.

[32]Gene M. Smith and Henry K. Beecher, "Amphetamine Sulfate and Athletic Performance. I. Objective Effects," *Journal of the American Medical Association*, 170 (May 30, 1959), 542.

[33]William R. Pierson, "Amphetamine Sulphate and Performance: A Critique," *Journal of the American Medical Association*, 177 (August 5, 1961), 345.

[34]Bill W. Lovingood *et al.*, "Effects of d-Amphetamine Sulfate, Caffeine, and High Temperature on Human Performance," *Research Quarterly*, 38 (March 1967), 64.

[35]Michio Ikai and Arthur H. Steinhaus, "Some Factors Modifying the Expression of Human Strength," *Journal of Applied Physiology*, 16 (1961), 157.

phetamines. Casner *et al.*[36] had subjects take steroids during a progressive weight training program, and found that they gained significantly more weight than control subjects, but no changes occurred in muscular strength. Similar results were found by Fahey and Brown[37] during a ten week weight training program; neither dynamic nor isokinetic strength was different than that of a placebo group. Johnson and O'Shea[38] administered a steroid plus a protein supplement to subjects exposed to a weight training program and found significant increases in strength. When controls were established for steroid and exercise, Fowler and associates[39] failed to show gains in strength as a result of sixteen weeks of exercise. Finally, Strømme and others[40] received steroid during an eight week progressive weight training program. None of the gains in strength were significantly better than the control subjects. In summary, the effects of steroid ingestion seem of no value alone, but may be helpful when taken in conjunction with protein supplementation, as a means for increasing muscular strength.

Caffeine

Caffeine is known to stimulate the central nervous system, to produce a more rapid and clear flow of thought, and to delay drowsiness and fatigue. Whether or not there exists a real effect on voluntary muscular performance is questionable. Thornton and co-workers[41] found that administration of a placebo produced scores that equalled or excelled those for caffeine in three out of sixteen cases in which both isotonic and isometric handgrip tests were given. Blyth and others[42] found no helpful or deleterious effects of caffeine on muscular strength and fatigue, and Margaria *et al.*[43] failed to find a significant change in aerobic capacity or treadmill performance time from caffeine ingestion. Thus, the use of caffeine as a means for increasing performance can not be encouraged.

[36]S. W. Casner *et al.*, "Anabolic Steroid Effects on Body Composition in Normal Young Men," *Journal of Sports Medicine and Physical Fitness*, 11 (June 1971), 98.

[37]Thomas D. Fahey and C. Harmon Brown, "The Effects of an Anabolic Steroid on the Strength, Body Composition, and Endurance of College Males when Accompanied by a Weight Training Program," *Medicine and Science in Sports*, 5 (Winter 1973), 272.

[38]L. C. Johnson and J. P. O'Shea, "Anabolic Steroid: Effects on Strength Development," *Science*, 164 (May 1969), 957.

[39]William M. Fowler *et al.*, "Effect of an Anabolic Steroid on Physical Performance of Young Men," *Journal of Applied Physiology*, 20 (September 1965), 1038.

[40]S. B. Strømme, H. D. Meen and A. Aakvaag, "Effects of an Androgenic-Anabolic Steroid on Strength Development and Plasma Testosterone Levels in Normal Males," *Medicine and Science in Sports*, 6 (Fall 1974), 203.

[41]G. H. Thornton *et al.*, "The Effects of Benzedrine and Caffeine upon Performance in Certain Psychomotor Tasks," *Journal of Abnormal and Social Psychology*, 34 (January 1939), 96.

[42]Carl S. Blyth *et al.*, "Effects of Amphetamine (Dexedrine) and Caffeine on Subjects Exposed to Heat and Exercise Stress," *Research Quarterly*, 31 (December 1960), 553.

[43]R. Margaria *et al.*, "The Effect of Some Drugs on the Maximal Capacity of Athletic Performance in Man," *Int. Z. angew. Physiol. einschl. Arbeitsphysiol.*, 20 (1964), 281.

The three constituents of the diet are carbohydrates, fats, and proteins, with carbohydrates being the chief source of energy and fats second. Proteins, on the other hand, are composed of amino acids, and their synthesis accompanies muscular hypertrophy. A number of minerals and vitamins are required, but the usual diet seems to provide them in sufficient quantities. Body weight depends upon a balance between the caloric intake and energy expenditure; when an imbalance occurs, weight will either increase or decrease.

The respiratory exchange ratio (R), the ratio of carbon dioxide produced by the body to the oxygen consumed, is highest for carbohydrates and lowest for fats. It may increase in exercise, owing to the buffering of lactic acid, and decrease later in recovery when the lactic acid is oxidized and bicarbonate is being reformed. The respiratory exchange ratio may serve as an index of the involvement of lactic acid, which in the trained individual would tend to decrease R.

Mechanical efficiency is the ratio of external work done divided by the energy consumed. For the human body it varies from 20 to 25 percent; it may be increased if more work can be performed for the same energy cost, or if the energy cost is lowered for the same amount of work. The person with the lowest oxygen uptake for the performance of a standard task is the most efficient. Improving physical fitness can improve efficiency, as can adjusting the rate of work to an optimum level.

Body composition can be divided into lean and fat components. Body density, the key to understanding lean body weight and percent fat, can be estimated by immersion in water, by anthropometric measurement, or by determination of skinfold. The relative ratio of lean to fat tissue may make a contribution to athletic performance, for it seems advisable for body bulk to be composed of muscle rather than fat tissue. Controlling the development of adipose tissue and promoting lean tissue development depends on the caloric intake as compared with the caloric expenditure, and fat weight loss will occur when the expenditure is greater than the intake. Exercise is important, as is the diet, in controlling weight. Contrary to popular opinion, exercise does not seem to stimulate the appetite; obesity is more a product of sedentary living. Recent evidence indicates that obesity increases the number as well as the size of adipose cells. Obesity in childhood seems to precipitate a greater increase in cell number than obesity beginning later in life.

Exercise increases lean body mass and can lead to loss of fat weight through mobilization of the adipose tissue. Athletes seldom require food supplements to provide more energy, since ample nutrients usually appear in sufficient quantities in the average diet. The fuel for athletic performance usually does not depend on the previous meal, as some events are essentially anaerobic anyway. Distance running requires more energy and will need an ample supply of carbohydrate. Very little effect seems to be gained by using drugs to improve performance.

SELECTED REFERENCES

Åstrand, Per-Olof, and Kaare Rodahl, *Textbook of Work Physiology*. New York: McGraw-Hill Book Company, 1970, chap. 14.

Banister, E. W., and S. R. Brown, "The Relative Energy Requirements of Physical Activity," in Harold B. Falls, ed., *Exercise Physiology*. New York: Academic Press, 1968.

Behnke, Albert R., "Quantitative Assessment of Body Build," *Journal of Applied Physiology*, 16 (November 1961), 960.

————, and Jack H. Wilmore, *Evaluation and Regulation of Body Build and Composition*. Englewood Cliffs, N.J.: Prentice-Hall, Inc., 1974.

Bogert, L. Jean, George M. Briggs, and Doris Howes Calloway, *Nutrition and Physical Fitness*, 9th ed. Philadelphia: W. B. Saunders Company, 1973.

Brožek, Josef, ed., "Body Composition," parts I and II, *Annals of the New York Academy of Sciences*, 110 (September 26, 1963).

————, and A. Henschel, eds., *Techniques for Measuring Body Composition*. Washington, D.C.: National Academy of Sciences—National Research Council, 1961.

————, and A. Keys, "The Evaluation of Leanness-Fatness in Man: Norms and Interrelations," *British Journal of Nutrition*, 5 (1951), 194.

Costill, D. L., R. Bowers, and W. F. Kammer, "Skinfold Estimates of Body Fat Among Marathon Runners," *Medicine and Science in Sports*, 2 (Summer 1970), 93.

DeMoor, Janice C., "Individual Differences in Oxygen Debt Curves Related to Mechanical Efficiency and Sex," *Journal of Applied Physiology*, 6 (1954), 460.

Henry, Franklin M., *Physiology of Work: The Physiological Basis of Muscular Exercise*. Berkeley: Associated Students' Store, University of California, 1968, chap. 3.

Hirsch, Jules, and Jerome L. Knittle, "Cellularity of Obese and Nonobese Human Adipose Tissue," *Federation Proceedings*, 29 (July–August 1970), 1516.

Issekutz, B., and K. Rodahl, "Respiratory Quotient during Exercise," *Journal of Applied Physiology*, 16 (1961), 606.

Mayer, Jean, and Beverly Bullen, "Nutrition and Athletic Performance," *Physiological Reviews*, 40 (July 1960), 369.

————, Purnima Roy, and K. P. Mitra, "Relation Between Caloric Intake, Body Weight, and Physical Work: Studies in an Industrial Male Population in West Bengal," *American Journal of Clinical Nutrition*, 4 (1956), 169.

Oscai, Lawrence B., "The Role of Exercise in Weight Control," in Jack H. Wilmore, ed., *Exercise and Sport Sciences Reviews*, Vol. 1. New York: Academic Press, 1973, pp. 103–123.

nutrition and
performance

Passmore, R., and J. V. G. A. Durnin, "Human Energy Expenditure," *Physiological Reviews*, 35 (October 1955), 801.

Pollock, Michael L., *et al.,* "Effects of Walking on Body Composition and Cardiovascular Function of Middle-Aged Men," *Journal of Applied Physiology*, 30 (January 1971), 126.

Sloan, A. W., J. J. Burt, and C. S. Blyth, "Estimation of Body Fat in Young Women," *Journal of Applied Physiology*, 17 (November 1962), 967.

Van Itallie, Theodore B., Leonardo Sinisterra, and Fredrick J. Stare, "Nutrition and Athletic Performance," *Journal of the American Medical Association*, 162 (November 17, 1956), 1120.

Wilmore, Jack H., and Albert R. Behnke, "Predictability of Lean Body Weight through Anthropometric Assessment in College Men," *Journal of Applied Physiology*, 25 (October 1968), 349.

chapter
8

oxygen
and
carbon dioxide
transport

The preceding chapters have provided a basic knowledge of the mechanism for exercise. Not only have we been able to see how muscles contract, but the basis for the energy exchange has been reviewed with the objective to give a firm grasp of the metabolic processes involved in aerobic and anaerobic work. It should be clear at this point that the ability to perform endurance exercise is dependent upon the supply of oxygen to the muscle cells of the body. Therefore, an important concern in exercise physiology is the capacity to transport oxygen to and carbon dioxide away from the muscles. Both will be considered in this chapter.

GAS LAWS

One of the more difficult challenges in physiology is to understand the way in which gases behave and then to describe how gas transport is achieved in the human organism. One can see the blood and feel the muscles, but the factors controlling the distribution of gases such as oxygen and carbon dioxide into blood and the tissues must be accepted largely on faith. Yet, since gases obey physical laws, it may be helpful to review some of the underlying concepts that are basic to the whole field of respiratory physiology.

A gas is composed of individual molecules that engage in continuous random motion. When the pressure is low, the molecules are separated by relatively large distances, but in any case they will fill the available volume. The bombardment of the walls of a container by the molecules imparts to it a *pressure*, which will vary proportionately to a change in *temperature*, since heat will increase the speed with which the molecules move. Also, the *number* of molecules per unit volume will determine the gas pressure, as the more molecules the greater the bombardment on the walls of the container. Again, this change in pressure will be proportional to the number of moleclues present.

It is important to note that if two or more gases are mixed together, such as oxygen and nitrogen, for example, the molecules of each simply behave as if the other were not present, and intermingle, all molecules engaging in random motion. Thus, the total pressure becomes the sum of the individual pressures, and each gas then contributes its *partial pres-*

sure. This will be represented by the symbol *P* before the gas, such as P_{O_2}, the partial pressure of oxygen. The value for partial pressure will usually be expressed in millimeters of mercury (Hg). Pressure can be increased by pumping more molecules into the container, which has the effect of compressing the molecules, thus increasing the molecular contact with the container walls. If more oxygen is introduced to our mixture of oxygen and nitrogen, the total pressure will increase, as will the partial pressure of oxygen, but the partial pressure of nitrogen will remain the same. Remember that the air we breathe (atmospheric air) is under pressure, brought about by the weight of the air above the earth's surface.

If one surface of our container is a liquid, it can be expected that gas molecules will diffuse into the liquid in a manner that is *directly proportional to the pressure of the gas*, until there is equilibrium both inside and outside the liquid boundary. In other words, the gas will flow in a direction dictated by the *pressure gradient*, the numerical difference between the high and low pressures. Thus, knowledge of the partial pressures will explain the direction of gas flow. On this basis we can explain the transfer of gases between alveolar air and pulmonary capillary blood.

Another concept to be remembered is that gases will dissolve into liquids not only in proportion to the partial pressure, but also according to the *solubility* of the gas in the liquid. Solubility is defined as the amount of that solute (gas, in this case) which will dissolve in a given quantity of solvent to produce a saturated solution. The number of molecules of a gas entering solution will vary according to its solubility characteristics, which makes it possible for identical amounts of two gases to enter solution even though their pressure gradients may be different. This is a useful concept that will be applied subsequently to oxygen and carbon dioxide. Raising the temperature of a solution lowers the solubility, since gas molecules tend to leave solution when the temperature is increased. Also, a gas will enter and leave solution quite independent of the presence of other gases. The removal of one gas will lower the total pressure but will not alter the other gases present.

The following gas laws may be helpful in summarizing the behavior of gases:

1. *Boyle's law:* The volume of a given quantity of gas maintained at constant temperature is inversely proportional to the pressure to which it is subjected.

2. *Charles' law:* The volume of a given mass of gas is directly proportional to its absolute temperature when the pressure is held constant.

3. *Dalton's law:* The total pressure of a gas mixture is equal to the sum of the partial pressures of the component gases.

4. *Avogadro's law:* Equal volumes of all gases, measured at the same temperature and pressure, contain the same number of molecules.

5. *Henry's law:* The quantity of a gas that dissolves in a volume of liquid is directly proportional to the partial pressure of that gas, the pressure remaining constant.

Fortunately for the study of respiratory physiology, the composition of *atmospheric air*, the air we breathe, remains practically constant, and the values given in Table 8–1 can ordinarily be used in computations where the composition of inspired air is to be known. By far the largest component is nitrogen, but (like the rare gases) it does not participate in metabolic exchanges; it only becomes important when breathed under higher than normal pressures, such as in underwater diving. This will be

Table 8–1. Composition of Dry Atmospheric Air

	%	Partial Pressure (mm Hg)
Oxygen	20.93	159.1
Carbon dioxide	.04	.3
Nitrogen	79.03	600.6
TOTAL	100.00	760.0

NOTE: The total also includes traces of a number of so-called rare gases, such as argon, neon, helium, krypton, etc., but because they are inert with respect to gas exchange, they may be ignored.

discussed in greater detail in Chapter 12. The partial pressures are also given in the table, based upon a total *barometric pressure* of 760 mm Hg; we can calculate them by obtaining the product of the percentage and the total pressure. For example,

$$P_{O_2} = .2093 \times 760 = 159.1 \text{ mm Hg.}$$

Contrary to popular impression, the percentage composition of atmospheric air is relatively constant even at high altitude; what happens is that the barometric pressure decreases so that the partial pressures become reduced, resulting in decreased pressure gradients. Again, this will be discussed in Chapter 12.

COMPOSITION OF ALVEOLAR AIR

It is essential not to confuse atmospheric air with *alveolar air*, because alveolar air is actually what comes into contact with the pulmonary capillaries, where the blood-gas exchange takes place. The values are given in Table 8–2. By contrast with atmospheric air, alveolar air is considered

Table 8–2. Composition of Saturated Alveolar Air

	%	Partial Pressure (mm Hg)
Oxygen	13.6	104.0
Carbon dioxide	5.3	40.0
Nitrogen	74.9	569.0
Water vapor	6.2	47.0
TOTAL	100.0	760.0

saturated with water vapor at a body temperature of 37°C and has a partial pressure (P_{H_2O}) of 47 mm Hg. Since the total pressure is still 760 mm Hg, it reduces the proportion of the other gases, but primarily the changes are brought about because oxygen is entering the pulmonary capillaries and carbon dioxide is entering the alveoli. This brings the P_{O_2} down to approximately 104 mm Hg and the P_{CO_2} up to 40 mm Hg. Actually, these values will vary, and for convenience the P_{O_2} is frequently rounded off at 100 mm Hg. One important feature of alveolar air, however, is that it will remain relatively constant during variations in the respiratory cycle, which assures a smooth exchange of gas with the blood at all times.

GAS EXCHANGE BETWEEN LUNGS AND THE BLOOD

The blood pumped via the pulmonary artery to the lungs is mixed venous blood from all the tissues of the body. Consequently, it has a high P_{CO_2} (46 mm Hg) and low P_{O_2} (40 mm Hg), the values representing resting conditions. When it reaches the region of the lungs it is dispersed through a series of vessels that eventually ends in pulmonary capillaries surrounding the alveoli. The membrane that separates the two is only about .001 mm thick, and the human lung is so constructed that the total area available for gas exchange amounts to some 70 square meters, or 40 times the surface area of the entire body.[1] With some 300 million alveoli, the individual actually has more than sufficient capability for oxygen uptake, and for this reason it is concluded that the lungs are not limiting factors in exercise. More will be said about this in the next chapter.

As the blood flows through the pulmonary capillaries, it encounters differences in partial pressures of oxygen and carbon dioxide with the alveoli. In fact, the pressure gradient of 64 mm Hg (104 — 40 mm Hg) for oxygen and 6 mm Hg for carbon dioxide favors the flow of oxygen into the blood and carbon dioxide into the alveoli, and this takes place very efficiently, so that by the time the blood reaches the end of the capillaries

[1]Julius H. Comroe, "The Lung," *Scientific American*, 214 (February 1966), 56.

the net diffusion ceases as the alveolar and capillary partial pressures become approximately equal. The blood that leaves the lungs to return to the heart via the pulmonary vein is ready to be pumped into the systemic arteries. Arterial blood has a Po_2 of 96 mm Hg and a Pco_2 of 40 mm Hg, nearly the same as that of alveolar air. The partial pressure of arterial oxygen (Pao_2) is slightly less than the alveolar (Pao_2) because a small amount of the blood in the systemic arteries has actually bypassed the pulmonary capillaries in what is known as a "physiologic shunt" or a "venous admixture" of blood. At any rate, the blood is considered fully oxygenated, and it has also lost its excess CO_2, as reflected in the fact that the $Paco_2$ and $Paco_2$ are the same. The differences in pressure gradients for oxygen and carbon dioxide reflect differences in solubility for the two gases, resulting in a diffusing capacity some twenty times greater for CO_2. Therefore, the differences in pressure are entirely adequate for effective blood-gas exchange.

GAS EXCHANGE BETWEEN BLOOD AND THE CELLS

The arterial blood eventually enters capillaries throughout the body, and oxygen diffuses into the tissues in a manner essentially the reverse of the process that occurred in the lungs. The capillaries are separated from the interstitial fluid by a very thin, highly permeable membrane, which in turn is separated from intracellular fluid by cell membranes that are very permeable to oxygen and carbon dioxide. Muscle cells engaged in heavy work may have a Po_2 of 0–12 mm Hg, depending upon the extent of exercise and the type and rate of contraction. The pressure difference favors the diffusion of oxygen into the tissues, and it does so quickly, leaving the venous blood with a Po_2 of 40 mm Hg, although this value will be higher than the venous Po_2 of the vessels leading away from the muscles themselves. The Pco_2, on the other hand, will be high, perhaps as high as 50–80 mm Hg in working tissues, and will diffuse to the blood as it filters through the capillaries, resulting in the venous Pco_2 of 46 mm Hg. The relationship of these various factors of gas distribution are shown in Figure 63.

THE EFFECT OF EXERCISE ON PULMONARY DIFFUSING CAPACITY

The effect of exercise on pulmonary function will be discussed in Chapter 9, but it might be helpful to mention briefly a few important factors that bear on pulmonary diffusing capacity. As we know, there is an increase in ventilation during exercise as well as an increase in oxygen uptake by the blood. The latter factor is a result of the increase in diffusing capacity for oxygen, caused partly because a number of dormant pulmonary

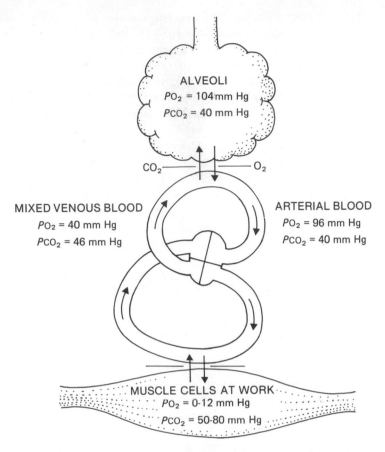

ALVEOLI
PO_2 = 104 mm Hg
PCO_2 = 40 mm Hg

CO_2 —— O_2

MIXED VENOUS BLOOD
PO_2 = 40 mm Hg
PCO_2 = 46 mm Hg

ARTERIAL BLOOD
PO_2 = 96 mm Hg
PCO_2 = 40 mm Hg

MUSCLE CELLS AT WORK
PO_2 = 0-12 mm Hg
PCO_2 = 50-80 mm Hg

Figure 63. Oxygen and Carbon Dioxide Pressures at Various Sites within the Body.

capillaries are suddenly opened up for use during exercise. Blood is now able to course over a larger surface area, providing a greater opportunity for oxygen diffusion. In addition, an increased dilatation of the capillaries already in use further enhances the surface area favoring blood-gas exchange. Both changes are over and above those that occur normally. Moreover, an additional factor operates to ensure the adequate oxygenation of the blood: the entry of oxygen into the blood is so rapid that even under normal exercise conditions adequate time is available for this exchange to take place. This, however, may not be true for endurance athletes, where reduced arterial oxygen saturation has been noticed.[2] The causative factors are difficult to identify, and, indeed, difficult to understand, since by the very nature of their performance, athletes have great capacities for ventilation, cardiac output, and oxygen uptake.

[2]Loring B. Rowell, Henry L. Taylor, Yang Wang, and Walter S. Carlson, "Saturation of Arterial Blood with Oxygen During Maximal Exercise," *Journal of Applied Physiology*, 19 (March 1964), 284.

The oxygen that diffuses into the blood can be carried in two ways. The first is by being *physically dissolved* in the water of the plasma, but because oxygen is relatively insoluble in water, only .3 ml can be dissolved per 100 ml of plasma—a very small amount. This contrasts with some 19–20 ml per 100 ml when oxygen enters into *chemical combination* with *hemoglobin*. Thus, the most important vehicle for oxygen is hemoglobin, since 97 or 98 percent of the total is carried in this manner when the P_{O_2} is approximately 100 mm Hg, as it is with alveolar air. The reverse is true at the tissue capillaries, where the P_{O_2} is low; in this instance the oxygen is released from the hemoglobin.

Hemoglobin is the primary constituent of the red blood cells, the erythrocytes, each red cell carrying about 280 million molecules of hemoglobin. Each molecule, in turn, is made up of about 10,000 atoms of hydrogen, carbon, nitrogen, oxygen, and sulfur, plus four atoms of iron.[3] This last item is of great interest, since each iron atom can take up two atoms of oxygen by combining with the heme portion in a reversible reaction:

$$Hb + O_2 \rightleftharpoons HbO_2. \tag{8–1}$$

The result is the formation of *oxyhemoglobin*, which becomes fully oxygenated when the four atoms of iron combine with four molecules (eight atoms) of oxygen according to the following equation:

$$Hb_4 + 4O_2 \rightleftharpoons Hb_4O_8. \tag{8–2}$$

This very loose relationship is determined by the P_{O_2} to which hemoglobin is exposed. When the P_{O_2} is low and the oxygen leaves the blood, it results in what is known as *reduced hemoglobin*.

OXYGEN DISSOCIATION CURVES OF HEMOGLOBIN

The way in which blood takes up and gives off oxygen can be described by employing what is known as the *oxygen dissociation curves*, as shown in Figure 64. They reveal the percentage of hemoglobin saturation (vertical axis) with varying partial pressures of oxygen (horizontal axis). Under normal circumstances there is enough hemoglobin (approximately 15 grams per 100 ml of blood) to combine with 19 ml O_2 per

[3]M. F. Perutz, "The Hemoglobin Molecule," *Scientific American*, 211 (November 1964), 64.

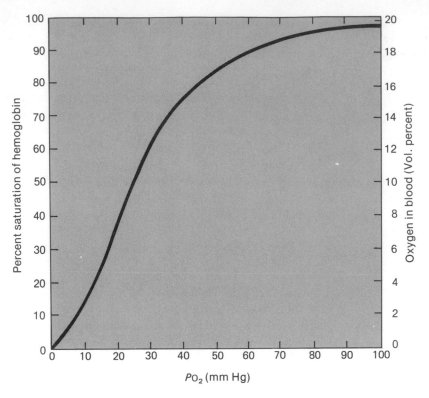

Figure 64. The Oxygen Dissociation Curves of Hemoglobin.

100 ml of blood, which is therefore considered *fully saturated* at approximately 97 percent, assuming a Po_2 of 100 mm Hg. At an oxygen tension of 40 mm Hg it is only about 70 percent saturated, which corresponds to an oxygen content of 14 ml per 100 ml. It should be clear that 19 ml per 100 ml of blood (usually called *volumes percent*) represents the oxygen saturation of arterial blood and 14 volumes percent represents the saturation of venous blood, since the Po_2 values correspond to those given earlier for both samples of blood. Thus, the blood while traveling throughout the body has given up approximately 5 volumes percent of oxygen to the tissues at rest.

An interesting feature of the oxygen dissociation curve is that this portion associated with arterial blood is rather flat. In fact, the Po_2 can drop to as low as 70 mm Hg and still result in some 90 percent saturation, which insures very nearly full saturation of the hemoglobin even if some changes should occur in alveolar Po_2. Moreover, the steep portion occurs over the range of oxygen tensions that will occur in the tissues, which is an important effect, since the blood will give up its oxygen in response to subtle changes in partial pressures caused by the demand for oxygen in the tissues.

Several factors bearing on the oxygen-hemoglobin dissociation should be considered. For one thing, increasing the acidity, by raising the Pco_2

to which the blood is exposed, shifts the dissociation curve to the right (Figure 65). This is accomplished by altering the hydrogen-ion concentration (lowering the pH), and it means that for a given partial pressure of oxygen the hemoglobin is *less* saturated with oxygen when it becomes more acidic. This is called the *Bohr effect*. Stated in another way, the change in blood toward acidity reduces the affinity of hemoglobin for oxygen. This is shown in Figure 65 for CO_2 and in the insert graph for pH.

Note that in the tissues where CO_2 is being produced, and consequently where the acidity is increased, the shifting of the oxygen dissociation curve downward and to the right means that less oxygen will remain bound to hemoglobin than otherwise would be the case. For example, with a Po_2 of 40 mm Hg and a Pco_2 of 40 mm Hg, the saturation of the blood is 13 volumes percent, whereas at the same Po_2, but with a Pco_2 of 80 mm Hg, the hemoglobin saturation is only 9.5 volumes percent. Thus, an additional 3.5 volumes percent have been given up to the tissues. It should also be mentioned that increasing temperature has a similar effect on hemoglobin desaturation, as shown in Figure 65. In

Figure 65. Effect of CO_2, pH, and Temperature on Oxygen-Hemoglobin Dissociation.

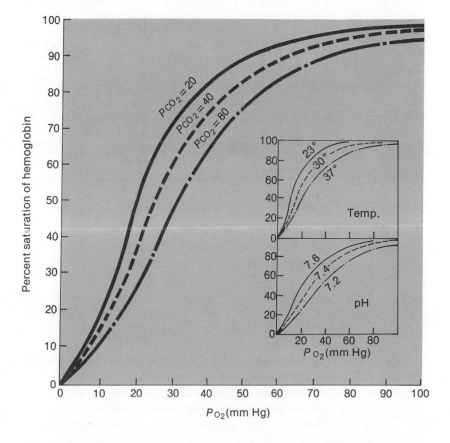

other words, active tissue, such as muscle during exercise, increases its temperature, which facilitates the release of oxygen from hemoglobin as the blood flows through muscle capillaries.

EXERCISE AND THE UTILIZATION OF OXYGEN

Exercise provides an environment for the increase in oxygen uptake from a basal value of 250 ml/min to some 4.5 l/min at maximum. Without considering the increase in blood flow itself that will take place, nor the vasodilation of the tissue capillaries, there still remains the fact that heavy exercise causes the interstitial fluid Po_2 to drop extremely low. If a value of 15 mm Hg is employed as an example, Figure 64 reveals that the amount of oxygen in the blood will drop from a resting value ($Po_2 = 40$ mm Hg) of 14 vol. percent to approximately 4 vol. percent. With the amount of oxygen available to the tissues in the incoming arterial blood of 19 vol. percent, this means that the amount given up to the tissues increases from 5 vol. percent to 15 vol. percent. We can express this as a *coefficient of oxygen utilization* by relating the amount of oxygen given up to the tissues to the amount available, according to the following equation:

$$\frac{O_2 \text{ content of arterial blood} - O_2 \text{ content of venous blood}}{O_2 \text{ content of arterial blood}}. \qquad (8\text{--}3)$$

The numerator is the amount of oxygen taken up by the tissues, which is 5 vol. percent at rest. When divided by 19 vol. percent, the resulting coefficient is .26 or 26 percent. However, during heavy work, the coefficient can increase to almost 80 percent (15/19 = .79 or 79 percent), which means the tissues become more than three times as efficient in their utilization of oxygen. Later on, it will be important for us to add in the fact that the number of capillaries participating in gas transfer increases, which enlarges the surface area and further facilitates gas exchange. Not only that, but the production of CO_2 and lactic acid and the increase in temperature that occur during exercise are very important in enabling the oxygen uptake to increase.

MYOGLOBIN

Myoglobin is an iron-containing protein found in muscles, especially those which are engaged in slow, repeated contractions, such as the leg muscles. As brought out in Chapter 2, myoglobin has the ability to combine with oxygen at low pressures more readily than does blood. The comparison with the usual dissociation curve can be seen in Figure 66. Even at a Po_2 of 40 mm Hg myoglobin is still 95 percent saturated. It begins to release large quantities of oxygen only when the Po_2 falls below 20 mm Hg, so that during mild exercise myoglobin presumably remains saturated. However, when severe exercise conditions prevail, the reduced intracellular

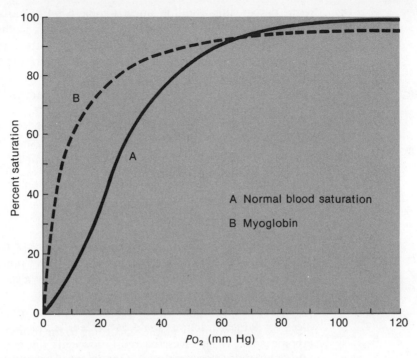

Figure 66. The Oxygen Dissociation Curves of Myoglobin.

Po_2 permits myoglobin to release its oxygen to the cytochrome oxidase system. Myoglobin thus acts as a temporary oxygen store, amounting maximally to probably no more than .5 liters, and useful to those muscles in which it is located only during strenuous exercise. Moreover, its effect may not be enhanced in prolonged and continuous isometric exercise where the Po_2 remains low; in such circumstances there would be limited opportunity for recharging myoglobin stores once the original supply was exhausted. In isotonic activity, on the other hand, the intermittent rest periods could conceivably permit recharging of the myoglobin by the blood during periods when the Po_2 had increased. Pattengale and Holloszy[4] have found that quadriceps and hamstring muscles undergoing training (white rats) increased their myoglobin content 80 percent more than muscles not employed in training, so an additional effect of training is to enhance the oxygen support of muscles by augmenting myoglobin.

TRANSPORT OF CARBON DIOXIDE IN THE BLOOD

The average resting Respiratory Exchange Ratio (R) is approximately .82 (see Chapter 7). If 5 ml of oxygen per 100 ml of blood are utilized

[4]Paul K. Pattengale and John O. Holloszy, "Augmentation of Skeletal Muscle Myoglobin by a Program of Treadmill Running," *American Journal of Physiology*, 213 (September 1967), 783.

by the tissues, this would mean that some 4 ml of carbon dioxide per 100 ml of blood must be transported from the tissues to the lungs. During exercise, when the R goes higher, approximately the same volume of CO_2 is produced for every volume of oxygen that is transported to the tissues. This is a major function of the blood.

As we found for oxygen, the amount of carbon dioxide that can be transported in the dissolved state in the plasma and red blood cells is small, probably not much more than .3 ml per 100 ml of blood, which is only about 7 percent of the total. In the plasma, the carbon dioxide combines slowly with water to form *carbonic acid* (H_2CO_3), according to the following reversible reaction:

$$CO_2 + H_2O \rightleftharpoons H_2CO_3. \qquad (8\text{--}4)$$

The carbonic acid thus formed dissociates into *hydrogen ions* (H^+) and *bicarbonate ions* (HCO_3^-), the resulting H^+ being buffered by the plasma buffering systems. Dissolved CO_2 in the plasma also reacts with various plasma proteins to form *carbamino compounds*.[5]

Most of the carbon dioxide, however, passes into the red blood cells, where the largest fraction, some 68 percent, combines with water to form carbonic acid. What gives the red blood cells the special ability to react with CO_2 is the fact that they contain the enzyme *carbonic anhydrase*, which catalyzes the reaction. The plasma does not contain this enzyme, which explains why it has such limited CO_2-carrying power. The formed carbonic acid in the red blood cells dissociates into H^+ and HCO_3^-, as shown in the following equation:

$$CO_2 + H_2O \overset{\text{carbonic anhydrase}}{\rightleftharpoons} H_2CO_3 \rightleftharpoons HCO_3^- + H^+. \qquad (8\text{--}5)$$

This tends to make the inside of the cell acid, but the resulting H^+ are buffered by the hemoglobin molecule, which leaves the concentration of HCO_3^- increased within the red blood cell. These excess HCO_3^- ions tend to diffuse out into the plasma, but can only do so if an equal number of Cl^- ions enter the red blood cells from the plasma, in what is known as the *chloride shift* (or Hamburger phenomenon, as it is sometimes called). Thus, electrical neutrality is preserved within the red blood cell.

A mechanism may now be seen for the increased dissociation of oxygen from hemoglobin in the presence of carbon dioxide, as discussed earlier. The majority of the H^+ reacts with oxyhemoglobin (HbO_2), forming HHb and releasing O_2, which diffuses out of the red blood cell to supply the tissue needs.[6] There remains a slight excess of H^+, and because of the outward diffusion of HCO_3^- the stage is set for the entry of

---

[5]N. Balfour Slonim and John L. Chapin, *Respiratory Physiology* (St. Louis: The C. V. Mosby Company, 1967), p. 71.

[6]Franklin M. Henry, *Physiology of Work: The Physiological Basis of Muscular Exercise* (Berkeley: Associated Students' Store, University of California, 1968), pp. 75–78.

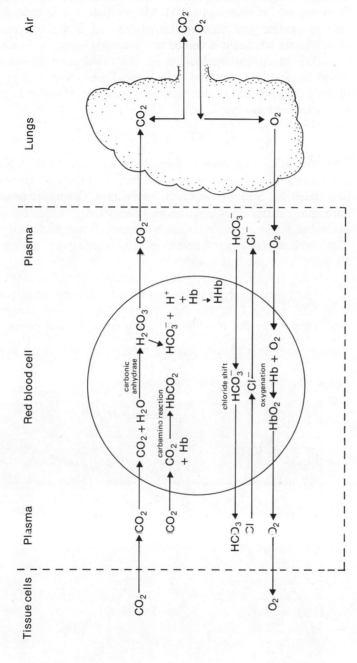

Figure 67. Summary of the Factors Contributing to Gas Transport by the Blood.

additional Cl^- from the plasma to restore ionic equilibrium. When the blood reaches the lungs the entry of oxygen into the red blood cell causes the hemoglobin to be more acid, which releases HCO_3^-. Also, Cl^- diffuses from the cell in exchange for HCO_3^-, which now is quickly converted to carbon dioxide and diffuses out of the red blood cell and to the lung alveoli, from whence it is voided to the atmosphere.

The remaining mechanism for the rapid combination of CO_2 in the blood is the direct reaction with hemoglobin. Approximately 25 percent of the CO_2 combines in this manner, forming *carbamino hemoglobin*, as in the following equation:

$$CO_2 + Hb \rightleftharpoons HbCO_2. \tag{8-6}$$

The carbon dioxide does not combine with the hemoglobin molecule at the same point as does oxygen, so both oxygen and carbon dioxide can be carried by hemoglobin at the same time. Reduced hemoglobin forms carbamino compounds much more readily than oxyhemoglobin, which explains why CO_2 transport in this manner is facilitated in venous blood. The several factors involved in CO_2 transport are summarized in Figure 67.

CARBON DIOXIDE DISSOCIATION CURVES

The oxygen dissociation curves described earlier involve the influence of carbon dioxide on the binding of oxygen to hemoglobin. The

Figure 68. The Carbon Dioxide Dissociation Curves.

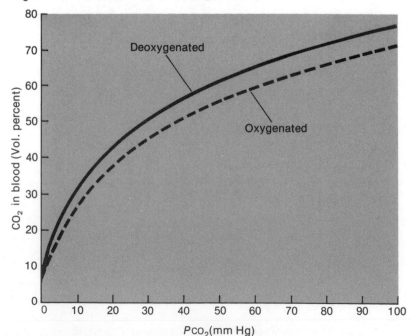

same concept can also be applied to the carbon dioxide transport in the blood, where the presence of oxygen causes the dissociation of carbon dioxide. This *Haldane effect* is illustrated in Figure 68. The two curves, one plotted for oxygenated blood and one for deoxygenated blood, reveal that there is greater reduction of CO_2 from the blood (vertical axis) when blood is oxygenated at any value for P_{CO_2} (horizontal axis). The physiologically important range for P_{CO_2} is from 40 to 46 mm Hg at rest and can be even higher during exercise. This can be seen as a helpful effect, for when venous blood enters the pulmonary capillaries, the entry of oxygen helps force carbon dioxide out of the blood. The essential reactions have already been described.

SUMMARY

Gases consist of molecules engaged in random movement, each imparting its own partial pressure, the magnitude of which will depend upon the temperature and the number of molecules per unit volume. Gases will diffuse into or out of a liquid, depending on the pressure gradient to which they are exposed and the characteristics of their solubility. The total pressure for atmospheric air is the barometric pressure, which remains relatively constant in percentage composition of oxygen, nitrogen, and carbon dioxide. However, the air that engages in reaction with the blood is alveolar air, which is saturated with water vapor.

The pressure gradient for oxygen permits the rapid flow of oxygen from the alveoli to the blood, and the flow of carbon dioxide from the blood to the alveoli, so that the arterial blood has a full complement of oxygen and has reduced its supply of carbon dioxide. At the site of the active tissues the opposite occurs, as the oxygen diffuses out of the blood and the carbon dioxide out of the tissues. Exercise increases the pulmonary diffusing capacity for oxygen, because of an increased surface area and an increased capillary dilatation.

Oxygen is carried in chemical combination with hemoglobin in the blood, which, when fully oxygenated, results in the formation of oxyhemoglobin. The relationship between the amount of oxygen held in hemoglobin and the partial pressure of oxygen is revealed in the oxygen dissociation curves, which show that the hemoglobin saturation remains extremely high even though the partial pressure of oxygen may drop some 25 percent. The Bohr effect reveals that more oxygen is given off to the tissues as they become more acidic. The coefficient of oxygen utilization relates the amount of oxygen given up to the tissues to the amount available; it averages approximately 25 percent at rest. This value can triple during heavy work, as the tissues extract proportionately more oxygen. Part of the muscle response to oxygen uptake is to myoglobin, which combines with oxygen at low pressures more readily than does blood. The quantity of muscle myoglobin may increase as a result of training.

Carbon dioxide is carried in amounts up to 7 percent in the dissolved state in the plasma by the formation of carbonic acid. However, some 68 percent combines with water in the red blood cells to form carbonic acid because of the enzyme carbonic anhydrase. The remaining portion forms carbamino compounds in the hemoglobin. The amount held by hemoglobin may be reduced (Haldane effect) because the entry of oxygen helps force carbon dioxide out of the blood.

SELECTED REFERENCES

Åstrand, Irma, Per-Olof Åstrand, E. H. Christensen, and Rune Hedman, "Myohemoglobin as an Oxygen-Store in Man," *Acta Physiologica Scandinavica*, 48 (1960), 454.

Best, Charles H., and Norman B. Taylor, *The Physiological Basis of Medical Practice*, 7th ed. Baltimore: The Williams & Wilkins Company, 1961, chap. 29.

Comroe, Julius H., "The Lung," *Scientific American*, 214 (February 1966), 56.

Guyton, Arthur C., *Textbook of Medical Physiology*, 4th ed. Philadelphia: W. B. Saunders Company, 1971, chap. 41.

Henry, Franklin M., *Physiology of Work: The Physiological Basis of Muscular Exercise*. Berkeley: Associated Students' Store, University of California, 1968, pp. 59–78.

Pattengale, Paul K. and John O. Holloszy, "Augmentation of Skeletal Muscle Myoglobin by a Program of Treadmill Running," *American Journal of Physiology*, 213 (September 1967), 783.

Perutz, M. F., "The Hemoglobin Molecule," *Scientific American*, 211 (November 1964), 64.

Slonim, N. Balfour, and John L. Chapin, *Respiratory Physiology*. St. Louis: The C. V. Mosby Company, 1967.

Vander, Arthur J., James H. Sherman, and Dorothy S. Luciano, *Human Physiology: The Mechanisms of Body Function*. New York: McGraw-Hill Book Company, 1970, chap .11.

chapter
9

respiration

The metabolic link with the atmosphere is established by the act of breathing. The oxygen uptake is totally dependent upon the maintenance of a free airway and the proper diffusion of gas from the alveoli to the pulmonary capillaries and then to the cells throughout the body. Pulmonary obstruction or other abnormality, either chemical or neural, that impairs the proper passage of air to the lungs will disturb the gas diffusion, and consequently can leave arterial blood with insufficient quantities of oxygen, at the same time failing to rid the circulation of carbon dioxide. Both conditions can severely limit the individual's ability to exercise by reducing the aerobic capacity and causing metabolic acidosis. Ordinarily, respiration proceeds extremely well and efficiently and, as pointed out in the previous chapter, is not a limiting factor in exercise. The present chapter will deal with the factors that control breathing and the regulation of respiration.

LUNG VOLUMES

It is customary in respiratory physiology to begin with the various subdivisions of lung volume, since they provide a basis for the study of pulmonary capacity. The following categories are illustrated in Figure 69,

Figure 69. Subdivisions of Lung Volume.

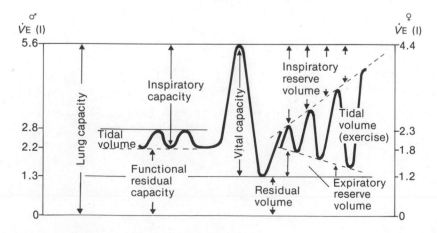

with the average values for ventilation ($\dot{V}$E) for both men and women given on the left and right vertical axes:

1. *Lung capacity.* Total *lung capacity* is the entire volume of air that can be contained in all the air passages.

2. *Vital capacity.* A pulmonary measure often used to represent the capacity of the lungs is *vital capacity.* As seen in Figure 69, it is a major fraction of the total lung capacity; it is defined as the largest volume of air that can be exhaled after the deepest possible inhalation. It probably represents a structural component of the body, similar to other anthropometric assessments of body size, since it is known to correlate well with a variety of strength tests in young boys.[1]

3. *Residual volume.* Beyond vital capacity, and completing the total lung capacity, is *residual volume.* It represents the air remaining in the lungs after a complete exhalation. The residual volume is stable and cannot be exhaled. We encountered it in the discussion of body composition in Chapter 7, where measurement of the amount of residual air was important in the calculation of body density.

4. *Tidal volume.* The amount of air breathed in and out in ventilation is termed *tidal volume.* This is small during rest, but will enlarge considerably during exercise, as illustrated in Figure 68.

5. *Expiratory reserve volume.* The amount of air that can still be exhaled following a normal exhalation of tidal volume is the *expiratory reserve volume.*

6. *Inspiratory reserve volume.* The *inspiratory reserve volume* is the volume of air that can be inspired after inhalation of tidal volume. Together, the tidal volume and the expiratory and inspiratory volumes make up the vital capacity.

7. *Functional residual capacity.* *Functional residual capacity* is the sum of the expiratory reserve volume and the residual volume.

8. *Inspiratory capacity.* The sum of the tidal volume and inspiratory reserve volume equals the *inspiratory capacity.* In other words, it is the greatest amount of air that can be inhaled following a normal tidal exhalation.

MECHANICS OF BREATHING

During quiet breathing the act of inspiration is an active one, and expiration is largely passive. According to Figure 69 only about .6 liter for men and .5 liter for women are involved in the tidal exchange of air, which contrasts with the average values of 4.3 and 3.2 liters, respectively, that comprise the vital capacities. Therefore, some 15 percent of the ventilatory capacity is involved with each respiration. This is accomplished primarily by action of the diaphragm, which on inspiration moves downward, expanding the longitudinal dimensions of the chest cavity, and also by contraction of the external intercostal muscles, which increases the

[1]William A. Tomaras, "The Relationship of Anthropometric and Strength Measures of Junior High School Boys to Various Arm Strength Criteria," microcard Doctoral Dissertation, University of Oregon, 1958.

anteroposterior diameter. The diaphragm is dominant, and the amount of energy is small, requiring only .5 ml of O_2 per liter of air inspired. Expiration, on the other hand, is brought about primarily by relaxation of the act of inspiration. The stretching of the elastic tissues of the lungs and thorax is now followed by recoil, which is essentially a passive process.

Heavy breathing is accomplished by the involvement of several groups of muscles. Inspiration, for example, can be assisted by the other muscles about the neck and thorax, such as the sternocleidomastoid and the scaleni, as well as the trapezius, which may be used to raise the shoulders as a secondary gesture to assist in the free flow of air. An athlete in respiratory distress may even bend over at the waist to relieve the pressure of gravity on the chest. Expiration may now involve the active contraction of internal intercostal and abdominal muscles.

INTRAPULMONARY PRESSURES

It is important to remember that the lungs themselves have no skeletal muscles, so the increase in volume must be accomplished by movement of the external chest wall or by descent and ascent of the diaphragm. The lungs are suspended in the thorax and are covered by the *visceral pleura*, a serous membrane that is in close contact with the *parietal pleura*, the lining of the interior wall of the thorax and diaphragm. The two surfaces are kept moist by means of a pleural fluid, so the lungs may glide easily over the inner surface of the thorax, yet are in so intimate contact that when the thorax expands, the lungs will also expand. During inspiration, the pressure within the alveoli becomes negative with respect to the pressure of the atmosphere by approximately -5 to -10 mm Hg, and air flows inward. The normal expiration, however, is accompanied by a rise in intraalveolar pressure of some $+3$ to $+5$ mm Hg over atmospheric pressure, and air flows outward. These rather small pressures during quiet breathing can be magnified several times; a strong sucking effort can reduce the intrapulmonary pressure from -60 to -80 mm Hg, and with a forced expiration the pressure rise can be well over 100 mm Hg.

ALVEOLAR VENTILATION

As pointed out in Chapter 8, the essential ingredient in respiration is the ventilation of the alveoli by air from the atmosphere, a process known as *alveolar ventilation* ($\dot{V}$A). The amount of air moved in respiration is the *respiratory minute volume* (RMV), and is not the same as the alveolar ventilation. The most obvious reason is that a great portion of the air inhaled simply fills the respiratory passages that lead to the alveoli. Upon exhalation, this is the first air breathed out before alveolar air is ventilated, and so in order to calculate the alveolar ventilation, the amount of this *dead-space air* must be subtracted from the tidal volume. It amounts to approximately 150 ml for men and 100 ml for women, increases slightly with age, and because of pulmonary expansion may amount to 35–40 percent more during exercise.

The alveolar ventilation is equal to the rate of respiration times the tidal volume less the dead-space volume. The individual with a tidal volume of 500 ml (.5 liter, according to Figure 69), a dead space of 150 ml, and breathing at the rate of 12 per minute will have an alveolar ventilation equal to $12 \times (500 - 150)$, or 4200 ml/min. The total pulmonary ventilation ($\dot{V}$E) equals the rate of breathing times the tidal air, or $12 \times 500 = 6000$ ml/min. Thus, the alveolar ventilation is 4.2 l/min and the pulmonary ventilation is 6.0 l/min, the amount of dead space air being a fairly substantial proportion of total ventilation. However, when the tidal air increases appreciably, the fraction that is dead-space air becomes smaller, and for all practical purposes the alveolar ventilation is equal to the pulmonary ventilation. Now, if we assume for the time being that the heart is delivering approximately 5 liters of blood per minute to the lungs, and the resting alveolar ventilation is 4.2 liters per minute, it is possible to calculate a ratio of alveolar ventilation to pulmonary capillary blood flow. This *ventilation-perfusion ratio* (4.2:5.0) has a value of approximately .82 at rest. With exercise there is a disproportionate change in ventilation and cardiac output. While the cardiac output may increase some five times over rest, the ventilation increases about fifteenfold, an effect which triples the ventilation-perfusion ratio.

REFLEX REGULATION OF RESPIRATION

The center that controls respiration, which is located in the brainstem, from the upper *pons* to lower *medulla*, adjusts the rate of alveolar ventilation within very close limits imposed by the demands of the body. These demands vary from sea level to high altitude and with exercise. The rhythmic nature of respiration causes it to continue while the individual is sleeping, so although there is a voluntary control, there must also be an inherent rhythmicity (but not automaticity) to provide an uninterrupted supply of fresh air to the alveoli.

The respiratory center consists of a grouping of neurons that, however elegantly integrated, is rather well dispersed in the brainstem and thus does not correspond to the usual definition of a center. The motor neurons descending to innervate the diaphragm, the *phrenic nerve*, originate at levels C_3, C_4, and C_5 of the spinal cord; the *intercostal nerve*, which innervates the intercostal muscles, originates at T_1 to T_6. They are served by neurons which descend within the spinal cord from the medulla. The respiratory center is monitored by sensory neurons of the *vagus nerve,* which inhibit the spontaneous activity of the inspiratory center.

Medullary Respiratory Center

The center that controls the rhythmic nature of respiration is located in the medulla and contains what is usually referred to as the *inspiratory center* and the *expiratory center* or simply the *medullary respiratory center*. Increased activity here accompanies the acts of inspiration and expiration; neurons which produce the respiratory response are portions of the descending excitatory areas of the reticular formation.[2] A diagram illustrating the nervous control of respiration is shown in Figure 70. The cyclical innervation of the phrenic and intercostal nerves, then, is governed by the medullary respiratory center, but in order to obtain the type of control that permits an adequately smooth pattern, a variety of signals are received from other sources.

Apneustic Center

Located in the posterior portion of the pons, the *apneustic center* has a stimulating effect on the inspiratory center. Impulses stimulate inspiration and, if unmodified, lead to what is known as inspiratory "cramps" —that is, a prolonged period of inspiration (apneusis), lasting perhaps 20–30 seconds, followed by a shortened period of expiration.

Pneumotaxic Center

The *pneumotaxic center*, in the anterior portion of the upper pons, has the overall function of inhibiting impulses from the apneustic center— that is, changing inspiratory activity into rhythmical activity of normal respiration. It causes a slowing and deepening of respiration.

Pattern of Respiration

The inspiratory activity of respiration is brought about by a gradually increased firing of the neurons in the inspiratory center, supported strongly by the apneustic center.[3] Impulses from the inspiratory center ascend to the pneumotaxic center and bring about excitation. At the same time, there is an increase in the frequency of impulses originating from stretch receptors in the lungs (to be discussed below), which, at the height of inspiration, causes inhibition of the inspiratory center by acting through the apneustic center. Expiration follows, and there is a gradual lessening of the inhibitory effect so that the cycle may begin once again. Thus, by reflex action, there is rhythmicity and a cyclic response of the nervous mechanisms involved in respiration.

[2]N. Balfour Slonim and John L. Chapin, *Respiratory Physiology* (St. Louis: The C. V. Mosby Company, 1967), p. 109.

[3]Hugh Davson and M. Grace Eggleton, eds., *Principles of Human Physiology*, 14th ed. (Philadelphia: Lea & Febiger, 1968), p. 452.

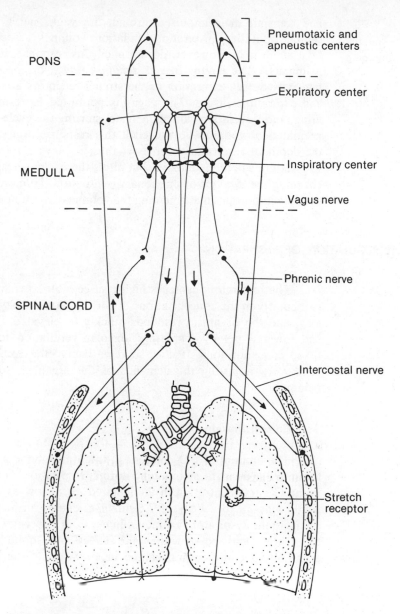

Figure 70. Diagram of the Primary Nervous Connections for the Control of Respiration. [C. H. Best and N. B. Taylor, *The Physiological Basis of Medical Practice*, 7th ed. Baltimore: The Williams & Wilkins Company (1961), p. 490.]

THE HERING-BREUER REFLEXES

The *Hering-Breuer inflation reflex* protects the lungs from overdistention. Nerve endings in the bronchioles become stimulated upon inflation and transmit their impulses through the vagus nerve to the respiratory center, inhibiting inspiration. Inflation volumes associated with resting tidal air in man, however, do not elicit this response, in contrast to other mammals.[4] The *Hering-Breuer deflation reflex*, on the other hand, comes into play during expiration as the stretch receptors are relieved of stretch and expiration ensues. The vagus is permitted to resume a low level of firing, and inspiration can begin again, starting the cycle once more. Again, normal tidal volumes do not elicit this response, but it does ensue when the depth of respiration increases; thus, it plays a role in the rhythm of respiration, as outlined above, but alters the *cycle* of respiration more than changing the *amount* of pulmonary ventilation. Humoral factors seems to be more important in augmenting the volume of ventilation.

HUMORAL REGULATION OF RESPIRATION

The respiratory center is highly susceptible to changes in body fluids, particularly in the concentrations of carbon dioxide, oxygen, and hydrogen ions; and the organism responds quickly to elevated P_{CO_2}, reduced P_{O_2}, and lowered pH by increasing alveolar ventilation to maintain normal tissue concentrations. It does so remarkably effectively under almost all conditions, adjusting the demands of the organism so that changes are minimal.

Carbon Dioxide

The amount of CO_2 present in the atmospheric air (0.04 percent) is too small to assist in maintaining normal respiration. However, an increase in the CO_2 concentration in the inspired air as low as one percent, which would amount to a P_{CO_2} of 7.6 mm Hg, causes an increase, even though small, in the respiratory minute volume. Four percent would nearly double the RMV, and beyond that the effects are quite pronounced, until eventually unconsciousness can occur, or worse. An increase with alveolar P_{CO_2} of only 1.6 mm Hg can double the RMV.

Hydrogen Ion

It is usual to think of increased P_{CO_2} and increased hydrogen ions together as representing changes in acidity, but it is becoming clear that the role of hydrogen ions is an extremely important one by itself. In fact, decreased pH, which means an increase in hydrogen ion concentration, can increase RMV to nearly the same extent as does the increase in P_{CO_2}, provided other factors remain the same. Other factors do not remain the same, and in such a case an increase in CO_2 is dominant.

[4]A. Guz *et al.*, "Studies on the Vagus Nerves in Man: Their Role in Respiratory and Circulatory Control," *Clinical Science*, 27 (1964), 293.

Mechanism for the PCO_2 and pH Effect on Respiration

The combined effect of Pco_2 and pH is important in the control of respiratory minute volume. In fact, the mechanism for the increase in RMV suggests that the two effects are actually additive; that is, that their summed effect is greater than either taken by itself. H^+ and CO_2 in the blood reach the area of the medullary respiratory center and react not with the respiratory center directly, but with chemosensitive receptors (called *central chemoreceptors*) on the ventrolateral surface of the medulla and other locations on the brainstem,[5] which are associated with the cerebrospinal fluid and with arterial blood. These chemoreceptors are especially sensitive to changes in hydrogen ion concentration, and CO_2 reaching the area of the central chemoreceptors reacts with water of the cerebrospinal fluid, forming carbonic acid (H_2CO_3), in a reaction described in Chapter 8. The H_2CO_3 dissociates into HCO_3^- and H^+, and the H^+ ions thus formed excite the chemoreceptors. It may be helpful to point out that the barrier between the blood and the cerebrospinal fluid (the blood-brain barrier) is not penetrated by H^+ in the blood itself, but is permeable to the CO_2 molecule, so that the reaction described above can occur. Therefore, the control of respiration at rest is directed chiefly at the regulation of the hydrogen ion concentration in the brain.

Oxygen

It may seem paradoxical that the role played by decreased Po_2 does not achieve more prominence in the discussion of respiratory regulation. The fact is, however, its influence is not generally considered as important as the changes in Pco_2 and hydrogen ion concentration just described. The reason is primarily that the other influences are noncritical, and the ventilation is adjusted so that arterial Po_2 is not reduced. That is not to say, however, that a reduction in arterial oxygen concentration can not become a factor if great enough. In fact, though, the drop in arterial Po_2 must fall below 70 mm Hg before there is an appreciable effect on alveolar ventilation.

This may be clearer if we refer to the oxygen dissociation curves presented in Chapter 8 (Figure 65); the arterial blood does not become significantly desaturated until about this point. When this occurs, the effect of decreased Po_2 is not sensed by the respiratory center directly, but by the peripheral chemoreceptors, the *carotid* and *aortic bodies*. As illustrated in Figure 71, the carotid bodies are located at the bifurcations of the carotid arteries, and the aortic bodies are located along the arch of the aorta. Within them are chemoreceptors, nerve endings specialized to respond to changes in chemical composition of the arterial blood. Nerve fibers pass to the medulla, where the respiratory center is stimulated.

[5]Richard A. Cozine and S. H. Ngai, "Medullary Surface Chemoreceptors and Regulation of Respiration in the Cat," *Journal of Applied Physiology*, 22 (1967), 117.

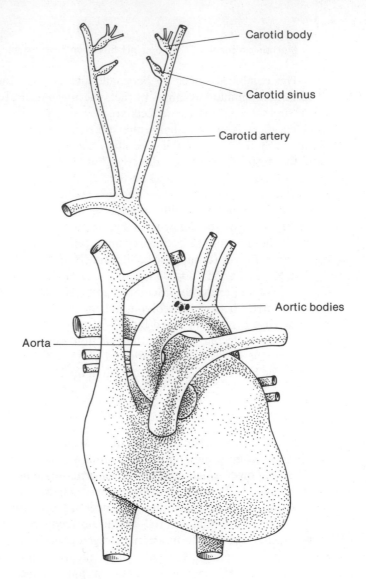

Carotid body

Carotid sinus

Carotid artery

Aortic bodies

Aorta

Figure 71. The Carotid and Aortic Bodies. [A. J. Vander *et al., Human Physiology: The Mechanisms of Body Function.* New York: McGraw-Hill Book Company (1970), p. 326.]

THE EFFECT OF EXERCISE ON PULMONARY VENTILATION

The relationship between exercise oxygen uptake ($\dot{V}_{O_2}$) and pulmonary ventilation ($\dot{V}_E$) is shown in Figure 72. Respiration as a result of muscular exercise can increase from a resting value of approximately 8

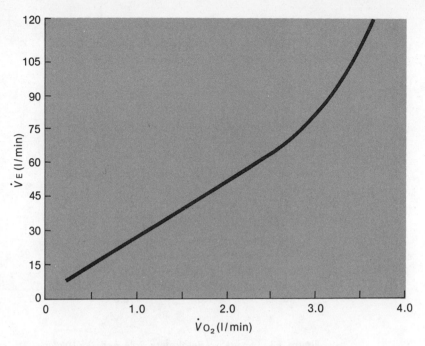

Figure 72. Relationship Between Oxygen Consumption and Ventilation during Exercise. [R. Margaria and P. Cerretelli, "The Respiratory System and Exercise," in H. Falls, *Exercise Physiology*. New York: Academic Press (1968), p. 73.]

liters per minute to over 100 in severe work. Values as high as 150 liters per minute have been observed in certain endurance-trained athletes for short periods of maximal work. It appears certain that the lungs are actually capable of moving vast quantities of air when the demand arises. The respiratory rate goes from some 12 to 15 per minute to over 30, and the tidal volume goes from .6 to 3.5 liters, although each does not change at the same rate, as illustrated in Figure 73. If tidal volume can represent depth of respiration, then it is clear that both contribute to the total respiratory minute volume, but the depth of breathing rises more rapidly and then seems to plateau at moderately heavy work values. On the other hand, the rate of breathing changes much more slowly during light to moderate exercise, then accelerates in heavy exercise. The maximal ventilation is reached when the ability to increase respiratory frequency has occurred without diminishing the tidal volume.

The pulmonary ventilation increases approximately linearly with the increase in oxygen consumed up to $\dot{V}_{O_2}$ values of 2.5 to 3.0 l/min (Figure 72), after which the ventilation increases more rapidly for a given increment in metabolic work. This increase in alveolar ventilation has been referred to as the *hyperpnea* of exercise.

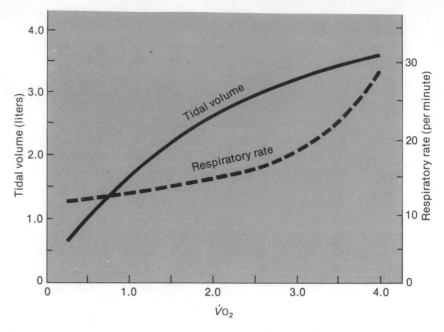

Figure 73. Changes in Respiratory Rate and Tidal Volume. [H. Davson and M. G. Eggleton, eds., *Principles of Human Physiology*, 14th ed. Philadelphia: Lea & Febiger (1968), p. 485.]

MECHANISMS THAT CONTROL PULMONARY VENTILATION IN EXERCISE

The search for mechanisms that can adequately account for all the changes seen in pulmonary ventilation during exercise has been surprisingly difficult. It is clear *what* happens: the organism increases its need for oxygen and the respiratory system responds by generating an increase in the volume of air moved. The problem is to justify *how* this takes place. From preceding sections of this chapter, one might conclude that the respiratory center responds to increased production of CO_2. However, such a justification is untenable, since the PCO_2 of arterial blood ($PaCO_2$) fails to increase during light exercise, and during heavy exercise may even fall as excess CO_2 is blown off. This is shown in Figure 74.

Much the same can be said of arterial hydrogen ion concentration, for during mild and moderate exercise (curve portion A of Figure 74) no appreciable change occurs, nor does a change occur in lactic acid production. As anticipated, the arterial PO_2 does not change either, so with the organism experiencing about a fourfold change in ventilation, known stimuli fail to change in a manner commensurate with such an increase. It is clear that the increase in respiration during exercise of mild and moderate intensity cannot be due to increased acidity of the blood.

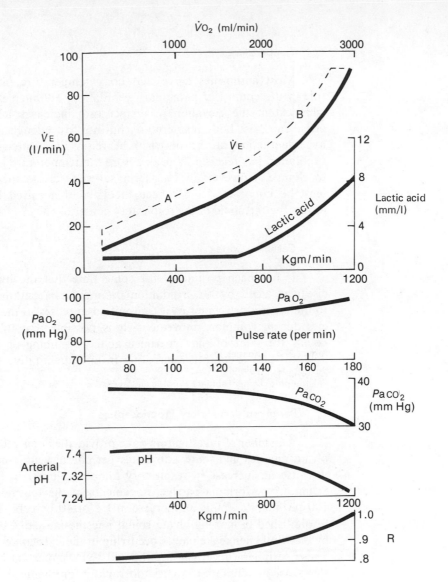

Figure 74. Relationships of Various Metabolic Factors to Pulmonary Ventilation in Exercise. [M. B. McIlroy, "The Respiratory Response to Exercise," *Pediatrics*, Part II, 32 (October 1963), p. 681.]

During severe exercise (curve portion B of Figure 74) the upward rise in ventilation is even more pronounced and is considered disproportionate. Again, the known stimuli fail to support such an intensity of ventilation. The lactic acid increases and the pH goes down as the organism becomes more acid, but even this change is not sufficient to explain all of the respiratory behavior during heavy exercise. Therefore, other factors must be examined.

Temperature

Most authorities agree that body temperature plays an important role in the control of pulmonary ventilation, although it is not known to what extent the elevation in temperature increases RMV. Clearly, exercise can raise body temperature, but not fast enough to account for the hyperventilation at the onset of exercise. In steady-state exercise, the ventilation has reached its peak before the temperature has quite had time to change. However, in long-term severe exercise the temperature rise must be important. It has been theorized that raised body temperature lowers the threshold of the respiratory center to CO_2.[6]

Cerebral Cortex

It has been postulated for some time that the hyperpnea of exercise was aided by the irradiation of impulses from the cerebral cortex to the respiratory center as it transmitted impulses to the contracting muscles during voluntary movement. It is possible that this mechanism accounts for some of the hyperpnea at the beginning of exercise, but it is doubtful that it controls ventilation in any quantitative way over a range of work loads.

Peripheral Ventilatory Proprioceptors

A number of investigators have provided evidence that the movement of the muscles and joints stimulates peripheral ventilatory proprioceptors to cause an increase in respiratory minute volume. In fact, Comroe and Schmidt,[7] performing passive movements of the lower leg at the rate of 100 per minute, found an increase in $\dot{V}E$ of 40 percent. This response can be abolished in man by giving spinal anesthesia, and it can be augmented by the local chemical changes occurring in the extremities during exercise.[8] These peripheral receptors are thought to be important because the initial sharp rise in ventilation occurs too rapidly for chemical changes to occur, so it seems reasonable to consider a neurogenic factor. Also, isometric exercise causes little ventilatory change due to the restricted range of movement, while running and cycling, with their relatively large limb and joint motion, cause large changes. Just where these receptors are located seems somewhat obscure, but fairly recently muscle spindle receptors

[6]R. G. Bannister and D. J. C. Cunningham, "The Effects on the Respiration and Performance During Exercise of Adding Oxygen to the Inspired Air," *Journal of Physiology*, 125 (1954), 118.

[7]J. H. Comroe and Carl F. Schmidt, "Reflexes from the Limbs as a Factor in the Hyperpnea of Muscular Exercise," *American Journal of Physiology*, 138 (1943), 536.

[8]Pierre Dejours, John C. Mithoefer, and Yvette Labrousse, "Influence of Local Chemical Change on Ventilatory Stimulus from the Legs During Exercise," *Journal of Applied Physiology*, 10 (1957), 372.

have been cited as the locus of effect in animals,[9] causing increased ventilation when they become stimulated mechanically during muscular contraction.

Stretch Reflex

The presence of muscle spindles in the intercostal muscles, and to a lesser extent in the diaphragm, brings up a mechanism that was discussed in Chapter 4. The reader may wish to review the basic stretch reflex response. As applied to the respiratory process, it is postulated[10] that upon inflation of the lungs, the muscle spindles increase their rate of firing and thereby facilitate muscle contraction. This leads to an increase in the respiratory minute volume.

THE WORK OF BREATHING

The energy expenditure for the act of breathing is usually ignored in energy cost studies. It is reasonably clear, though, that sufficient ventilation takes place during exercise to justify the concept that the muscular work of breathing can be fairly substantial. Think what must be involved in moving 100 liters of air or so per minute in and out of the lungs. Slonim and Chapin[11] estimate the oxygen cost of breathing to be about .5 to 1 ml/liter of ventilation at rest, and to increase disproportionately as the respiratory minute volume increases. At maximal levels, the cost of ventilation may increase as much as tenfold. This is illustrated in Figure 75. The exercise task in this example consisted of pedalling a bicycle ergometer at a work rate of 1080 kgm/min for 10 minutes, followed by a 15-minute recovery period. The large curve reflects the total $\dot{V}O_2$, and the small curve represents the fraction attributed to the oxygen cost of ventilation. It will be recalled in Chapter 6 that the term *oxygen deficit* was used to define the difference between the observed oxygen uptake and that which would have occurred had the rate of uptake instantly achieved a steady state. The O_2 cost of ventilation in Figure 75 accounted for approximately 20 percent of this deficit and reduced the recovery oxygen uptake by 11 percent. The cost of ventilation, then, exerts about twice as great an effect on the oxygen uptake during exercise than during recovery.

TRAINING

The effect of training on ventilation can best be described as one of improving the efficiency of breathing. The trained individual reduces the

[9]H. Gautier, A. Lacaisse, and P. Dejours, "Ventilatory Response to Muscle Spindle Stimulation by Succinylcholine in Cats," *Respiration Physiology*, 7 (1969), 383.

[10]M. Corda, G. Eklund, and C. v. Euler, "External Intercostal and Phrenic α Motor Responses to Changes in Respiratory Load," *Acta Physiologica Scandinavica*, 63 (1965), 391.

[11]Slonim and Chapin, *op. cit.*, p. 43.

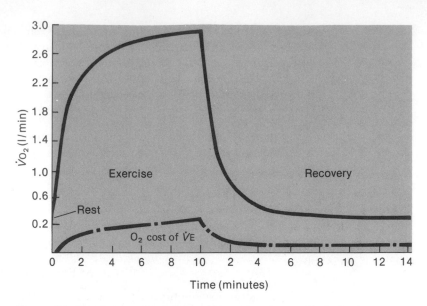

Figure 75. The Oxygen Cost of Exercise and Ventilation. [F. I. Katch, R. N. Girandola, and F. M. Henry, "The Influence of the Estimated Oxygen Cost of Ventilation on Oxygen Deficit and Recovery Oxygen Intake for Moderately Heavy Bicycle Ergometer Exercise," *Medicine and Science in Sports*, 4 (Summer 1972), p. 72.]

rate of breathing and increases the depth, yet for a given level of sub-maximal exercise he is able to achieve a $\dot{V}o_2$ with less overall respiration. This means that he is able to extract a greater proportion of oxygen from the air he breathes than the untrained person. The air is now able to reach a wider alveolar area at rest and during exercise; in short, there is an increased *aeration* as a result of training.

SUMMARY

Total lung capacity can be divided into vital capacity, residual volume, tidal volume, inspiratory and expiratory reserve volumes, functional residual capacity, and inspiratory capacity. The quiet inspiration of tidal air occurs because of the downward movement of the diaphragm, assisted by the external intercostal muscles. Expiration is more passive, following a recoil of the elastic tissues of the lungs and thorax. Heavy breathing during exercise requires the recruitment of additional musculature. Alveolar ventilation, equal to the tidal volume less the dead-space air, is a rather substantial portion of the respiratory minute volume at rest. During exercise, when the total ventilation is increased, it becomes smaller and may be ignored. The ratio of alveolar ventilation to pulmonary capillary blood flow is the ventilation-perfusion ratio.

The respiratory center is located in the brainstem, from upper pons to lower medulla. The medullary respiratory center contains neurons that give rhythmic inspiration and expiration. The apneustic center, located in the pons, stimulates inspiration, while the pneumotaxic center inhibits the apneustic center, causing a slowing and deepening of respiration. The Hering-Breuer inflation and deflation reflexes seem more important in the control of other mammals than in man, and other factors account for respiratory control. The respiratory center is highly susceptible to changes in concentrations of carbon dioxide, oxygen, and hydrogen ions, with carbon dioxide the most potent stimulus. Next comes pH and then oxygen, although the oxygen tension must fall considerably to become an effective stimulus.

The lungs seem capable of moving large quantities of air during exercise. The increase at first comes as a result of deeper breathing, but in heavy exercise the augmentation in rate of breathing becomes important. A search for the factors responsible for the hyperpnea of exercise has been difficult, because ventilation increases in mild exercise in excess of some known causative factors, including carbon dioxide, hydrogen ion concentration, and oxygen tension. Factors that may help explain the increase in ventilation during heavy exercise include lactic acid, increased body temperature, impulses radiating from the cerebral cortex during voluntary movement, peripheral ventilatory proprioceptors, and intercostal muscle spindles. Training reduces the rate of breathing and increases the depth, improving ventilatory efficiency.

SELECTED REFERENCES

Comroe, Julius H., *Physiology of Respiration*. Chicago: Year Book Medical Publishers, Inc., 1965.

———, "The Lung," *Scientific American*, 214 (February 1966), 56.

———, and Carl F. Schmidt, "Reflexes from the Limbs as a Factor in the Hyperpnea of Muscular Exercise," *American Journal of Physiology*, 138 (1943), 536.

Davson, Hugh, and M. Grace Eggleton, eds., *Principles of Human Physiology*, 14th ed. Philadelphia: Lea & Febiger, 1968, chap. 19.

Dejours, Pierre, "Neurogenic Factors in the Control of Ventilation During Exercise," *American Heart Association Monograph* No. 15 (1967), 147.

———, *Respiration*. New York: Oxford University Press, 1966.

———, John C. Mithoefer, and Yvette Labrousse, "Influence of Local Chemical Change on Ventilatory Stimulus from the Legs During Exercise," *Journal of Applied Physiology*, 10 (1957), 372.

McIlroy, Malcolm B., "The Respiratory Response to Exercise," *Pediatrics*, Part II, 32 (October 1963), 680.

Slonim, N. Balfour, and John L. Chapin, *Respiratory Physiology*. St. Louis: The C. V. Mosby Company, 1967.

chapter

10

central circulation

The individual engaging in exercise must supply significant amounts of blood to the active muscular tissues to meet metabolic demands. Since the total amount of blood will remain approximately the same, the requirement must be met by increasing the rate at which blood is dispersed throughout the body. The importance of cardiac output is now emphasized, especially since we have already learned that the amount of oxygen carried by the blood changes very little at rest or during exercise (Chapter 8). Assuming that the respiratory process is adequate, then we must turn our attention to factors controlling the central circulation in an effort to determine the characteristics of the heart and the regulation of cardiac output.

THE CARDIAC CYCLE

The *cardiac cycle* represents the sequence of events from the end of one contraction of the heart muscle to the end of the next. Each cycle begins by the spontaneous generation of an action potential in the *S-A node*. The action potential travels very quickly throughout both atria and through the *A-V node* into the ventricles. A delay of .10 sec for the passage of this impulse through the atria and then into the ventricles allows enough time for the blood to be pumped from the atria and into the ventricles prior to their contraction and the subsequent distribution of the blood throughout the body. It must be remembered that the sole function of the heart is to pump blood to the various organs. Set up for this task is an orderly process of depolarization of the heart muscle, the events of which were described in Chapter 1.

The electrocardiogram (ECG), as shown in Figure 76, represents the electrical excitation of the heart which precedes the actual cardiac muscle contraction. The cardiac cycle, then, begins with a spread of depolarization through the atria and is represented by the *P wave*. This causes an increase in pressure (note the change in atrial pressure in Figure 76) as the atria contract. This state of depolarization lasts for about .15 sec. After approximately .16 sec the ventricles are depolarized, an event which appears in the ECG as the *QRS complex*, causing the ventricular pressure to rise. The third major segment, the *T wave*, represents the repolarization of the ventricles as their muscle fibers relax. Thus the heart undergoes

175

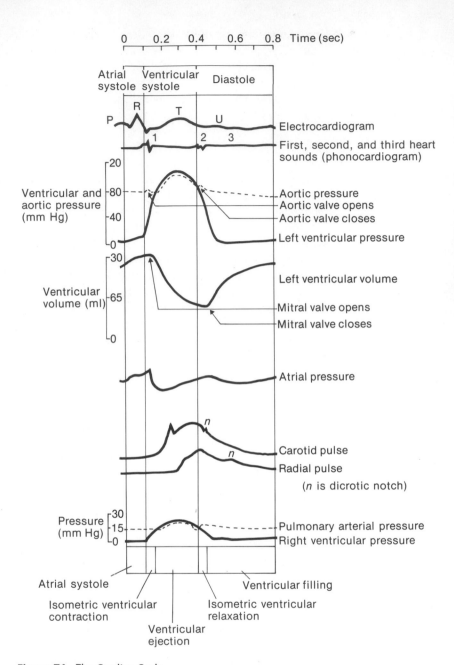

Figure 76. The Cardiac Cycle.

periods of relaxation and contraction; the former is called *diastole* and the latter *systole*. Right after the conclusion of the ventricles' contraction the atria are beginning to fill with blood, raising the pressure; this, together with the reduced pressure in the ventricles, permits the *atrioventricular* (AV) *valves* to open. The blood flows rapidly into the ventricles during this period of diastolic filling of the heart, as shown in Figure 76. The fill-

176

ing occurs very rapidly at first, then levels off, achieving its greatest volume just before the ventricles contract. The period of emptying during ventricular contraction is the systolic phase, and the strength of this contraction not only forces the AV valves shut but at the same time opens the *semilunar valves*, as blood is ejected into the aorta and pulmonary artery. The amount of blood ejected by each ventricle varies from 70 to 90 ml, leaving approximately 50 ml of blood in each ventricle at the end of systole —the *end-systolic ventricular blood volume*. Following contraction of the ventricles there is an immediate fall in ventricular pressure which, combined with an elevated pressure in the large arteries, forces blood back toward the ventricles, closing the aortic and pulmonary valves. This permits the cardiac cycle to begin once again.

A schematic illustration that represents the subdivisions of ventricular volume is shown in Figure 77. We can see the similarity with the subdivisions of lung volume (Figure 69). The *total ventricular volume* represents the total amount of blood that can be contained in the ventricle under the most favorable circumstances. During rest the *stroke volume* is a modest fraction of the total volume, but during exercise the stroke volume increases substantially, employing increasingly greater amounts of the *diastolic reserve volume* and the *systolic reserve volume*. Thus, *maximal stroke volume* represents the events that permit diastolic filling of the ventricle and its subsequent emptying. As with pulmonary ventilation, there is a *functional residual capacity*, and a small *residual volume* of blood remains in the heart chamber after ventricular contraction. The quantitative nature of these divisions will be discussed in this chapter.

Exercise and Training

When an individual engages in *exercise*, the time available for the cardiac cycle decreases considerably. In fact, as we will learn later, the heart rate conceivably can triple in going from rest to maximum exercise, which now means that the cardiac cycle time will be decreased by one-third. But the time components of the left ventricle do not all change to the same degree during exercise. Instead, there is an increase in the percentage of the cycle time given to the ejection phase, with a decrease in the percentage of diastole.[1] Three to five months of vigorous physical *training,* on the other hand, three to five times per week for an hour each time, increases the resting and postexercise time of systole, as measured from the onset of ventricular contraction to the end of ejection. Training also increases diastole, which is the time from the end of ejection to the onset of excitation of the left ventricle.[2] Thus, the increase in diastole permits

[1]Jack F. Wiley, B. Don Franks, and Sandor Molnar, "Time Components of the Left Ventricle During Work," *New Zealand Journal of Health, Physical Education and Recreation*, 2 (November 1969), 67.

[2]B. Don Franks and T. K. Cureton, "Effects of Training on Time Components of the Left Ventricle," *Journal of Sports Medicine and Physical Fitness*, 9 (June 1969), 80.

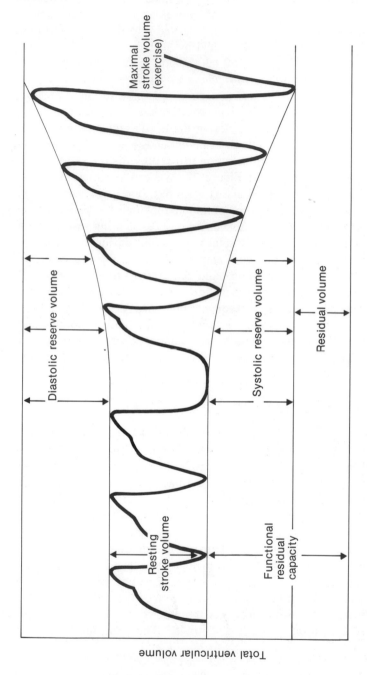

Figure 77. Subdivisions of Ventricular Volume. [G. A. Brecher and P. M. Galletti, "Functional Anatomy of Cardiac Pumping," in W. F. Hamilton, ed., *Handbook of Physiology*, Section 2: *Circulation*. Washington, D.C.: American Physiology Society (1963), p. 783.]

more time for the resting phase per beat, which allows greater time for blood to flow into the ventricles, plus a special bonus—an increase in blood circulation in the heart muscle itself due to the increased resting time.

CARDIAC OUTPUT

A matter of great concern to the exercise physiologist is the amount of blood ejected from the heart in a given period. This *cardiac output* ($\dot{Q}$) is the product of the amount of blood ejected per beat, termed *stroke volume* (SV), and the number of beats per minute, or *heart rate* (HR); thus $\dot{Q} = \text{SV} \times \text{HR}$, usually given in liters per minute. Stroke volume can be calculated as $\text{SV} = \dot{Q}/\text{HR}$. It may be of interest to learn something of the way in which cardiac output is determined at rest and during exercise. Several procedures (and others not mentioned) have evolved over the years.

The Fick Principle

The most basic of all the procedures for the determination of cardiac output involves the *Fick principle*. It requires knowledge of the difference between the oxygen content of arterial and mixed venous blood and the total quantity of oxygen consumed over a given period of time. A calculation can be made of the volume of blood which has passed through the lungs during that interval. The variables that must be determined in this case are the oxygen content of arterial blood, the oxygen content of mixed venous blood, and the oxygen consumption ($\dot{V}_{O_2}$). The following equation illustrates the calculations for cardiac output:

$$\dot{Q} = \frac{\dot{V}_{O_2}}{\text{A-V oxygen difference in ml/100 ml blood}} \times 100. \qquad (10\text{-}1)$$

For example, if an individual has a $\dot{V}_{O_2}$ of 250 ml/min at rest and an arterial oxygen saturation of 19 ml of oxygen per 100 ml of blood with a mixed venous oxygen content of 14 vol. percent, which gives an arterio-venous oxygen difference of 5 vol. percent, then

$$\dot{Q} = \frac{250}{19 - 14} \times 100 = 5,000 \text{ ml/min} = 5 \text{ l/min}.$$

Thus, resting cardiac output is 5 l/min.

The use of the Fick principle requires the simultaneous determination of the oxygen content in both arterial and mixed venous blood. The blood for the arterial sample can be obtained from any artery in the body, since all arterial blood is mixed before it leaves the heart and therefore will have the same oxygen concentration everywhere. The difficulty in applying the principle is in obtaining the accurate determination of venous oxygen concentration, as it is necessary to sample blood directly from the right ventricle where blood has been brought by the major veins of the body, or preferably from the pulmonary artery. This is important, because venous blood will reflect the activity of the region of the body from which it is found and may not be representative of the body as a whole. In order to obtain venous blood that is truly mixed it is necessary to insert a catheter, which is a small flexible sampling tube, into a brachial vein of the arm and thread it centrally down through the subclavian vein and into the right atrium, coming to rest finally in the right ventricle or pulmonary artery. At this point a sample of blood may be withdrawn for analysis. The oxygen intake is obtained in the usual way at the same time by collecting expired air and analyzing its content to determine $\dot{V}_{O_2}$.

The Dye Dilution Technique

It has become increasingly more common to employ an indicator dilution (*dye dilution*) procedure, in which a small amount of dye is injected into a vein. The venous blood distributes the dye through the right side of the heart, through the pulmonary artery to the lungs, back to the left side of the heart and from there into the arterial blood system. Subsequently, if a sample of arterial blood from a peripheral artery is obtained, the concentration of the dye may be measured. The procedures for the determination of cardiac output take note of the amount of dilution of the dye in the blood, which permits calculation of the quantity of blood that this amount of dye must have contacted.

Radioisotopes

More recently, *radioisotopes* have been substituted for dyes, in which case measurement of the cardiac output can be obtained by employing an external detector directed over the heart. The recording of radioactivity may be achieved with a digital counter and other associated instruments. Dilution curves may be plotted and interpreted in a manner similar to that of the dye dilution techniques in calculating cardiac output.

Carbon Dioxide Rebreathing Procedure

The difficulty with some of the other tests for cardiac output is that they must sample blood or they require the injection of a substance into the circulation. A nonblood technique employed in recent years involves *carbon dioxide rebreathing*, which avoids some of the difficulties of these other tests and apparently gives comparable results. The method is based on the measurement of the difference in CO_2 concentration between mixed venous and arterial blood and the rate of CO_2 output. This corresponds with the original Fick principle, employing the following equation:

$$\dot{Q} = \frac{\dot{V}_{CO_2}}{\text{A-V } CO_2 \text{ difference}}. \tag{10-2}$$

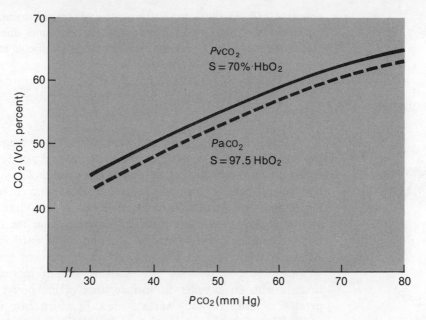

Figure 78. Standard CO_2 Dissociation Curves for Mixed Venous and Arterial Blood. [J. R. Magel and K. L. Anderson, "Cardiac Output in Muscular Exercise Measured by the CO_2 Rebreathing Procedure," in H. Dobelin *et al.*, eds., *Ergometry in Cardiology*. Freiberg: Boehringer Mannheim GmbH. (1968), p. 148.]

Therefore, we need to know the amount of CO_2 output in ml/min ($\dot{V}CO_2$), the milliliters of CO_2 per liter of mixed venous blood, and the milliliters per liter of arterial blood.[3] One of the differences with the Fick principle is that the concentration of CO_2 in arterial blood is calculated by multiplying the percentage of CO_2 in end-tidal gas (which would be the alveolar CO_2) by the barometric pressure, the result being equivalent to the arterial PCO_2 ($PaCO_2$). This is then converted to CO_2 content in vol. percent by use of the CO_2 dissociation curve for arterialized blood, as given in Figure 78. Calculation of the percentage of CO_2 in mixed venous blood requires breathing in and out of a bag containing 5 to 10 percent CO_2, which results in an equilibrium in the lung-bag system with the mixed venous blood. An analysis is then made of the CO_2 content, and the percentage is multiplied by the barometric pressure to give the venous PCO_2 ($PvCO_2$). Using CO_2 dissociation curve for mixed venous blood (Figure 78) results in determination of the CO_2 content in volumes percent. Substitution in

[3]John R. Magel and K. Lange Anderson, "Cardiac Output in Muscular Exercise Measured by the CO_2 Rebreathing Procedure," in H. Dobeln *et al.*, eds., *Ergometry in Cardiology* (Freiberg: Boehringer Mannheim GmbH., 1968), 147.

equation (10–2) gives cardiac output in liters per minute. This technique is valid for measuring cardiac output at rest and during exercise when steady-state conditions prevail, but it becomes difficult to accomplish when maximal exercise is performed.

CARDIAC INDEX

Calculation of cardiac output reveals the average value to be approximately 5.0 l/min, without regard to age, sex, or body size. However, it should be reasonably clear that large individuals will also have large body components. Thus, the heart may be expected to be larger in the larger male and smaller in the smaller female. Children's hearts obviously will be smaller than adult hearts. This means that the cardiac output will differ depending upon heart size. Therefore, the cardiac output in normal active men is closer to 6 l/min, about 10 percent greater than that of women of the same body size. Cardiac output increases approximately linearly with an increase in surface area of the body, so it may be expressed in terms of body surface area, in which case it is called *cardiac index*. Thus, an individual weighing 154 lb (70 kg) has a body surface area of approximately 1.7 m^2, which results in an average value for cardiac index of 3.0 l/min.

CARDIAC HYPERTROPHY

It has long been a matter of interest that the heart itself enlarges as a result of physical training. This *cardiac hypertrophy* in the past has been referred to as "athlete's heart" to differentiate it from a diseased heart enlarged because of some pathological state. During training it is possible for the heart to enlarge as much as 15 percent,[4] which helps an athlete to increase cardiac output from 5 l/min at rest to 20–25 l/min during maximal exercise. This compares with only 12–15 l/min that can be achieved by a nonathlete. Since cardiac output is the product of stroke volume and heart rate, the increased strength of contraction would be reflected in some increase in stroke volume. The increased capacity of the heart to exercise appears to be the result of an increase in the ratio of heart weight to body weight.[5] Such hypertrophy thus is associated with an increase in the capacity to supply blood to the working muscles. The changes in volume of the heart in relation to the maximal oxygen uptake in response to a five-week training program can be seen in Figure 79.

[4]K. Lange Andersen, "The Capacity of Aerobic Muscle Metabolism as Affected by Habitual Physical Activity," in Martti J. Karvonen and Alan J. Barry, eds., *Physical Activity and the Heart* (Springfield, Ill.: Charles C. Thomas, 1967), pp. 16–17.

[5]L. B. Oscai *et al.*, "Cardiac Growth and Respiratory Enzyme Levels in Male Rats Subjected to a Running Program," *American Journal of Physiology*, 220 (1971), 1238.

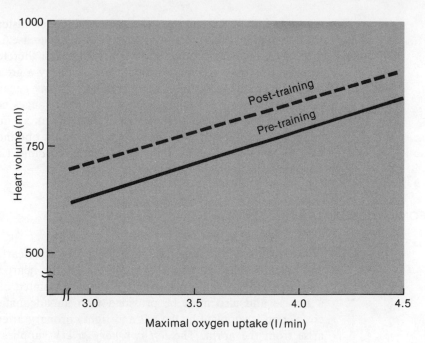

Figure 79. Relationship between Cardiac Output and Maximal Oxygen Uptake. [K. L. Andersen, "The Cardiovascular System in Exercise," in H. Falls, ed., *Exercise Physiology*. New York: Academic Press, Inc. (1968), p. 120.]

STROKE VOLUME: STARLING'S LAW OF THE HEART

A factor which controls cardiac output is the amount of blood that enters the heart from the veins, the *venous return*. The heart cannot pump what it does not receive, and so over a given period the input and the output must be approximately equal. For a long time it was assumed that the venous return was the *controlling* factor—that the cardiac output was wholly dependent upon the rate at which blood returned to the heart. This relationship, put forth as *Starling's law of the heart*, stated that the energy of contraction was proportional to the initial length of the cardiac muscle fibers. This means that the greater the filling during diastole the greater the amount of blood that is distributed into the aorta, and that the incoming blood will stretch the walls of the atria, causing a larger contraction. If the heart wall is distended, it will increase the length of the heart muscle fiber, much as the skeletal muscle increases its contractile force when placed on a slight stretch.

This theory requires an increased diastolic volume of the heart in order for the systolic output to increase. Recent data have cast some doubt on the theory as a normal mechanism to account for cardiac function. Using a technique of X-ray kymography, it would appear that the size of the heart at the end of diastole is not increased during exercise over that which occurs at rest. This represents the size on filling, so instead of enlarging, its size is essentially the same or at least does not increase.[6] Not only that, but the endsystolic size decreases as well. It appears, therefore, that the slight increase in stroke volume is brought about not by a greater diastolic filling but by a greater systolic emptying.[7] There seems general agreement that the increase in stroke volume during exercise changes no more than some 50 to 60 percent over rest, which is just about as much as the stroke volume in recumbency increases over the amount obtained in moving to an upright position. A more important factor causing a change in cardiac function is an increase in heart rate.

CORONARY CIRCULATION

Because of the important role played by the heart, not only in exercise but in disease as well, the circulation of the heart itself has taken on new and added significance. Again it must be pointed out that the heart is a muscle and also must be provided with an adequate blood flow. This circulation is supplied by the left and right coronary arteries, both of which arise from the aorta. The *left coronary artery* supplies primarily the left ventricle and atrium and the *right coronary artery* is the main supplier of the right ventricle and atrium. The arrangement of blood-vessel distribution is reflected in Figure 80. The left coronary artery is predominant in most people, so that more blood flows through this vessel than flows through the right side. Some 10 to 20 percent have the opposite, the right coronary artery being dominant, and still others have coronary arteries of approximately the same size. The two coronary arteries of an adult albino rat are shown in Figure 81. Note the extensive branching.

The coronary arteries infiltrate the myocardium, giving off branches which eventually provide a complete circulatory network. After passage through the capillary beds most of the venous blood flow that emanates from the left ventricle leaves by way of the *coronary sinus;* conversely, most of the blood from the right ventricle returns by way of the *anterior coronary veins*. A small amount of the coronary blood flow returns to the heart by means of the *thebesian veins*, which arise from capillaries and veins and primarily enter the right ventricle.

The flow of blood through the coronary vessels is subject to fluctuation during the cardiac cycle, based upon the activities of the cardiac muscle itself. For example, the flow of blood through the left coronary artery and capillaries of the left ventricle decreases during systolic contraction as tension in that portion of the heart increases. During diastole, when the muscle relaxes, the blood flows more freely. In the coronary arteries on the

[6]Robert F. Rushmer and Orville A. Smith, "Cardiac Control," *Physiological Reviews*, 39 (January 1959), 41.

[7]George M. Andrew, Carole A. Guzman, and Margaret R. Becklake, "Effect of Athletic Training on Exercise Cardiac Output," *Journal of Applied Physiology*, 21 (March 1966), 603.

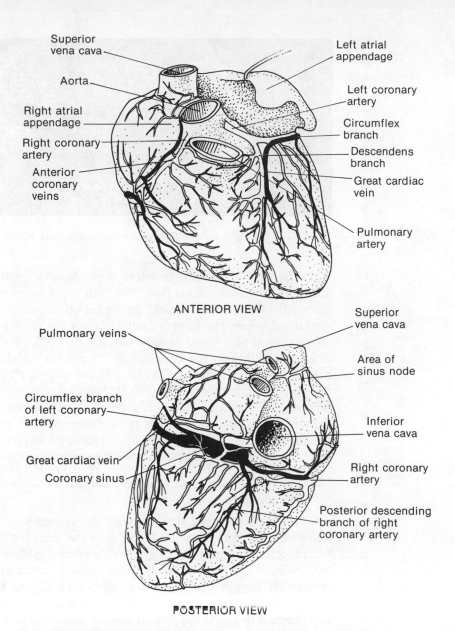

Figure 80. Blood Vessel Distribution on the Anterior and Posterior Surfaces of the Heart. [R. M. Berne and M. N. Levy, *Cardiovascular Physiology*. St. Louis: The C. V. Mosby Company (1967), p. 199.]

right side of the heart, right ventricular contraction is not as strong as on the left side. It will be recalled that right ventricular contraction supplies the pulmonary artery, and left ventricular contraction supplies the aorta. Thus, the coronary flow in diastole is several times the flow recorded during systole.

185

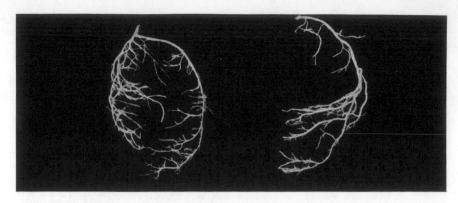

Figure 81. The Right and Left Coronary Arteries of a Male Albino Rat.

The heart's function therefore depends to a great extent upon its ability to increase its blood flow. This will occur in general proportion to the needs of the cardiac muscle for increased nutrients. As it is a rather specialized organ, the heart actually receives far greater blood flow than does the body as a whole. As illustrated earlier (Chapter 8) the coefficient of oxygen utilization is approximately 26 percent for the total body, calculated according to formula (8–3): the A-V oxygen difference divided by the oxygen content of arterial blood. When this is applied to the heart, however, the coefficient becomes about 75 percent, based on the fact that the venous oxygen content drops from a normal of 14 volumes percent to 5 volumes percent. The myocardial extraction of oxygen, consequently, is some three times greater than that for the systemic circulation.

Exercise

The rate of blood flow through the coronary system is regulated almost directly in response to the needs of the heart for oxygen. When the heart accelerates during exercise, there is an increased flow of blood through the coronary vessels. The relationship between coronary blood flow and myocardial oxygen consumption is shown in Figure 82. It should be pointed out that the data presented in this figure were obtained employing experimental dogs. At any rate, it reveals that there is a four- to five-fold increase in coronary blood flow. Thus, the heart seems to be under control of a local *autoregulation* of blood flow in very much the same manner that occurs in skeletal muscle. These additional factors will be discussed in Chapter 11. The heart is also regulated by hormonal factors, particularly *epinephrine* and *norepinephrine*, secreted by the adrenal medulla. Just prior to and during exercise they are released by stimulation of the sympathetic nervous system and serve to increase coronary blood flow and reinforce the strength of contraction.[8]

[8]Lucien Brouha and Edward P. Radford, "The Cardiovascular System in Muscular Activity," in Warren R. Johnson, ed. *Science and Medicine of Exercise and Sports* (New York: Harper & Row, 1960), p. 195.

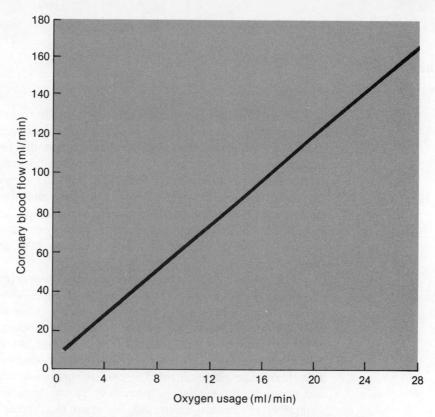

Figure 82. The Relationship between Coronary Blood Flow and Myocardial Oxygen Consumption. [See J. C. Scott, "Physical Activity and the Coronary Circulation," *Canadian Medical Association Journal*, 96, (March 25, 1967), p. 858.]

Training

Intensive physical training increases the capacity of the heart to meet increased demands for oxygen. In part this is accomplished by an increased rate of coronary blood flow. Several mechanisms are responsible for this adjustment to long-term systematic activity. One of the most important, perhaps, is an increase in the amount of collateral coronary blood vessels, causing a more favorable circulatory system for the heart. The coronary arterioles respond more adequately to physical and chemical influences and because of better coronary vasodilation offer less resistance to blood flow. The lumen of the coronary artery is also increased in experimental animals subjected to daily and intermittent exercise.[9] The great distance runner Clarence DeMar had coronary arteries two or three times the normal size.[10] This serves to ensure an adequate blood supply to the cardiac muscle.

[9]Arthur S. Leon and Colin M. Bloor, "Effects of Exercise and Its Cessation on the Heart and Its Blood Supply," *Journal of Applied Physiology*, 24 (April 1968), 485.

[10]Arlie V. Bock ,"The Circulation of a Marathoner," *Journal of Sports Medicine and Physical Fitness*, 3 (1963), 80.

Under normal resting conditions the heart is controlled primarily by the autonomic nervous system, where parasympathetic and sympathetic effects balance each other. In the normal adult the heart rate averages approximately 70 beats per minute, but during various periods of emotional excitement or muscular activity it may rise considerably. It is not uncommon for excitement to elevate the heart rate above 100 beats per minute, and of course violent exercise can drive it close to 200. Conversely, an individual in deep sleep may find the resting rate reduced. As we shall see, the athlete in training develops a resting rate considerably below average.

The sympathetic system, represented by the *accelerator nerve*, exerts a facilitory influence upon the rhythmicity of the S-A node; the parasympathetic fibers, represented by the *vagus nerve*, cause an inhibitory effect on heart rate. Acceleration of rate is actually produced by a reduction in parasympathetic activity, along with an increase in sympathetic activity, whereas deceleration results from the opposite causes. Parasympathetic tone seems to be predominant. The cardiac center is located in the medulla, and consequently resides in proximity to the area designated for the respiratory rhythmicity center, as discussed in Chapter 9. The following mechanisms are mainly responsible for cardiac control.

Baroreceptor Reflex

Raising the arterial blood pressure can cause a slowing of heart rate. This is the result of a *baroreceptor reflex*, sometimes called *Marey's law*, which states that the pulse rate varies inversely with the arterial pressure. The mechanism is based upon stretch receptors in the carotid sinus and aortic arch. The increased blood volume in the arterial system causes an increase in the neural impulses passing from the baroreceptors, which in turn results in excitation of the cardioinhibitory center and inhibition of the cardioaccelerator center. Consequently, there is a slowing of the heart, preventing an increase in blood pressure. At the same time there is a vasodilation of the systemic arterioles, decreasing peripheral resistance and facilitating the flow of blood into the peripheral tissues of the body.

Respiratory Reflex

Fluctuations in the respiratory cycle have an effect on the pattern of heart rate. During inspiration the heart accelerates and during expiration it decelerates, a condition called *sinus arrhythmia*. The vagus nerve is primarily responsible for controlling this cardiac variation.[11] During inspiration the intrathoracic pressure decreases, which permits a greater venous return to the right side of the heart. This eventually leads to an increase in left ventricular output as the blood circulates to the lungs and back to the heart, producing a rise in arterial blood pressure. This effect recedes during the period of expiration. During heavy breathing, the increased activity of the abdominal muscles increases abdominal pressure, transmitting the pressure to the veins and promoting venous flow into the thorax, resulting in a so-called *respiratory pump*.

Valsalva Maneuver

There is a situation, however, where *increased* intrathoracic pressure, if severe enough, can actually *decrease* blood flow by bringing into play the *Valsalva maneuver*. Straining against a closed glottis may cause sufficient positive pressure to be imparted against the large veins and atria to impede the flow of blood into the heart. This results in a fall in arterial pressure, owing to decreased blood volume to the heart, with a concomitant rise in venous pressure in the extremities and head. In order to counteract the reduced blood flow the heart rate increases. As soon as the expiratory effort has subsided, the accumulated blood in the veins rushes into the right ventricle, causing the heart to increase its output and raise arterial pressure. This evokes a baroreceptor response and a brief decline in heart rate until prior conditions are reestablished. This maneuver can be invoked by coughing, defecation, playing a muscial instrument, or straining during the lifting of a heavy weight. The results are ordinarily transient, and not dangerous, unless the individual is suffering from congestive heart failure, in which case it could be fatal. Weight lifters can modify the response by maintaining a normal rhythmic respiration during the concentric and eccentric phases of movement and trying to avoid holding the breath.

Chemical Factors

There is some controversy concerning the manner in which changes in blood chemistry alter the activity of the heart. Anoxia accelerates the heart, but probably not because of its action on the carotid or aortic chemoreceptors. Rather, the increase is probably due to the effect of lack of oxygen on the S-A node. It is not expected that this would affect heart rate under normal conditions, although the effects at altitude may be more pronounced (Chapter 12). In a similar manner the increase in blood carbon dioxide will also cause an increase in heart rate. For example, CO_2 inhalation and lactic acid production cause elevated heart rates, although it is possible that this effect is associated with the increase in respiration in response to these chemical changes, as described above.

[11]Robert M. Berne and Matthew N. Levy, *Cardiovascular Physiology* (St. Louis: The C. V. Mosby Company, 1967), p. 139.

Another factor that increases heart rate is the hormone epinephrine (adrenalin) liberated from the adrenal medulla. It induces glycogenolysis in the heart and other tissues, enhances contractility of the individual cardiac muscle cells, and increases cardiac excitability and conductivity.

Bainbridge Effect

It is appropriate here to discuss the *Bainbridge effect*, one of the longest-standing factors in cardiac function found in the literature. In fact, Bainbridge demonstrated in 1915 that intravenous infusions of blood into the venous return of an anesthetized animal suddenly caused the heart rate to increase. This increase, called *tachycardia*, is typically found when the initial heart rate is slow. The reflex was attributed to the fact that this increased blood volume caused a distention of the large veins and right atrium, resulting in a rise in pressure, owing to stimulation of vagal sensory neurons in the venous (right) side of the heart. The afferent impulses were thought to pass by way of the vagus nerve to bring about cardiac acceleration, which would be a response to reduction in vagal tone. This effect has not received much support in recent years when experiments have been repeated. In fact, stimulation of the vegal receptors in the right atrium and the atriocaval region does not cause an increase in heart rate but a decrease (called *bradycardia*). It is the point of view here that other factors cause an increase in heart rate, thereby modifying the increase or the distention that might occur in the right side of the heart during venous return. It seems likely that other factors are more important than the Bainbridge effect.

Cerebral Cortex

When an individual begins exercise, and even slightly before, there is an acceleration of the heart. The anticipatory rise is due to anxiety or excitement and involves activation of the corticohypothalamic fibers of the hypothalamus, which discharge impulses to the cardioaccelerator center in the medulla inhibiting activity of the cardioinhibitory area. Thus, signals are transmitted directly into the sympathetic nervous system causing an increase in heart rate. How important this actually is in increasing cardiac output during exercise is not entirely clear, for other factors once again seem to predominate.

Muscle Pump

One of the important factors in exercise is the effect on blood flow caused by the intermittent contraction and relaxation of skeletal muscles. Because peripheral veins contain one-way valves, preventing the backward flow of blood, the compression of the muscles surrounding the veins causes the milking of the blood toward the heart—sometimes referred to as the milking action of muscles or simply the *muscle pump.* This results in an increase in the mean systemic pressure which serves to move the blood from the peripheral areas of the body toward the heart, causing an increase in cardiac output due to the increase in cardiac input.

The opposite effect occurs in upright standing, in which the pull of gravity causes a pooling of blood in the lower extremities. In fact, individuals in occupations that require periods of prolonged standing frequently develop an overdistention of the veins and an impairment of the valves. This may lead to a condition known as *varicose veins.* The pooling effect can be demonstrated by employing a tilt table and a volume recorder for one of the lower limbs. Tilting to the upright position results in an increased volume of fluid in the legs and an increase in heart rate to compensate for this reduction of fluid to the heart. When this is followed by rhythmic muscular contractions there is an emptying of blood from the lower extremities and consequently a reduction in heart rate. Pooling of blood has even been known to result in fainting (*syncope*), which is one reason why soldiers are instructed to contract and relax their leg muscles rhythmically while standing at attention. This is more important during hot weather, because of the shunting of blood to the surface of the body in an effort to maintain thermal balance.

Heart Suction

There is increasing evidence[12] that the heart not only acts as a pressure pump, dependent entirely on other factors to cause return of blood to the atria and ventricles, but also that the activity of the heart actively draws blood towards itself, thus acting as a suction pump as well. The mechanism that explains this finding is that during ventricular systole the atrioventricular junction descends, thereby enlarging the capacity for blood storage of the atria and vena cavae. During this pistonlike downward movement the heart itself attracts a greater amount of blood from the veins into the atria, a condition called ventricular systolic suction. Furthermore, when the atrioventricular valves open during diastole, there results a rapid increase in atrial pressure, causing acceleration of venous blood into the atrium. This is known as *ventricular diastolic suction.* Clearly, venous return may be accelerated, both during systole and during diastole. The relative balance in filling during systole and diastole depends upon the heart rate itself. At a relatively slow rate of 85 beats per minute, when a greater time for diastolic filling is available, there is a fairly even balance in the amount of blood entering the atrium during systole as during diastole. However, at a high heart rate, the great preponderance of blood enters during systole and only a small amount during diastole. Therefore, the heart is not entirely dependent for its filling on the available time during diastole.

[12]Hugh Davson and M. Grace Eggleton, eds., *Principles of Human Physiology* (Philadelphia: Lea & Febiger, 1968), pp. 149–151.

Although cortical reflexes may bear a role in increased cardiac output, as described above, there seems to be even greater reflex arising from the working muscles. The increase in heart rate at the beginning of exercise occurs too quickly for it to be of chemical origin. Experiments on humans have shown that when the muscles of the legs are caused to contract by direct electrical stimulation,[13] rather than by normal excitation, there is an increase in heart rate. Stimuli from the working muscles are transmitted via some peripheral sensory nerves to the cardiac center. The nature of these peripheral receptors has not been fully explained, but they are clearly not muscle spindles, nor are they chemoreceptors in the muscles.

EFFECTS OF EXERCISE ON CARDIAC OUTPUT

Of all the stressors that may be faced by an individual, exercise produces the greatest challenge to the function of the cardiovascular system. As we have already seen, the resting cardiac output is approximately 5 liters per minute. For the well-trained athlete in maximal exercise, this may go as high as 40 liters per minute. The increased cardiac output is due to several factors, as the organism strives to supply the exercising muscles. It does so by increasing both stroke volume and heart rate. The relationship of these factors in response to increased oxygen uptake is shown in Figure 83.

Several features of this illustration are of interest. The slope of the line for cardiac output ($\dot{Q}$) is approximately linear for increasing work loads up to values slightly in excess of 25 l/min. Stroke volume increases slightly during exercise, especially during the early phase of activity, and is most pronounced during fairly mild exercise. The literature indicates that the increase in stroke volume is likely not to be more than 50 percent over resting values and may well stabilize at some value early in the work curve. On the other hand, a more important factor is the heart rate itself. This is clearly dominant in the figure and reflects a linearity with increased metabolic cost, up to a value of 185 beats per minute, considered maximal for untrained adults. The heart rate can even triple in some individuals during exercise. The finding of linearity between heart rate and $\dot{V}O_2$ has led to a number of interesting attempts to predict one variable from the other, and since the heart rate is so easily obtained, and oxygen uptake so difficult, it has become fashionable to try to estimate $\dot{V}O_2$ max from a measure of heart rate during exercise. This will be discussed in Chapter 14.

Thus, the cardiac output is dominated by the change in heart rate during successive work loads, whether shown by some value of work done

[13]E. Asmussen, M. Nielsen, and G. Wieth-Pedersen, "On the Regulation of Circulation during Muscular Work," *Acta Physiological Scandinavica*, 6 (1943), 353.

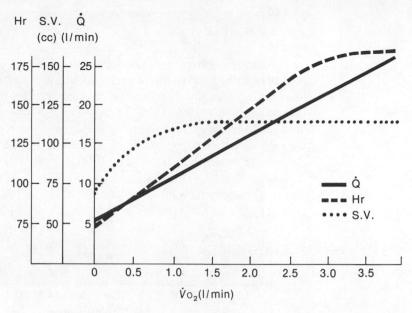

Figure 83. Relationship between Cardiac Output, Stroke Volume, and Heart Rate as a Function of Oxygen Uptake.

or as in Figure 83, by $\dot{V}_{O_2}$. Eventually the cardiac output reaches its maximal value and stabilizes, just as other metabolic factors reach their upper limits, causing the tissues to achieve their maximal oxygen uptake. When all of these factors have participated to the fullest extent, the individual has reached *crest load* and no further aerobic increase in work capacity can be accomplished.

The heart, like the body as a whole, has a given *mechanical efficiency*. The term that describes the ratio of work accomplished to energy utilized is given in formula (7–1). When applied to the work of the two ventricles, the net efficiency turns out to be much the same as for skeletal muscles (20–25 percent). The energy expended in cardiac metabolism that does not actively contribute to the work involved in propelling blood through the body is lost as heat. Berne and Levy[14] point out that efficiency improves with exercise, since with little change in mean blood pressure the cardiac output and work increase considerably, without incurring the same kind of increase in myocardial oxygen consumption.

The increase in cardiac output can also be appreciated when one examines the Fick principle. Formula (10–1) shows the ratio of oxygen intake to A-V oxygen difference in the calculation of $\dot{Q}$, showing that the relative balance of $\dot{V}_{O_2}$ to A-V O_2 difference can be used to calculate the amount of blood ejected by the heart per minute. The relationship of $\dot{V}_{O_2}$ and A-V O_2 difference is reflected in Figure 84 for both men and women

[14]Berne and Levy, *op cit.*, p. 207.

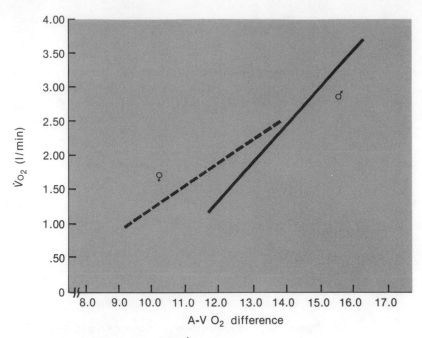

Figure 84. Relationship between $\dot{V}O_2$ and A-V Oxygen Difference for Men and Women. [Data from P.-O. Åstrand *et al.*, "Cardiac Output during Submaximal and Maximal Work," *Journal of Applied Physiology,* 19 (March 1964), p. 268.]

over increments in work approaching maximum. In both instances the A-V O_2 difference increases linearly with an increase in metabolic cost ($\dot{V}O_2$). For men, there is a threefold increase in $\dot{V}O_2$, but only a 1.4-fold increase in A-V O_2 difference. In other words, the $\dot{V}O_2$ change was approximately twice as great as the A-V O_2 difference, resulting in an increase in $\dot{Q}$. Actually, as shown in Table 10–1, the cardiac output for men increased from 10.2 to

Table 10–1. Values for Oxygen Uptake, A-V Difference, and Cardiac Output for Men and Women

	Men			*Women*		
	$\dot{V}O_2$ (l/min)	A-V O_2 diff (ml/100 ml)	$\dot{Q}$ (l/min)	$\dot{V}O_2$ (l/min)	A-V O_2 diff (ml/100 ml)	$\dot{Q}$ (l/min)
Rest	.35	6.94	5.1	.26	4.97	5.3
1.	1.21	11.83	10.3	.90	9.06	10.0
2.	1.80	12.66	14.3	1.48	10.79	13.8
3.	2.86	14.67	19.6	2.09	12.39	17.0
4.	3.71	16.26	22.9	2.50	13.81	18.2
5.	4.31	17.34	24.8	2.78	15.7	17.7

Data summarized from Åstrand, Per-Olof, *et al.*, "Cardiac Output During Submaximal and Maximal Work," *Journal of Applied Physiology*, 19 (March, 1964), 268.

22.9 l/min over the range of values shown for $\dot{V}_{O_2}$ and A-V O_2 difference, which is not necessarily maximal for all subjects. For women, the cardiac output ranged from 10.0 to 18.2 l/min. Values for rest are also shown in the table. Thus, the tissues absorb a greater proportion of oxygen from the blood that circulates through them during exercise, a fact we considered in Chapter 8 when discussing the coefficient of oxygen utilization.

Emphasis so far has been placed on exercise involving endurance work, such as would occur with extended running or cycling, where a large muscle mass is involved and the exercise persists for 5 to 6 minutes, a time sufficient for the individual to have achieved a steady state or perhaps a maximal level of cardiac stress. However, what about activities such as weight lifting? What are the differences if one is performing maximal repetitions with heavy weights? Usually, these are performed in sets involving anywhere from 5 to 15 repetitions, lasting but a few seconds. Nevertheless, it is quickly observed that an increment in heart rate occurs. This is shown in Figure 85, where heart rates of approximately 120 beats per minute were observed during the bench press, and even higher during back and leg exercises. From what we learned earlier, the energy for this form of activity would not make use of increased oxygen delivered by the circulatory system. Clearly, weight lifting is an anaerobic task, employing energy from intracellular stores at ATP and creatine phosphate. Yet, the heart responds to the exercise stimulus reflexly by increasing in rate—in anticipation, perhaps, of continued demands to be made on the circulation. Instead, the exercise bout terminates, leaving the performer to recover from the circulatory and metabolic demands imposed by the exercise.

TRAINING

Considerable interest has been displayed in the results of training on the cardiovascular system, and in particular, on the heart itself. The primary training stimulus is endurance exercise carried out over an extended period of time, in activities such as endurance running, swimming, cycling, cross country skiing, orienteering, and others. Strength training, on the other hand, such as weight lifting and activities that tax the aerobic capacity in only a limited way, is generally not very successful in improving cardiovascular function. Weight trainers that combine exercises to improve the cardiovascular system find that muscular hypertrophy occurs, but also that other changes in cardiac function appear as well.

It is beyond the scope of this chapter to review all the possibilities for training routines that can be undertaken to provide the proper stimulus for a training effect. Undoubtedly there are wide individual differences in this based on age, sex, level of initial physical fitness, and other factors, so it is difficult to generalize as to the type of exercise needed or its intensity. Various programs for the development of exercise regimens, particularly for those subpar in the basic physical fitness elements, can be found else-

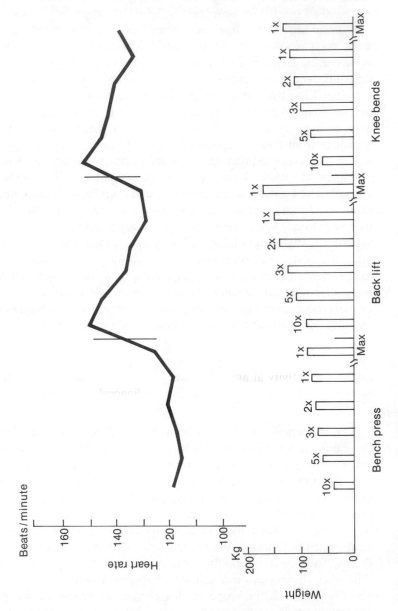

Figure 85. The Response of Heart Rate to Weight Lifting. [Adapted from J. Kuel, "The Relationship between Circulation and Metabolism during Exercise," *Medicine and Science in Sports, 5* (Winter 1973), p. 210.]

where.[15] Because the intensity of exercise is usually difficult to determine accurately, the heart rate can be employed as a general index. If the exercise program elicits a heart rate in excess of 150 beats per minute for at least 5 minutes, gains in aerobic endurance will probably result, although optimal results will be obtained if the exercise brings the heart rate to within 10 beats of maximum during successive work bouts of 3 to 5 minutes' duration.[16]

Heart Rate

A very noticeable change associated with training is the reduction in resting heart rate. This *bradycardia* may result in resting values for the athlete as much as 20 to 30 beats per minute slower than for an untrained person. When this is coupled with a larger stroke volume and a more efficient extraction of oxygen from the blood by the tissues, a more efficient circulation occurs. Moreover, and perhaps more importantly, the endurance-trained athlete enjoys a lower heart rate for any given work load, when compared with his untrained counterpart. In other words, the metabolic change that occurs during any level of work is accomplished with a smaller increase in heart rate. Moreover, some studies indicate that the *maximum* heart rate of athletes is lower than that of sedentary subjects,[17] which again may attest to the increased pumping capacity of the heart in response to training. It has recently been suggested[18] that the bradycardia of training results from two factors: a decrease in the intrinsic firing of the S-A node, and an increase in tonic vagal cardioinhibitory activity. As Hall[19] points out, training also reduces the intensity of several other mechanisms known to cause cardiac acceleration, such as the intensity of muscular activity at any given workload, a diminution in the production of acid products of exercise, and a cardioaccelerator effect that might be experienced reflexly from respiration.

Stroke Volume

If it is true that the heart rate increase to maximum is about the same for athletes and nonathletes, without considering the differences in

---

[15]H. Harrison Clarke and David H. Clarke, *Developmental and Adapted Physical Education* (Englewood Cliffs, N.J.: Prentice-Hall, Inc., 1963), chap. 7.

[16]Clayne R. Jensen and A. Garth Fisher, *Scientific Basis of Athletic Conditioning* (Philadelphia: Lea & Febiger, 1972), chap. 6.

[17]K. Lange Andersen, "The Cardiovascular System in Exercise," in Harold Falls, ed., *Exercise Physiology* (New York: Academic Press, 1968), chap. 3.

[18]C. P. Bolter, R. L. Hughson, and J. B. Critz, "Intrinsic Rate and Cholinergic Sensitivity of Isolated Atria from Trained and Sedentary Rats," *Proceedings of the Society for Experimental Biology and Medicine*, 144 (October 1973), 364.

[19]Victor E. Hall, "The Relation of Heart Rate to Exercise Fitness: An Attempt at Physiological Interpretation of the Bradycardia of Training," *Pediatrics*, 32 (October 1963), 723.

work that can be performed, then an understanding of the increased car-diac output may well hinge on the changes in stroke volume. Maximum values for stroke volume may be above 175 ml/beat for highly trained individuals engaged in maximal exercise,[20] while it is more customary to see values around 120 ml/beat for nontrained subjects (Figure 83). Resting values are lower for sedentary people, but there seems to be a parallel in-crease in stroke volume during the progress of exercise. There is an im-mediate response to exercise by an increase during the lighter work loads, but after reaching values at work loads corresponding to 30 to 40 percent of $\dot{V}O_2$ max,[21] the stroke volume stabilizes, as the cardiac output is influ-enced now by changes in heart rate.

Cardiac Output

Summarizing what we know, training strengthens the heart, particu-larly when employing activity such as endurance running. This results in an increased stroke volume, made possible by the heart's emptying its con-tents more completely than it does in the untrained state. The heart beats less frequently, both at rest and during comparable work loads, but be-cause of other circulatory changes accompanying training, more physical work can actually be accomplished. Musshoff[22] indicates that athletes have a higher resting A-V oxygen difference, which would mean that they would actually have a smaller cardiac output at rest; that is, with the increased ability of the tissues for extracting oxygen from the circulation, less blood volume is required. Athletes also have a greater A-V oxygen difference at the highest levels of work, and together with a high $\dot{V}O_2$ max they have a greater cardiac output in maximum exercise. Thus, in order to transport 4 liters of oxygen from the lungs to the muscles, 34 liters of blood are required; since the volume of blood in the body is approximately 5 liters, the blood must circulate seven times a minute in order to meet this require-ment. This is a sizable task, and requiring the careful coordination of a large number of physiological factors.

Obviously, a normal individual would be unable to exercise for long periods at or even near his $\dot{V}O_2$ max. This would even be true for many athletes. Protracted exercise can be maintained in a *steady state*, as ex-plained in Chapter 6, where not only is the oxygen uptake below maximal, but the heart rate, and thus cardiac output, is submaximal as well. The key to success in such activities as marathon running is probably largely deter-mined by the ability of the individual to utilize a higher percentage of the

[20]Björn Ekblom and Lars Hermansen, "Cardiac Output in Athletes," *Journal of Applied Physiology*, 25 (November 1968), 619.

[21]Andersen, *op cit.*, p. 122.

[22]K. Musshoff, H. Reindell, and H. Klepzig, "Stroke Volume, Arterio-Venous Difference, Cardiac Output and Physical Working Capacity, and their Relationship to Heart Volume," *Acta Cardiologica Brux.* 14 (1959), 427.

$\dot{V}O_2$ max. According to Costill,[23] marathon runners may employ 75 percent or more of their $\dot{V}O_2$ max during a contest that lasts over two hours, and at the same time use about 92 percent of their maximal cardiac output and 95 percent of their maximal stroke volume during peak periods of stress. The stroke volume gradually declines after the first few minutes, during which time the heart rate increases, leaving cardiac output to increase only slightly during the main period of running.

SUMMARY

The cardiac cycle represents the series of events that transpires during the contraction of the heart muscle. The action potential spreads throughout the heart and is represented by the electrocardiogram. The period of filling is called diastole; the period of emptying, systole. Exercise results in an increased time for ejection, with a decrease in time for filling, but training increases the time available for diastole, which permits more time for filling and promotes an increase in coronary blood flow.

Cardiac output is a product of stroke volume and heart rate and can be calculated by such means as the Fick principle, dye dilution techniques, radioisotopes, or the carbon dioxide rebreathing procedure. Cardiac index is the relationship of cardiac output to body surface area. Endurance training may lead to cardiac hypertrophy, sometimes referred to as athlete's heart, reflecting an increased strength of contraction. Starling's law of the heart says that the increase in cardiac output would be due to an increased filling on diastole, thus stretching the cardiac muscle fibers. Recent evidence does not confirm this finding but instead reflects a slightly greater systolic emptying.

The heart itself is provided with a circulation by means of the left and right coronary arteries, which arise from the aorta. During the heart cycle, coronary flow is greater in diastole than in systole. The coefficient of oxygen utilization for the heart is approximately 75 percent, equivalent to three times that of the systemic circulation. During exercise there is a four- to five-fold increase in coronary blood flow, suggesting a local autoregulation. Training brings about increased coronary circulation, owing to an increase in collateral blood vessels, and an increase in size of the lumen.

The heart is controlled by the autonomic nervous system, where sympathetic and parasympathetic factors balance each other. A number of mechanisms regulate the activity of the heart. The baroreceptors respond to increased arterial pressure and slow the heart, at the same time causing peripheral vasodilation. The changes in intrathoracic pressure during res-

[23]David L. Costill, "Physiology of Marathon Running," *Journal of the American Medical Association*, 221 (August 28, 1972), 1024.

piration promotes blood flow to the heart, and changes in blood chemistry will also have an accelerating effect. The Bainbridge effect of increased volume of venous return may have variable effects on heart rate; it is not considered an important factor. The transmission of nervous impulses to the cardioaccelerator center from the higher nervous centers may elevate heart rate, even prior to the beginning of exercise. The muscles during exercise help to milk the blood back toward the heart and promote blood return, and the heart itself may have an aspirating action, acting somewhat like a suction pump.

During exercise cardiac output is increased by a slight increase in stroke volume and a more important rise in heart rate. The efficiency of the heart is approximately the same as for the skeletal muscles. During training there is a decrease in resting heart rate, called bradycardia, and a lower heart rate for all levels of submaximal exercise. The maximum heart rate may also be lower. The stroke volume is larger in the athlete; consequently the cardiac output is also greater.

SELECTED REFERENCES

Andersen, K. Lange, "The Cardiovascular System in Exercise, " in Harold Falls, ed., *Exercise Physiology*. New York: Academic Press, 1968, chap. 3.

Andrew, George M., Carole A. Guzman, and Margaret R. Becklake, "Effect of Athletic Training on Exercise Cardiac Output," *Journal of Applied Physiology*, 21 (March 1966), 603.

Asmussen, Erling, and Marius Nielsen, "Cardiac Output During Muscular Work and Its Regulation," *Physiological Reviews*, 35 (October 1955), 778.

Asmussen, E., M. Nielsen, and G. Wieth-Pedersen, "On the Regulation of Circulation during Muscular Work," *Acta Physiologica Scandinavica*, 6 (1943), 353.

Åstrand, Per-Olof, T. Edward Cuddy, Bengt Saltin, and Jesper Stenberg, "Cardiac Output During Submaximal and Maximal Work," *Journal of Applied Physiology*, 19 (March 1964), 268.

Berne, Robert M., and Matthew N. Levy, *Cardiovascular Physiology*. St. Louis: The C. V. Mosby Company, 1967.

Bock, Arlie V., "The Circulation of a Marathoner," *Journal of Sports Medicine and Physical Fitness*, 3 (1963), 80.

Brouha, Lucien, and Edward P. Radford, "The Cardiovascular System in Muscular Activity," in Warren R. Johnson, ed., *Science and Medicine of Exercise and Sports*. New York: Harper & Row, 1960, chap. 10.

Costill, David L., "Physiology of Marathon Running," *Journal of the American Medical Association*, 221 (August 28, 1972), 1024.

Davson, Hugh, and M. Grace Eggleton, eds., *Principles of Human Physiology*. Philadelphia: Lea & Febiger, 1968, chap. 10.

Ekblom, Björn, and Lars Hermansen, "Cardiac Output in Athletes," *Journal of Applied Physiology*, 25 (November 1968), 619.

Franks, B. Don, and T. K. Cureton, "Effects of Training on Time Components of the Left Ventricle," *Journal of Sports Medicine and Physical Fitness*, 9 (June 1969), 80.

Guyton, Arthur C., Thomas G. Coleman, and Harris J. Granger, "Circulation: Overall Regulation," *Annual Review of Physiology*, 34 (1972), 13.

Hall, Victor E., "The Relation of Heart Rate to Exercise Fitness: An Attempt at Physiological Interpretation of the Bradycardia of Training," *Pediatrics*, 32 (October 1963), 723.

Keul, Joseph, "The Relationship between Circulation and Metabolism during Exercise," *Medicine and Science in Sports*, 5 (Winter 1973), 209.

Musshoff, K., H. Reindell, and H. Klepzig, "Stroke Volume, Arterio-Venous Difference, Cardiac Output and Physical Working Capacity, and their Relationship to Heart Volume," *Acta Cardiologica Brux.*, 14 (1959), 427.

Reeves, John T., Robert F. Grover, Giles F. Filley, and S. Gilbert Blount, "Cardiac Output in Normal Resting Man," *Journal of Applied Physiology*, 16 (March 1961), 276.

Rushmer, Robert F. and Orville A. Smith, "Cardiac Control," *Physiological Reviews*, 39 (January 1959), 41.

Scott, J. C., "Physical Activity and the Coronary Circulation," *Canadian Medical Association Journal*, 96 (March 25, 1967), 853.

chapter 11

peripheral circulation

At the other end of the circulatory system are the tissue capillaries. The heart is the central pump and the various blood vessels are the conduits through which the blood must be delivered to the working tissues. The mechanisms which control the flow of blood are important, since the delivery of oxygen is crucial in exercise physiology. The blood vessels become smaller and smaller, in order that the most microscopic distribution is possible for the exchange of nutrients. As we shall see, this takes place in the capillary bed of the muscle and other tissues. This means that the heart and blood vessels must be very precisely coordinated so that a sufficient return of blood occurs to the heart in order that the proper output of blood can be moved from the heart. During exercise the needs of the tissues multiply many times, yet essentially the same amount of blood must be used by the body. In order to achieve this, there is a redistribution of blood, and the body does this primarily by reducing the amount of blood flow to the splanchnic region of the body and at the same time causing an increased flow to those tissues that are in the greatest need. The blood flow to muscle at rest is very minimal, but it will increase some twenty or thirty times to meet the demands imposed by severe muscular activity.

DESCRIPTION OF THE PERIPHERAL CIRCULATORY SYSTEM

Arteries

Arteries are designed to withstand high pressures and to transport blood to the tissues. The walls of the arteries are strongly vascular and conduct blood rapidly toward the periphery.

Arterioles

In the tissues the arteries narrow to become arterioles. They have strong muscular walls which makes it possible for them to control the amount of blood that is to pass through them.

Capillaries

203   The function of the capillaries is to exchange nutrients between the

blood and the active tissues. The capillaries are extremely small and have permeable membranes to permit the passage of molecular substances.

Venules

After the blood leaves the capillaries it collects into gradually enlarging blood vessels called venules.

Veins

The veins serve as the major conduits by which the blood returns to the heart. In contrast to the arteries, veins are subject to very low pressures, so their walls are rather thin.

CHARACTERISTICS OF THE SYSTEMIC CIRCULATION

The blood is unevenly distributed in the various components of the circulation at any one time.[1] Only about 9 percent is located in the heart itself, with about 12 percent in the pulmonary vessels. The remainder, some 79 percent, is distributed about the systemic circulation, with 59 percent in the veins, 15 percent in the arteries, and 5 percent in the capillaries. It may be surprising to find such a small amount of the total volume of blood in the capillaries, and conversely, so large an amount in the veins. The venous system plays an important role in the storage of blood, and in fact the total cross-sectional area of the veins is approximately four times that of the arteries.

The velocity of blood flow is inversely proportional to the cross-sectional area: the greater the cross section, the slower the blood flow. Therefore, the velocity of flow is rather high in the aorta (33 cm/sec), but in the capillaries, which have an estimated total area of 2,500 cm^2, the velocity is only about .3 mm/sec.

The advantage in such a system can be quickly realized: the blood needs to be moved from the heart quickly, and so the pressure is highest in the aorta, averaging approximately 100 mm Hg. Since the pulsatile flow from the heart is intermittent, the pressure fluctuates from a high of 120 mm Hg, called *systolic pressure*, to a low of 80 mm Hg, called *diastolic pressure*. The difference of 40 mm Hg is called the *pulse pressure*. The term *mean arterial pressure* refers to the average pressure throughout the cardiac cycle, but because systole is slightly shorter than diastole, the mean pressure is somewhat less than half the difference between systolic and diastolic pressures. As an approximation, it is equal to diastolic pressure plus one-third of the pulse pressure. As the blood vessels become smaller, the blood encounters increasingly greater resistance to flow, and the pressure has dropped to approximately 85 mm Hg by the time it has reached the arterioles. Nevertheless, this is sufficient to force blood into the capillary bed, where the pressure has now been reduced to some 30 mm Hg,

[1]Arthur C. Guyton, *Textbook of Medical Physiology*, 4th ed. (Philadelphia: W. B. Saunders Company, 1971), chap. 19.

and by the time it has passed through the capillaries it will be lowered still further, to 10 mm Hg. As the blood is moved centrally to the vena cavae, the pressure may eventually become nearly 0 mm Hg by the time the blood enters the right atrium.

The pressure in the veins of the feet in the upright position may be as high as 90 mm Hg in order to overcome the hydrostatic pressure brought about by the influence of gravity, to provide the required blood flow to the heart. We learned in Chapter 10 that veins possess one-way valves, but it should be clarified here that while this is true of veins of the limbs, it is not true of the thoracic and abdominal veins. Thus, blood filtering through exercising muscles is massaged centrally, being prevented from backward flow not only by the valves, but by the pressure from the capillaries as well. The valves do serve an important role by breaking up the blood column into segments small enough to prevent overdistention of the thin-walled vessels. Yet, the veins are rather freely distensible, and the walls are equipped with some smooth muscle so that *venoconstriction* is possible by action of *adrenergic nerves* and chemical agents such as norepinephrine.

Thus, the veins can serve as a reservoir, in a sense holding blood for distribution to the heart. As we noted in the last chapter, the heart itself can act as a suction pump, and the changing intrathoracic pressure also may transmit subtle effects to the central venous pressure, forcing blood toward the heart. It is important, therefore, to bear in mind that the veins serve a vital role in the regulation of cardiac output by constricting and enlarging, storing blood to make it available when required by the circulation.

The arteries have relatively thick walls, more so than their corresponding veins, and the walls impart an elasticity that permits them to stretch in response to the driving force of the blood during systole. They return to original size during diastole, but do not collapse as do the veins. In addition, arteries are equipped with muscular layers which are contractile. When stimulated, the lumen of the vessel narrows, restricting the flow of blood. This *vasoconstriction* reduces the amount of blood permitted to flow to the peripheral vessels, just as relaxation of the muscle widens the lumen in a condition called *vasodilation*, permitting an increased blood flow. In the arterioles, a single muscle cell may wrap around the vessel two or three times. Arterioles are usually in a state of partial constriction as a result of tonic discharge from *sympathetic vasoconstrictor nerves*; the amount of this constriction can be augmented or lessened, depending upon the discharge from these nerves. The degree of tone of the arterioles constitutes *peripheral resistance*.

THE CAPILLARY SYSTEM

Blood reaches the capillaries from the arterioles by passing through a series of *metarterioles*, which have a structure halfway between an arteriole and a capillary. The capillaries themselves permeate every tissue of the body, being some 7 to 9 microns in diameter, which is barely large enough for a red blood cell to squeeze through. It has been estimated that

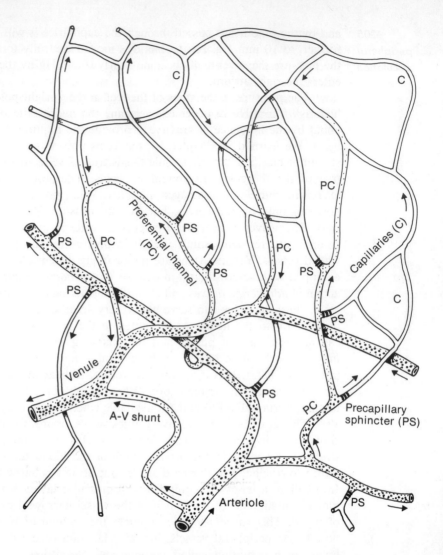

Figure 86. Microcirculation of the Capillary Bed. [B. W. Zweifach, "The Microcirculation of the Blood," *Scientific American*, 200 (January 1959), p. 56.]

it would take 1 cc of blood from 5 to 7 hours to pass through a single capillary; yet, so many capillaries are present in the body that their total length is nearly 60,000 miles, making them theoretically the largest organ in the body.[2]

Some of the capillaries are large and are called *preferential channels,* while others are small, called *true capillaries.* As shown in Figure 86, a ring of smooth muscle encircles the capillary at the point of entry. This *precapillary sphincter* controls the flow of blood into the capillary bed, since the capillaries themselves have no muscle cells. Each preferential

[2]Benjamin W. Zweifach, "The Microcirculation of the Blood," *Scientific American,* 200 (January 1959), 54.

channel may give rise to as many as 20 to 30 true capillaries. Also present is a channel, an *arteriovenous anastomosis*, which can shunt the blood directly from the arterial system to the venous system when necessary. Shunts are located primarily in the skin and represent a nonnutritive blood flow, bypassing the normal route for exchanging nutrients with the tissues. These A-V anastomoses provide a means of promoting an influx of arterial blood into the veins of the skin, causing a warming effect.

During conditions of rest the great majority of capillaries are closed, but during exercise those present in muscle dilate and are filled with blood, thereby enlarging the cross-sectional area considerably. This serves to bring blood flow into contact with an increasingly greater portion of muscle, enhancing the exchange of gases at the tissue level. Blood flow to the skin may also increase during exercise as a response to general body heating, in an effort to dissipate internal temperature increases.

MEASUREMENT OF BLOOD FLOW

The measurement of blood flow is not a simple procedure, as the reader might well imagine. Some success has been attained through the use of *electromagnetic flowmeters*, in which the blood vessel is positioned between the poles of an electromagnet. When the blood moves through a magnetic field at right angles to the lines of force, it will induce a voltage proportionate to the rate of flow. The voltage generated can be recorded using an appropriate meter or electronic recorder.

It is more likely, however, than an instrument such as a *plethysmograph* will be used, especially in studies of human blood flow. A number of such devices are available, based in one way or another on the principle that changes in the volume of an extremity reflect changes in the caliber of the indwelling blood vessels—that is, on the amount of blood and interstitial fluid within it. It is usual to employ the forearm, although the lower extremities have been used, and encase the limb in a watertight chamber (Figure 87). Some system is then devised to measure water displacement caused by the influx of blood; for this purpose, a mechanical unit consisting of a tambour, writing pen, and kymograph can be employed, or some sort of pressure transducer or strain gauge with electronic recorder. To determine the velocity of blood flow, *venous occlusion plethysmography* is employed. This requires that two pressure cuffs be used, one below the plethysmograph and one proximal to it, as shown in Figure 87. In measuring forearm blood flow, for example, an arterial cuff at the wrist is inflated to approximately 180 mm Hg to eliminate blood flow through the hand; for the upper arm, the pressure should be sufficient to permit arterial inflow to the forearm but great enough that the venous outflow is prohibited (some 40 to 80 mm Hg). Thus the essence of the venous occlusion technique is to suddenly inflate the cuffs and for a period of a few seconds record the increase in volume that results from the inflow of arterial blood. Plotting this rate of increase from the kymograph record

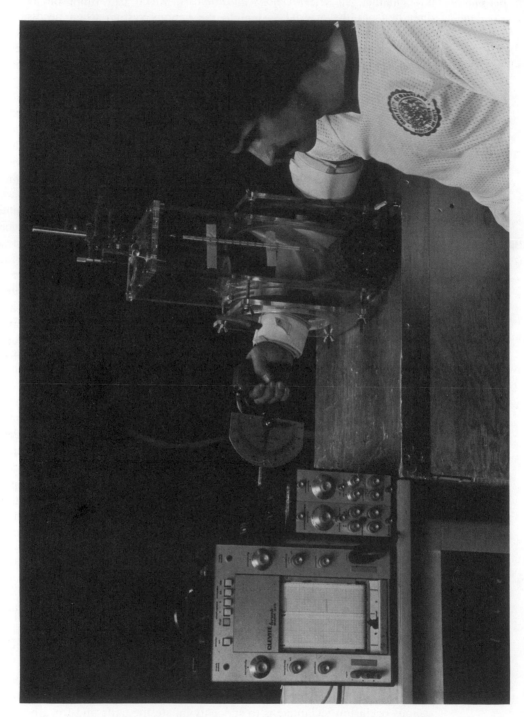

Figure 87. The Plethysmograph.

will lead to calculation of blood flow in ml/100 cc of arm volume per minute, provided that the system has been calibrated properly. At rest, blood flow through muscle is only about 1 to 3 ml/100 cc per min.

VASOMOTOR CONTROL OF PERIPHERAL CIRCULATION

Most blood vessels are provided with some means to respond quickly to stimulation by the central nervous system. The fibers responsible for control of the muscular sheet of the small arteries and arterioles form part of the autonomic nervous system and are known as vasomotor nerves. They are divided into *vasoconstrictors*, which are mainly sympathetic fibers, and *vasodilators*, which are parasympathetic fibers. The vasodilators play a minor role in the regulation of circulation and do not exert a tonic effect on blood vessels. Stimulation of the vasoconstrictors, on the other hand, causes a narrowing of the bore of the vessels, and this is apparently a tonic role played by the central nervous system in controlling blood flow. These fibers originate in the *vasomotor center* of the medulla and can take effect within two or three seconds to provide a means for rapid adjustment in peripheral circulation should the need arise. As we shall learn, the control of blood pressure is extremely important, and is monitored largely through the degree of peripheral resistance, so raising or lowering the blood pressure can be accomplished by raising or lowering the blood flow to major elements of the circulation.

LOCAL CONTROL OF SKELETAL MUSCLE BLOOD FLOW

Although the rate of blood flow in skeletal muscle is very low at rest, during exercise it has the capacity to increase as much as 20 times, so instead of demanding a small percentage of the total cardiac output (15 to 20 percent), the peripheral blood flow may suddenly jump to 80–85 percent during heavy work (Table 11–1). A number of factors responsible for the shift in circulation will be discussed briefly.

Autoregulation

The concept that skeletal muscle can maintain a constant blood flow even when there are wide variations in blood pressure can be demonstrated by use of an experimental animal, the cat.[3] If the arterial blood pressure is reduced to about 50 mm Hg, the muscle vascular resistance increases slightly at first, but after a few minutes the vascular resistance falls, permitting the smooth muscle tone to adjust to this new level of pressure. Restoring the arterial pressure suddenly to normal gradually restores the

[3]Hugh Davson and M. Grace Eggleton, eds., *Principles of Human Physiology,* 14th ed. (Philadelphia: Lea & Febiger, 1968), p. 281.

Table 11–1. Distribution of Total Blood Volume to Various Organs during Rest and Heavy Exercise

	Rest	% of Total	Light Exercise	% of Total	Strenuous Exercise	% of Total	Maximal Exercise	% of Total
Splanchnic	1,400	24	1,100	12	600	3	300	1
Renal	1,100	19	900	9	600	3	250	1
Cerebral	750	13	750	8	750	4	750	3
Coronary	250	4	350	4	750	4	1,000	4
Skeletal muscle	1,200	21	4,500	47	12,500	72	22,000	88
Skin	500	9	1,500	16	1,900	12	600	2
Other organs	600	10	400	4	400	2	100	1
Cardiac output (ml)	5,800	100	9,500	100	17,500	100	25,000	100

Adapted from D.L. Wade and J.M. Bishop, *Cardiac Output and Regional Blood Flow.* (Oxford: Blackwell Scientific Publications, 1962).

vascular resistance to normal. Thus, the muscles enjoy an important auto-regulatory ability to maintain normal blood flow. In other words, if the arterial pressure decreases, local factors in the tissues automatically dilate the arterioles and precapillary sphincters in an attempt to prevent a decrease in blood flow. Conversely, higher than normal arterial pressures cause automatic vasoconstriction, maintaining normal local blood flow.

Metabolites

One of the most pronounced effects on local circulation can occur as a result of the production of metabolites. Chemical changes in the muscles dilate the arterioles, metarterioles, and precapillary sphincters by direct action on the smooth muscles of these vessels. Thus, the production of CO_2 raises the tissue P_{CO_2}, perhaps causing a reduction in pH as the tissues become more acidic, at the same time leading to a decrease in P_{O_2}. All of these cause vasodilatation, as the local tissues endeavor to bring in more oxygen and eliminate waste products. Other metabolites, such as lactic acid, adenosine phosphate compounds, and so on, have been suggested as having vasodilating properties on skeletal muscle.

Humoral Agents

A number of substances contained in the body fluids serve to regulate blood flow locally. Probably the most important of these is *aldosterone,* secreted by the adrenal cortex. Aldosterone is a hormone that helps in the regulation of salt and water balance in the extracellular fluid, and thus assists in the regulation of blood volume. Should the blood volume or the sodium concentration fall, the aldosterone acts on the kidney to cause increased reabsorption of sodium, which leads to the increased reabsorption of chloride ions and water, thus increasing the extracellular fluid volume and blood volume.

Epinephrine and *norepinephrine* secretions are also very important in the control of local blood flow. Epinephrine causes vasodilation in the blood vessels of skeletal muscle, while norepinephrine produces vasocontriction and is said to maintain tone of the blood vessels.

Temperature

Exercise raises the body core temperature, and the blood vessels of the skin dilate so that blood may transport the heat to the surface of the body in order to maintain thermal balance. Much less seems known about the effect produced by changes in muscle temperature, except that the blood flow decreases with lowering of temperature and increases with raising of the temperature. The effect is less pronounced than that which occurs in the skin. Temperature regulation will be discussed more thoroughly in Chapter 12.

Reactive Hyperemia

When there is a temporary occlusion of the blood flow to a limb, and then this occlusion is withdrawn, there follows a compensatory increase in the blood flow through the extremity, due mainly to dilatation of muscle arterioles and capillaries. This *reactive hyperemia* parallels the deficit in the tissues for oxygen during the period of occlusion.

REFLEX CONTROL OF SKELETAL MUSCLE BLOOD FLOW

We learned in Chapter 10 that a number of factors serve to control the heart rate. It should be emphasized here that some of these factors, in order to be properly integrated, will also exert an influence on the peripheral resistance, to maintain blood pressure at proper levels.

Baroreceptor Reflex

The increase in arterial blood pressure excites the baroreceptors of the carotid sinus and aortic arch and transmits signals to the central nervous system to inhibit the vasomotor center of the medulla and excite the vagal center. This leads to a reduction in heart rate and a vasodilation throughout the systemic circulatory system, decreasing peripheral resistance, and consequently leading to a decrease in arterial pressure.

Chemoreceptor Reflex

Changes in chemical composition of the blood, when sufficiently pronounced, can exert an effect on the vasomotor center, but because of other factors, particularly those involved with respiration, the body maintains a fairly stable blood chemistry. Nevertheless, a high Pco_2 can increase the mean arterial pressure by affecting the vasomotor center, causing vasoconstriction. The increased arterial pressure assists the tissues by helping to drive the blood through the vascular system. The same effect is found when the Po_2 in arterial blood falls, and the carotid and aortic bodies become excited. The impulses are transmitted to the vasomotor center, elevating arterial pressure in an effort to provide increased blood and thus oxygen to the tissues.

Bainbridge Effect

The precise nature of the *Bainbridge effect* has been difficult to elucidate, as pointed out in Chapter 10, although increased pressure in the atria that might lead to an increased heart rate would also result in a slight increase in arterial pressure.

EFFECT OF EXERCISE ON PERIPHERAL CIRCULATION

It is difficult to formulate definitive statements about the circulatory effects of exercise, since the type of activity itself can be so variable, and because the form that exercise takes will ultimately make a difference in the blood flow. The idea that rhythmic exercise promotes blood flow and hastens venous return has been discussed before. This requires that there be a brief period of rest between muscular contractions so that there is time for blood to enter the capillary bed of the muscle. This can be illustrated as in Figure 88, where brief hand-grip contractions are followed by rest intervals of the same length. Contraction of the muscles causes a decrease in limb volume as the intramuscular veins are emptied by the mechanical compression, but as soon as the tension is released the volume progressively increases. This is due to the dilation of arterioles and capillaries responding to the action of locally formed metabolites. As Figure 87 shows, the subsequent contraction and relaxation further increase the blood volume after first causing a temporary reduction. Eventually, a full vasodilation would occur.

The unmistakable conclusion is that during maximal sustained or isometric contractions the intital period of exercise is associated with

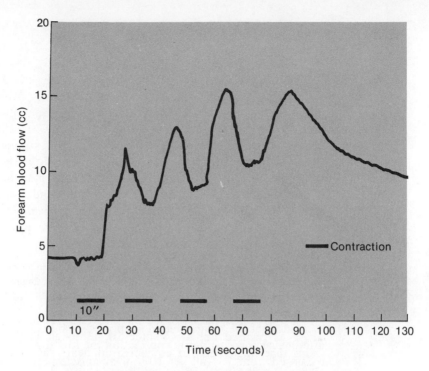

Figure 88. Effect of Rhythmic Contractions on Peripheral Blood Flow.
[R. T. Grant, "Observations on the Blood Circulation in Voluntary Muscle in Man," *Clinical Science*, 3 (April 1938), p. 166.]

occlusion of the blood flow, which will persist until the intramuscular tension declines to some 60 to 70 percent of maximum. Royce[4] performed two maximum isometric contractions, once with normal circulation and once with circulation mechanically occluded by an arterial pressure cuff. Blood flow seemed to be reinstated in the normal limb after the tension reduced to 60 percent, but at first both the intramuscular tension and the mechanical occlusion effectively reduced intramuscular blood flow. To examine this question further, Humphreys and Lind[5] had subjects perform sustained hand-grip contractions at 30, 40, 50, 60, and 70 percent of their maximum strength. At all values there was actually an increased rate of blood flow, although some difficulty was experienced at 70 percent; apparently, by this time the increase in blood flow had begun to subside.

Indirect evidence of blood-flow obstruction during isometric contractions is the finding of an increased oxygen debt from that form of exercise,

[4]Joseph Royce, "Isometric Fatigue Curves in Human Muscle with Normal and Occluded Circulation," *Research Quarterly*, 29 (May 1958), 204.

[5]P. W. Humphreys and A. R. Lind, "The Blood Flow Through Active and Inactive Muscles of the Forearm during Sustained Hand-Grip Contractions," *Journal of Physiology* (London), 166 (1963), 120.

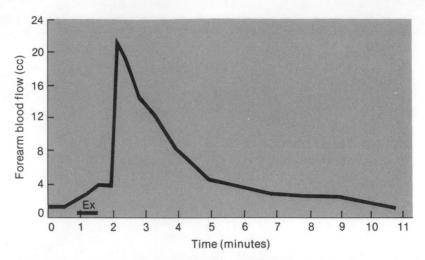

Figure 89. Forearm Blood Flow during Sustained Muscular Contraction and Recovery. [R. T. Grant, "Observations on the Blood Circulation in Voluntary Muscle in Man," *Clinical Science*, 3 (April 1938), p. 162.]

meaning that the oxygen-blood supply was inadequate.[6] Grant[7] found that after a sustained hand-grip contraction the forearm blood flow immediately increased from 1–4 ml per 100 ml of muscle per minute to above 20 ml per 100 ml, gradually subsiding over the next 10 minutes (Figure 89). In other words, a *blood-flow debt* is incurred during isometric exercise that is paid after exercise is over in the recovery period. Grant also employed rhythmic exercises of various durations and found that after 4 minutes the blood flow had increased to 33 ml per 100 ml, equivalent to 30 times the resting value. It is interesting to note the similarities between the muscular strength debt (Chapter 3), the oxygen debt (Chapter 6), and the blood-flow debt. Even blood flow is characterized by fast and slow phases of recovery,[8] as are the other functions. Since the common denominator is the metabolic process of the exercise itself, it is clear that these factors are all involved in one way or another with supplying nutrients, removing waste products, or simply reflecting the recuperation of the active muscle cells.

EFFECT OF TRAINING ON BLOOD FLOW

The individual who engages in training may expect to find circulatory changes reflecting increased efficiency of blood flow. One of the earlier

[6]David H. Clarke, "Energy Cost of Isometric Exercise," *Research Quarterly*, 31 (March 1960), 3.

[7]R. T. Grant, "Observations on the Blood Circulation in Voluntary Muscle in Man," *Clinical Science*, 3 (April 1938), 157.

[8]Jack H. Wilmore and Steven M. Horvath, "Alterations in Peripheral Blood Flow Consequent to Maximal Exercise," *American Heart Journal*, 66 (September 1963), 353.

studies[9] found that there was an increased capillarization in trained dogs, the number of capilaries increasing by 40 to 50 percent. Some hypertrophy of existing capilaries was also found. Resting blood flow does not seem to change as a result of physical training, but individuals who undertake muscular endurance training can expect to find the blood-flow debt (during recovery) to be reduced per unit of exercise effort.[10] This means that training of this sort makes it possible for the vascular bed to open up to a greater extent than normal in response to exercise. Increased blood flow has also been found in training for swimming,[11] but in this case blood flow was observed during exercise rather than during the postexercise recovery period. The swimmers' forearm blood flow increased progressively through training, reaching a peak during the fifth week and tapering off during the detraining period.

EFFECT OF EXERCISE ON BLOOD PRESSURE

In order to provide a mechanism to increase blood flow through the active tissues during exercise, the arterial blood pressure increases, sometimes achieving systolic levels in excess of 180 mm Hg during maximal work.[12] The diastolic pressure increases less, to approximately 110 mm Hg, so the pulse pressure increase is attributed more to a change in systolic than diastolic pressure. The peripheral vascular resistance decreases owing to the vasodilation of the skeletal muscle blood vessels, which should be expected to modify the blood pressure, but the increase in cardiac output nevertheless causes the blood pressure to rise.

The values for blood pressure are higher when work is performed with the arms as compared with the legs at a given submaximal $\dot{V}o_2$.[13] Perhaps the smaller vascular bed in the smaller muscles offers greater resistance to systemic blood flow. Åstrand and Rodahl[14] point out the potential hazard for individuals with heart damage to work with the arms in activities such as snow shoveling and digging, as contrasted with rhythmic leg

[9]T. Petrén, T. Sjöstrand, and Bengt Sylvén, "Der Einfluss des Trainings auf die Häufigkeit der Capillaren in Herz- und Skeletmuskulatur," *Arbeitsphysiologie*, 9 (1936), 376

[10]Ellen R. Vanderhoof, Charles J. Imig, and H. M. Hines, "Effect of Muscle Strength and Endurance Development on Blood Flow," *Journal of Applied Physiology*, 16 (1961), 873.

[11]Frank D. Rohter, Rene H. Rochelle, and Chester Hyman, "Exercise Blood Flow Changes in the Human Forearm during Physical Training," *Journal of Applied Physiology*, 18 (July 1963), 789.

[12]Per-Olof Åstrand, B. Ekblom, R. Messin, B. Saltin, and J. Stenberg, "Intra-Arterial Blood Pressure during Exercise with Different Muscle Groups," *Journal of Applied Physiology*, 20 (March 1965), 253.

[13]J. Stenberg, P.-O. Åstrand, B. Ekblom, J. Royce, and B. Saltin, "Hemodynamic Response to Work with Different Muscle Groups, Sitting and Supine," *Journal of Applied Physiology*, 22 (January 1967), 61.

[14]Per-Olof Åstrand and Kaare Rodahl, *Textbook of Work Physiology* (New York: McGraw-Hill Book Company, 1970), p. 168.

exercises such as walking or cycling. From previous discussions of the difference in circulation when isometric exercise is compared with isotonic, it should come as no surprise that blood pressure increases are greater during the isometric contractions.

SUMMARY

The peripheral circulatory system consists of arteries, arterioles, capillaries, venules, and veins, where nearly 80 percent of the circulation is distributed. Over half of the blood is located in the veins, emphasizing the role of the venous system for the storage of blood. The velocity of flow is high in the aorta and very low in the capillaries. This means that the blood pressure is highest in the aorta, and it will have dropped nearly to zero by the time the blood enters the right atrium. The flow of blood is directed centrally because the veins have one-way valves. Vasoconstriction reduces blood flow and vasodilation promotes blood flow; the degree of tone of the arterioles is called peripheral resistance. Blood reaches the capillaries by passing through the arterioles and then the metarterioles. At the point of entry to the capillary there is a muscular ring called a precapillary sphincter, controlling the flow of blood. The amount of blood flow in extremities can be measured with a plethysmograph.

Blood vessels may be stimulated by the autonomic nervous system, as vasoconstrictor fibers exert a tonic effect on the peripheral circulation. Local control is performed by autoregulation, the production of metabolites and humoral agents, temperature, and a compensatory reactive hyperemia. Reflex control may be exerted by baroreceptor and chemoreceptor reflexes.

Isometric exercise occludes peripheral circulation and isotonic exercise promotes blood flow. Contraction of the muscles first squeezes out blood; then the volume steadily increases owing to dilation of arterioles and capillaries. The recovery of blood flow after exercise reflects a blood-flow debt similar to the muscular strength debt and the oxygen debt. Training may lead to an increased capillarization and a reduction in blood-flow debt. The vascular bed opens up more than it does in the nontrained state. Systolic blood pressure increases to a greater extent during exercise than does diastolic pressure, and it is even higher when work is performed with the arms as compared with the legs.

SELECTED REFERENCES

Åstrand, Per-Olof, and Kaare Rodahl, *Textbook of Work Physiology*. New York: McGraw-Hill Book Company, 1970.

Carlsten, Arne, and Gunnar Grimby, *The Circulatory Response to Muscular Exercise in Man.* Springfield, Ill.: Charles C. Thomas, 1966.

Davson, Hugh, and M. Grace Eggleton, eds., *Principles of Human Physiology*, 14th ed. Philadelphia: Lea & Febiger, 1968.

Grant, R. T., "Observations on the Blood Circulation in Voluntary Muscle in Man," *Clinical Science*, 3 (April 1938), 157.

Guyton, Arthur C., *Textbook of Medical Physiology*, 4th ed. Philadelphia: W. B. Saunders Company, 1971.

Hudlická, O., ed., *Circulation is Skeletal Muscle*. New York: Pergamon Press, 1968.

Humphreys, P. W., and A. R. Lind, "The Blood Flow Through Active and Inactive Muscles of the Forearm during Sustained Hand-Grip Contractions," *Journal of Physiology* (London), 166 (1963), 120.

"Peripheral Circulation in Man," *British Medical Bulletin*, 19 (May 1963), 97.

Rohter, Frank D., Rene H. Rochelle, and Chester Hyman, "Exercise Blood Flow Changes in the Human Forearm during Physical Training," *Journal of Applied Physiology*, 18 (July 1963), 789.

Vanderhoof, Ellen R., Charles J. Imig, and H. M. Hines, "Effect of Muscle Strength and Endurance Development on Blood Flow," *Journal of Applied Physiology*, 16 (1961), 873.

Zweifach, Benjamin W., "The Microcirculation of the Blood," *Scientific American*, 200 (January 1959), 54.

chapter 12

environmental physiology

Man in action is frequently exposed to environmental conditions that might be classified as atypical, if not abnormal. The physiological concepts discussed until now have dealt with the body's response to normal exercise and training. But optimal conditions do not always prevail; the day may be excessively hot and humid, or cold; the clothing or uniform may be inadequate; or the individual may journey into unusual environmental circumstances, such as high altitudes or under water.

In all such situations the organism must adjust to a set of conditions that tends to alter normal physiology in significant ways. The performer finds that without acclimatization—a period of adjustment to the rigors of the environment—his performance may be impaired. The body has a remarkable ability to compensate either wholly or partially to environmental conditions if given the opportunity. This does not mean that complete success will always be experienced. While it might be argued scientifically that a slight impairment may not be particularly significant, to the athlete in competition it might well be the difference between winning and losing a contest. Morever, there may be an additive effect when the performer competes in extended running, swimming, cycling, or the like, as compared with shorter events. Thus, the potential length of exposure is an important factor when considering the effects of adverse environmental conditions. This chapter will discuss the more prominent factors in environmental physiology.

ALTITUDE

Recent advances in space technology and the burgeoning participation in international sporting events around the world have brought into the limelight some of the acute effects of altitude. Beginning with the early experimentation with balloon flights and continuing with mountain climbing, man (and woman, too) has gained notoriety and considerable respect by such feats as the dramatic ascent to the summit of Mount Everest, an elevation of 29,028 feet above sea level. The 1968 Olympic Games, held in Mexico City at an altitude of 7,347 feet above sea level, focused attention on the potential reduction in physical performance that can accrue from exercising at altitude, and also pointed clearly to the role of acclimatization as a means for adjusting physiologically to these rigors.

219

Gas laws, and in particular the laws governing partial pressures, were reviewed in Chapter 8. It was learned that approximately one-fifth of the atmospheric air consists of oxygen, which has a partial pressure of 159.1 mm Hg. Further, the Po_2 in the alveoli is reduced to some 104 mm Hg. which is the partial pressure to which incoming blood is exposed as it circulates through the pulmonary capillaries. Because the venous blood Po_2 is 40 mm Hg, the pressure gradient is quite satisfactory for the movement of oxygen into the blood. At altitude the problem is not that the percentage of the gas has changed, but that the column of air has been reduced so the total barometric pressure becomes less. This means that the Po_2 will be reduced according to the altitude to which one is exposed, and consequently the pressure gradient between the alveoli and the blood will be reduced, with the result that arterial blood will not be fully saturated.

It is common to think of a thinner atmosphere at high elevations. The reason is that there are fewer gas molecules per unit of space, a condition of reduced density. The number of molecules above ground is what imparts atmospheric pressure, so that the individual, when inspiring, is unable to bring the same number of oxygen molecules into the lungs as would be possible at sea level. In an effort to compensate for this, he may increase his pulmonary ventilation, a condition called *hyperventilation*. For example, at 20,000 feet the barometric pressure will be reduced slightly more than half, as shown in Table 12–1. This will result in a drop in Po_2 of atmospheric air to 73 mm Hg, and cause an alveolar Po_2 of 40 mm Hg and an arterial oxygen saturation of 70 percent. Compare this with 10,000 feet, where the Pao_2 becomes 67 mm Hg, but the arterial oxygen saturation drops only to 90 percent.

Even with a steady ascent to high altitude with its systematic reduction in barometric pressure, the effect on arterial oxygen saturation is somewhat modified. In other words, the drop in alveolar Po_2 of 37 mm Hg at 10,000 feet causes but a slight decline in the arterial blood saturation, as compared with the more precipitous reduction at 20,000 feet. This can be understood better by referring to Figure 64 (in Chapter 8), the oxygen-hemoglobin dissociation curves. As pointed out, the arterial end of these curves is quite flat, which means that with a reduction in Po_2 the percentage of oxygen bound to hemoglobin remains high, and it may actually

Table 12–1. Effect of Altitude on Various Gas Pressures

Altitude (ft)	Barometric Pressure	Atmospheric Po_2	Alveolar Po_2	% Arterial Saturation	Alveolar Pco_2
0	760	159	104	97	40
10,000	525	110	67	90	36
20,000	350	73	40	70	24

change the oxygen-hemoglobin dissociation curve, as will be discussed below. At any rate, the affinity of hemoglobin for oxygen works in favor of the individual and helps explain why relatively slight elevations above sea level (up to several thousand feet) can be handled with ease.

Hypoxia

The lack of oxygen at the tissue level, called *hypoxia*, is the result of the decreased Po_2 and the subsequent fall in arterial oxygen saturation. The body cells may simply not receive sufficient oxygen. At about 60 mm Hg, however, the drop in alveolar Po_2 provides enough drive to stimulate the peripheral chemoreceptors of the carotid and aortic bodies (see Chapter 9) to increase ventilation. The resultant hyperventilation may reduce the alveolar Pco_2, as shown in Table 12–1, producing a respiratory alkalosis and shifting the oxygen-hemoglobin dissociation curve to the left, permitting a greater affinity of hemoglobin for oxygen. This assists the individual in moving more oxygen from the lungs to the blood, and whereas it might also diminish slightly the transferrence of oxygen to the tissues, it may still remain a beneficial factor.

Cardiac Output. In order to counteract the hypoxia, it has been shown that the circulation increases as a result of increased cardiac output. The major shift is a result of changes in resting heart rate, which rises fairly directly with an increase in altitude. Whether or not systematic changes occur in stroke volume are open to some conjecture because of difficulties in measurement.

Pulmonary Ventilation. As has been pointed out, one of the effects of altitude is to cause hyperventilation, although the elevation must be sufficiently great for the hypoxia to activate chemoreceptors of the carotid sinus and aortic bodies.

Blood Pressure. Balke[1] indicates that blood-pressure changes at altitude are marked by individual differences, but a drop in peripheral resistance may cause a fall in diastolic pressure. Sudden exposure to acute hypoxia (26,000 feet) may also raise systolic pressure, and when this occurs diastolic pressure will probably increase slightly.

Oxygen Consumption. Exposure to hypoxic environments does not increase the oxygen consumption at rest; in other words, *cellular* metabolism does not alter as a result of altitude.

Lactic Acid Production. The amount of blood lactate at rest has been found to increase in subjects exposed to an altitude of approximately 12,500 feet.[2]

[1]Bruno Balke, "Variation in Altitude and Its Effects on Exercise Performance," in Harold B. Falls, *Exercise Physiology* (New York: Academic Press, 1968), p. 246.

[2]Pierre De Jours, Ralph H. Kellog, and Nello Pace, "Regulation of Respiration and Heart Rate Response in Exercise during Altitude Acclimatization," *Journal of Applied Physiology*, 18 (January 1963), 10.

As expected, altitude impairs exercise capacity and athletic performance, and generally in the direction one would anticipate. Keep in mind that the magnitude of the effects depends upon the extent of the elevation above sea level. If more specific detail is required, the reader should consult references listed at the end of the chapter.

Heart Rate. The heart-rate response to exercise is higher than at sea level during low and moderate intensities of work. Just as the resting value is elevated, each level of submaximal work elicits correspondingly increased heart rates. However, it is interesting to note that maximal heart rate is *lower* than at sea level, according to most accounts. It may be as much as 40 beats per minute lower for some subjects exposed to acute hypoxia, and it is achieved at lower work loads than at sea level.

Stroke Volume. Stroke volume has been found to increase at moderate and maximum work at altitude (14,000 feet). It is suggested[3] that the heart-rate and stroke-volume changes are initiated and controlled by stimuli arising from the peripheral vascular bed, which undergoes marked vasodilation to facilitate blood flow. Moreover, stroke volume may take on a greater proportion of the cardiac output at higher work intensities than heart rate.

Cardiac Output. Ascent to altitude thus causes an elevated cardiac output at rest and during most levels of work. The maximum cardiac output, however, is reduced. Whether this is due to a hypoxic myocardium (lack of oxygen to the heart muscle) or a decreased firing of the sinoauricular node (pacemaker of the heart) is not clear. More peripheral factors may be ultimately responsible for the reduced maximum capacity of the heart.

Blood Pressure. The change in blood pressure seems to be somewhat inconsistent, for large individual differences apparently exist in the response of subjects exposed to acute hypoxia. The reduction in peripheral resistance may lower systolic and diastolic pressures slightly up to about 18,000 feet.

Pulmonary Ventilation. The response of pulmonary ventilation during exercise is to become elevated over sea-level values, especially as maximum oxygen intake is approached.[4]

Oxygen Uptake. The aerobic capacity of individuals exercising at altitude is reduced. Maximum oxygen uptake is lowered, and each submaximal

[3]James A. Vogel and James E. Hansen, "Cardiovascular Function During Exercise at High Altitude," in *The Effects of Altitude on Physical Performance* (Chicago: The Athletic Institute, 1967), p. 47.

[4]L. G. C. E. Pugh, M. B. Gill, S. Lahiri, J. S. Milledge, M. P. Ward, and J. B. West, "Muscular Exercise at Great Altitudes," *Journal of Applied Physiology*, 19 (May 1964), 431.

work load requires higher $\dot{V}_{O_2}$ values than at sea level. This means that physical work capacity is reduced, since the $\dot{V}_{O_2}$ max will be attained at lower work loads.

Anaerobic Performance. Some forms of anaerobic work will not be adversely affected by altitude. Tests of strength, explosive power, and such athletic events as shot putting and short dashes are completed so quickly that they are not dependent upon oxygen uptake but instead rely on intracellular stores of ATP and phosphocreatine. Moreover, because the density of the air is reduced at altitude, some anaerobic events (such as sprinting and discus throwing) may even be enhanced. Anaerobic processes will be invoked sooner during exhaustive work, as the aerobic processes reach their limit. If the level of $\dot{V}_{O_2}$ could be equated, the production of lactic acid should not be different, but standard *work* performance at altitude causes a greater rise in lactate than equivalent performance at sea level. While this may be the case for isolated tasks, athletes may experience cumulative fatigue as a result of previous trials and thus find a gradual deterioration. Shephard[5] offers the theory that an increased flow of fluid from the tissues results from increased tissue hypoxia after exercise.

Acclimatization

Acclimatization refers to those circumstances by which the human organism adjusts to the rigors of the environment. In the case of altitude the acclimatization process involves a variety of compensatory mechanisms such that repeated exposure to potentially hypoxic conditions lessens the subsequent effect. Individuals upon first ascending to altitudes of 7,000 feet or more commonly experience symptoms of acute mountain sickness, including weakness, dizziness, headache, nausea, and vomiting. Their severity and the specific altitude at which they are first noticed may vary widely according to the individual. The leading cause of mountain sickness is the hyperventilation, which washes CO_2 out of the blood, disturbing its acid-base balance. Other factors are undoubtedly important.

A period of acclimatization not only relieves symptoms of mountain sickness but at the same time improves work performance. Consider for a moment how important such adjustments are. Acute exposure to 25,000 feet would permit the average person less than ten minutes of consciousness, and perhaps only twenty to thirty minutes of life. Yet, a person can acclimatize in such a manner that he could live for several days at this altitude.

A number of processes serve to acclimatize the individual by restoring the oxygen pressure of the cells toward normal. One of the first changes is an increase in pulmonary ventilation, as the alveolar air is brought closer

[5]R. J. Shephard, "A Possible Deterioration in Performance of Short-Term Olympic Events at Altitude," *Canadian Medical Association Journal*, 97 (December 2, 1967), 1414.

in composition to atmospheric air, raising P_{AO_2}, or at least preventing its decline as the altitude increases. This hyperventilation may result in some fluid loss from the blood, causing a greater blood viscosity and raising the concentration of hemoglobin. Later, there is an increase in the actual amount of hemoglobin and the number of erythrocytes (red blood cells), so that the total amount of oxygen circulating in arterial blood increases toward normal, in spite of the lowered barometric pressure. In addition,[6] there is a gradual decrease in the alveolar-arterial gradient for oxygen, thereby improving the diffusing capacity for oxygen in the lungs. The increased ventilation, in lowering blood carbon dioxide, makes the blood more alkaline, raises the pH slightly, and shifts the oxygen-hemoglobin dissociation curve to the left. Thus a more alkaline blood hemoglobin exhibits an increased affinity for oxygen from the lungs. This results in a loss of base, as the kidney excretes additional bicarbonate. The loss of buffering capacity of the blood by a reduction in base thus causes the carbon dioxide content to fall, restoring blood pH to normal.

At the tissue level important changes occur as part of the acclimatization process at altitude. These include the increased capillarization of the muscle tissue, an increase in the storage of myoglobin, and an increase in activity of the enzymes involved in the respiratory-chain oxidations (Chapter 5) which facilitates the transference of electrons from NAD2H for regeneration of ATP.[7] The result is to normalize the efforts of exercise, making performance at altitude more nearly like that at sea level. Heart rates decline, both at rest and for each given intensity of submaximal exercise, as sea-level values of exercise are made possible once again. Maximal heart rate, on the other hand, increases in the acclimatized subject to a level more commensurate with sea-level attainment. Thus total cardiac output is enhanced.

The increase in oxygen availability does not affect the performance of short anaerobic activities, but it does improve the aerobic ones. The long endurance events benefit greatly, as $\dot{V}O_2$ max gradually improves[8] and the times for distance running events shorten. This means that more work can be accomplished before anaerobic energy sources must be employed, and with this comes the added ability to incur a lactic debt. Overall the total work performance improves.

The time duration for acclimatization once again is very individualistic; what will work for one person may not be effective for another. Indeed, some individuals seem to resist acclimatization altogether, profiting very little by prolonged exposure to altitude. It is clear, however, that two to three weeks are required for acclimatization at an altitude of 7,500 feet. Even then, some individuals may need four weeks before improvement

[6]Balke, *op. cit.*, p. 249.

[7]Wolf H. Weihe, "Time Course of Acclimatization to High Altitude," in *The Effects of Altitude on Physical Performance* (Chicago: The Athletic Institute, 1967), p. 33.

[8]K. Klausen, D. B. Dill, and S. M. Horvath, "Exercise at Ambient and High Oxygen Pressure at High Altitude and at Sea Level," *Journal of Applied Physiology*, 29 (October 1970), 456.

ceases. The period of acclimatization will be extended for higher elevations and will be lost relatively quickly after the return to sea level.

THE PHYSIOLOGY OF DIVING

The opposite environmental condition to altitude is found under water. Whereas altitude represents a *hypobaric* situation of reduced pressure, the individual who goes below sea level and under water enters a *hyperbaric* environment. Both affect the respiratory system, and because this then exposes one to subsequent changes in gas pressure, there are internal consequences as well. Sport diving has become an international activity of significant proportions, and manufacturers of equipment have placed the world under water at the disposal of nearly anyone. Underwater fishing, photography, and exploration place thousands of people annually below the water's surface in an environment that is different and potentially hazardous. Added to these are skilled professional and semiprofessional divers who may be required to go to great depths and stay there for an extended period, during which they may be engaged in some form of work.

Anyone contemplating diving with a self-contained underwater breathing apparatus (scuba) must receive a period of instruction from competent professionals, preferably an official course in scuba diving, before ever entering the water with the equipment. This pertains to a swimming pool as well as the ocean, for the hazards are not restricted to depth. The use of the equipment and its care must be approached properly, so that all limitations are thoroughly understood and the individual can proceed independently to care for himself. Once the basic physics and physiology of diving are understood, the diver then becomes a functioning physiological entity. His entire existence below the surface of the water is subservient to the steady flow of oxygen to the alveoli; interruption for only a brief period places him in immediate danger. Obviously, the whole point of diving is to rule out such an eventuality.

There are three general forms of diving. (1) In *skin diving* the individual is equipped with snorkel and face mask and engages in breath-hold dives. His range of activity is obviously limited, although he may descend quite far if pressure in the ear is properly neutralized. (2) *Scuba diving* permits the individual a free flow of air for an extended period. The equipment is not excessively heavy under water, and there is great mobility. (3) In *conventional diving*, so-called "hard-hat" diving, the individual is able to descend to great depths and work, receiving his air supply from a hose fed via a compressor on the surface.

The Physics of Diving

As reviewed earlier, the barometric pressure at sea level is approximately 760 mm Hg or 14.7 pounds per square inch (psi); this pressure is known as one atmosphere. It is based on the weight of air above the surface of the earth. It takes 33 feet of water to duplicate the atmospheric pressure of air, so at that depth the diver is actually under two atmospheres, one of air and one of water, and the total pressure is now 1,520 mm Hg. At 66 feet the absolute pressure is three atmospheres, and at approximately 100 feet it is four atmospheres. Thus, it doesn't take a very deep dive to alter the physical environment considerably.

Gas is compressible, but water is not. Therefore it is important to note what happens to a gas under pressure. A liter of air at sea level will compress to one-half liter at 33 feet, according to Boyle's law (Chapter 8), which states that the volume of a gas varies inversely with the pressure (temperature remaining constant). Thus, doubling the pressure reduces the volume by half. At 66 feet the volume is one-third liter, and at 100 feet it is one-fourth liter. Conversely, a liter of air at four atmospheres (100 feet) becomes 4 liters at sea level.

Since the number of molecules of various gases remains the same, the effect of the increased pressure is to increase proportionately the partial pressures of the constituent gases. Referring to Table 12–2, we can see that as the total pressure rises, so do the partial pressures of nitrogen and oxygen. At 33 feet the P_{O_2} rises to 320 mm Hg, and the P_{N_2} reaches 1,200 mm Hg. We know that the factor which controls the dissolving of gases into surrounding fluids is the partial pressure and the pressure gradients, so at 33 feet twice as much nitrogen and oxygen will be dissolved in the blood. The consequences of this situation will be discussed subsequently.

Water also exerts pressure on the body as a whole, compressing the chest and causing the lung volume to be reduced, unless there is counteracting internal pressure changes. Undoubtedly there are wide individual differences here, but eventually internal tissue damage could ensue, including pulmonary hemorrhage and compression fractures of the ribs. Some have concluded that 100 feet is approaching the physiological limits for a free dive, even though the attainment of greater depths is common. Other air-containing cavities of the body, such as the paranasal sinuses and the middle ears, cannot adapt as readily as the lungs to compression; if they are not equalized in some way, a relative vacuum will exist. This can cause extreme discomfort, rupture of the eardrum, or bleeding in sinuses.

Table 12–2. Gas Pressures at Various Depths

Depth (ft)	Total Pressure (mm Hg)	P_{N_2} (mm Hg)	P_{O_2} (mm Hg)
0 (sea level)	760	600	160
33	1,520	1,200	320
66	2,280	1,800	480
99	3,040	2,400	640

Nitrogen Narcosis

It has been pointed out that the deeper one goes below the surface of the water, the greater will be the partial pressure of nitrogen, and consequently the greater the amount that will be dissolved in the blood and tissue fluids. Nitrogen is not considered a metabolic gas, and it does not participate in energy production or exercise metabolism. But its presence in the dissolved state leads to a condition called *nitrogen narcosis*, or "raptures of the deep," producing symptoms similar to those experienced after the consumption of alcohol. The first mild symptoms are felt at 100 feet, where observers claim the sensation may be likened to one martini taken on an empty stomach. Thus, the martini rule has been formulated, which says that at 300 feet the result is similar to consuming four martinis.

Individual variations exist with respect to the narcotic effect, but symptoms of lethargy or euphoria, together with a slowing of the mental processes, make it a potentially hazardous condition for the diver. Nitrogen dissolves freely into the fats of the body and the neurons and, like gas anesthesia, it reduces nervous-system excitability, thereby diminishing sensitivity and judgment.

Decompression Sickness

The diver breathing air under pressure also faces the potential hazard inherent in making a rapid ascent after prolonged submersion. Once again, nitrogen is at fault, owing to its presence in the dissolved state in the tissues of the body. Time is required for it to dissolve back out of solution to be exhaled. The factors of importance here are the depth and duration of the dive and the speed of ascent. If the dive fits the criteria established for decompression, then it is imperative that the ascent be made under controlled conditions, with pauses at various levels to permit the nitrogen to dissolve out of the body.

Too rapid an ascent will cause the nitrogen to form bubbles as the pressure is reduced, resulting in circulatory blockage and damage to tissues. The condition is known as *decompression sickness*, or "the bends," and is characterized by pain, especially in joints. Bubbles in the venous blood may become lodged in the pulmonary capillaries, causing respiratory distress (the "chokes"), and bubbles passing through the pulmonary bed may obstruct the capillaries of such vital organs as the brain or heart. Symptoms will appear within four to six hours, or even within a few minutes in sudden cases of abrupt decompression.

The time factor involved in diving in relation to decompression is given in Figure 90. It shows that a diver can tolerate a descent of up to 30 feet indefinitely without having to undergo decompression or experiencing decompression sickness. Sixty feet can be tolerated safely for approximately one hour, leading to the "60–60" rule for scuba divers: 60 feet, 60 minutes.

227

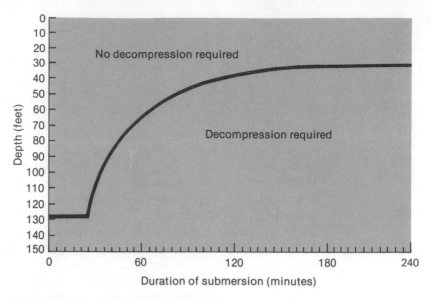

Figure 90. Time Table for Decompression at Various Depths. [From G. J. Duffner, "Medical Problems Involved in Underwater Compression and Decompression," *Clinical Symposia*, CIBA Pharmaceutical Products, Inc., 10 (July-August 1958), p. 112.]

One can stay at a depth of 100 feet for only about 30 minutes before decompression is necessary. Standard times of decompression should be consulted if extended dives using compressed air are contemplated. They will reveal the pattern of ascent required for effective decompression to take place. For this reason, the scuba diver must plan ahead so that sufficient air supplies are available for this phase. The pains of decompression sickness can be relieved by placing the individual in a decompression chamber and raising the pressure to reproduce the appropriate depth. He is then gradually brought back to sea-level values.

Oxygen Toxicity

Diving while using oxygen instead of air should be avoided, since breathing 100 percent oxygen under pressure for extended periods of time will lead to *oxygen toxicity*. In the final stages it can result in convulsions and coma. If the individual is under water at this point the danger is clear. Early signs depend upon the depth of dive and the duration of exposure, coupled with the susceptibility of the individual to toxicity. Such things as tingling in the fingers and toes, visual disturbances, confusion, muscle twitching, nausea, and dizziness may precede the convulsion stage. Of course, any early warning should be followed by surfacing as quickly as possible.

The amount of time that pure oxygen can be tolerated at various depths is shown in Figure 91. Very little effect is noticed up to a depth of

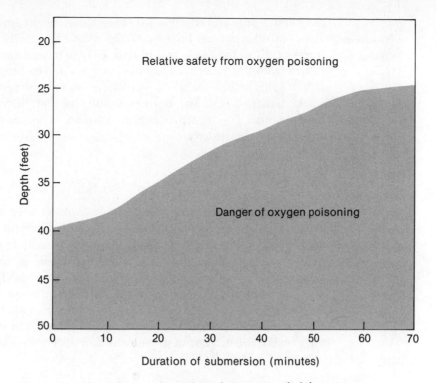

Figure 91. The Relation of Depth and Duration of Submersion to Oxygen Toxicity. [From G. J. Duffner, "Medical Problems Involved in Underwater Compression and Decompression," *Clinical Symposia*, CIBA Pharmaceutical Products, Inc., 10 (July-August 1958), p. 109.]

25 feet, and even at 30 feet there is relative safety for 40 minutes. Thereafter the individual runs the risk of toxic effects. Moreover, exercise tends to hasten the process, so sport diving and salvage operations should not be supported by a high-oxygen mixture. It is interesting to note that breathing pure oxygen at very low pressures (above 18,000 feet) even for extended periods does not lead to toxicity, and so it has been employed extensively in space exploration.

A search for the cause of oxygen toxicity has been somewhat elusive, but several concepts have been advanced.[9] (1) The amount of oxygen carried in physical solution in the blood, as compared with the oxyhemoglobin reaction, increases, so that the needs of the tissues for oxygen can be met from this source. This means that the oxygen bound to hemoglobin in the arterial blood remains unchanged as it circulates through the brain and other tissues, thereby changing the manner in which carbon dioxide is transported from the tissues, according to the Haldane effect (Chapter 8). (2) The high Po_2 may cause cerebral ischemia, owing to constriction of the cerebral blood vessels, although there is greater likelihood that the primary

[9]Hugh Davson and M. Grace Eggleton, eds., *Principles of Human Physiology* (Philadelphia: Lea & Febiger, 1968), pp. 504–506.

mechanism for this effect is the stimulation of respiration by increased P_{CO_2}. In other words, because of the reduced capacity of hemoglobin to transport CO_2, the tissue and plasma CO_2 is raised, and there is an interference with the buffer function of hemoglobin. The resulting hyperventilation would reduce the P_{CO_2} in arterial blood, bringing about cerebral vasoconstriction. (3) The third possibility is that there is a direct toxic effect of high P_{O_2} on tissue enzyme systems. This seems the most likely cause of oxygen toxicity.

Aerotitis

A common occurrence for most individuals is to experience pain or pressure in the ear upon diving. The increased pressure on the eardrum can be offset by equalizing the pressure behind it from the eustachian tube. Failing to do so can result in hemorrhaging in the middle ear and rupture of the eardrum. Sharp pain in the ear should be a warning of potential difficulty, and the dive should be terminated. Diving should not be attempted if the individual is suffering from an upper respiratory infection, because inflammation or edema occurring around the eustachian tube might make equalization of pressure difficult or impossible.

The Squeeze

The pressure of water against the body can be tolerated for the most part, but equipment worn about the head and face may predispose to a condition known as the *squeeze*. The difficulty is caused when areas of differential pressure are permitted to exist. A diver with a helmet must keep the air inside the helmet at the same pressure as that of the water outside. When this fails to happen, he risks the danger of literally being squeezed into his helmet. On a smaller scale the same may be said of the scuba diver wearing a face mask; he must remember to exhale into the mask during descent in order to equalize the pressure as he goes down. Failure to do so will usually result in very bloodshot eyes as extravasated blood is drawn to the surface of the conjunctiva. The use of goggles should be discouraged in diving because there is no way of equalizing pressure inside them.

Expansion of Air

Quite aside from the difficulties encountered as a result of decompression sickness, rapid ascent from any depth may be accompanied by still another problem: the expansion of air during decompression. Since the volume of a gas varies inversely with the pressure, as a person ascends there will be an increasing volume of air in his lungs. It is therefore imperative that he exhale continuously on the way up. Remember, if air is taken into the lungs at 100 feet it will expand four times in volume on the way up. If this were permitted to occur, alveoli would rupture and there would be immediate danger of *air embolism*, a condition characterized by the entry of bubbles of air into the bloodstream. The consequence is a blockage of blood flow to the heart or brain, causing the most serious results. Obviously, the diver must be aware of this possibility, ascend at a moderate pace, and exhale as he does so. Skin divers, on the other hand, who take a breath on the surface, will not be subject to the same difficulty, because the total volume will not increase on return.

Mammalian Responses to Diving

It has been known for some time that certain mammals, notably the seal, are enabled by various circulatory adjustments to undergo long dives with relative ease. Scholander *et al.*[10] point out that diving animals have considerably more blood, hemoglobin, and myoglobin than man, but not enough to explain the length of the dive. Apparently there is a tolerance to high P_{CO_2} and low P_{O_2}, but one of the most pronounced changes is a bradycardia (reduced heart rate). In the seal the heart rate may drop from a surface value of 80 beats per minute to 5 or 6 during a dive. In spite of this, the blood pressure remains normal, while vasoconstriction occurs at various sites. It has also been found that lactic acid increases in the muscles, but only a small amount enters the circulation until the animal reaches the surface and enters the recovery period.

Humans who dive have also shown circulatory adjustments.[11] Those who dive for food off the coast of Korea and Japan engage in breath holding of about a minute or less and descend to a depth of from 20 to 80 feet. Again, a noticeable bradycardia develops. Pearl divers have shown a similar slowing of heart rate, accompanied by normal blood pressure and followed by a sharp rise in blood lactates during recovery.

TEMPERATURE REGULATION

Each year a number of sports participants and others become fatalities as a result of exposure to excessive heat and subsequent dehydration. For the athlete, practice sessions that are held in the warm months with full equipment, as in football, are always subject to conditions that are potentially hazardous. With proper safeguards these dangers may be minimized. It is the purpose of this section to review some of the factors associated with temperature regulation and the possible mechanisms of acclimatization.

[10]P. F. Scholander *et al.*, "Circulatory Adjustments in Pearl Divers," *Journal of Applied Physiology*, 17(March 1962), 184.

[11]Suk Ki Hong and Herman Rahn, "The Diving Women of Korea and Japan," *Scientific American*, 216 (May 1967), 34.

Heat may be lost from the body in several ways—by radiation, conduction, convection, and evaporation.

Radiation.   Loss of heat from the body to cooler objects at a distance, as well as gain of heat by the body from warmer objects, can be accomplished by *radiation*. The magnitude of this loss or gain depends upon the difference in temperature between the skin and surrounding objects, but it has been estimated that a person at rest may lose 60 percent of his heat production by this process. The color of the skin makes some difference; the darker the skin, the greater will be the absorption of heat and the less the heat radiation. Thus, acquiring a tan does not protect one against heat absorption.

Conduction.   *Conduction* involves the loss of heat directly to surrounding objects. Ordinarily it accounts for only a small proportion of the body's total heat loss.

Convection.   If the surrounding temperature is lower than body temperature, heat will be lost by *convection*. The air immediately in contact with the skin becomes warmed and the molecules move away to be replaced by cooler ones, thus setting up a convection current. Increasing wind velocity hastens the process, but immersion in water is even more efficient.

Evaporation.   The conversion of one gram of water into water vapor results in the loss of .58 kcal of heat. This *evaporation* is the only method the body has of getting rid of heat when the surrounding temperature is greater than that of the skin. Thus, when 1 kg of water (about 1 liter) evaporates, 580 kcal of heat are lost from the body. Evaporation takes place from the lungs and the skin. In fact, a continual heat loss, averaging 15–20 kcal/hr, results from diffusion of water molecules through the skin and the lungs. This "insensible" perspiration (insensible because it cannot be felt) takes place rather uniformly regardless of environmental conditions, and represents some 600–800 ml per day, equivalent to about 400 kcal. On the other hand, sweating is the primary means of heat loss when body temperature rises.

When the humidity is high it is a common experience to note the presence of secreted sweat on the skin in the fluid state. According to gas laws, the evaporation into the atmosphere depends upon the amount of water vapor present, so on warm humid days when the atmosphere is already relatively saturated, sweat does not evaporate as readily as it does when the humidity is low. Since the evaporation provides the cooling, it follows that one feels more comfortable when the relative humidity is low, provided temperature remains the same. Thus, at times of high humidity, body temperature can continue to rise, even though copious sweating occurs.[12] This is the manner in which the steam bath or sauna works; the

[12]L. Brouha *et al.*, "Physiological Reactions of Men and Women during Muscular Activity and Recovery in Various Environments," *Journal of Applied Physiology*, 16 (January 1961), 133.

humidity is 100 percent, and all weight loss comes from the extracellular fluid. From discussion in Chapter 7 it should be clear that this loss of body weight does not come from the fat component.

It may be stated parenthetically at this point that in order to facilitate heat loss from the body by evaporation the type of clothing worn is important. Athletic shirts that are lightweight and porous permit evaporation and thus help regulate body temperature. Rubberized suits or clothing that become saturated with water prohibit this evaporation and thus trap the heat inside. This procedure, although a favorite way for wrestlers and other athletes to lose body weight quickly, presents a certain health hazard, just as a distance running event would do in the middle of a hot and humid day.

Sweating

Sweating is the primary mechanism for protecting the body from overheating in a hot environment or during exercise. Sweat glands themselves are of two types: eccrine and apocrine. *Eccrine* sweat glands are distributed widely over the body, secreting a dilute solution containing sodium chloride, urea, and lactic acid; the salt concentration ranges from .1 to .37 g percent. These glands are located principally in the palms of the hands and soles of the feet and in the head, although some may occur on the trunk and extremities. They are under control of cholinergic fibers of the sympathetic nervous system and are the primary means of controlling body temperature. *Apocrine* sweat glands develop mainly around hair follicles and are found primarily in the axillary and pubic regions. They are stimulated by thermal elevation, or by adrenaline, and can be produced by emotional stress. The strong odor characteristic of apocrine sweat is not due to the sweat itself, which is odorless, but to subsequent bacterial action.

The onset of sweating occurs on the nude person when the environmental temperature reaches approximately 88°F, or 84°F if wearing light clothing. Above this *set point*[13] there is a proportional increase in sweating with elevation in body temperature. The increase continues until a maximum point is reached, beyond which further increases in body temperature do not produce corresponding increases in rate of sweating. The maximum amount of sweat loss is approximately 1.5 1/hr in a person not accustomed to the hot environment, and may rise to 3.5 1/hr. in an acclimatized individual. More will be said about the acclimatization process later. Exposure to the sun for a six-hour period will cause a normal individual to lose approximately 2400 cc of sweat, and marathon runners may lose four to five liters of fluid during a race, amounting to 6 to 10 percent of the athlete's body weight.

[13]F. N. Craig, "Sweat Mechanisms in Heat," in Mohamed K. Yousef, Steven M. Horvath and Robert B. Bullard, eds., *Physiological Adaptations: Desert and Mountain* (New York: Academic Press, 1972), p. 53.

Regulation of Body Temperature

Regulation of body temperature is complex, yet it is possible to maintain temperature within a normal range of 97° to 100°F even though the temperature of the environment may vary from 70° to 125°F. The body is able to accomplish this both by *cutaneous receptors*, responsive to temperature changes such as involved in sweating or shivering, or by thermal mechanisms in the *anterior hypothalamus*, responsive to increased temperature of the blood. In addition, falling temperature is sensed by the *posterior hypothalamus*. Thus, stimulation of the anterior hypothalamus increases the rate of heat loss in the body by stimulating sweat glands to increase the cooling due to evaporation, and at the same time sending impulses to the vasodilator nerves of the skin, bringing the blood closer to the body surface for heat dissipation.

The activity of the posterior hypothalamus is to protect against cold, and it does so primarily by vasoconstriction, pulling the blood flow from the periphery toward the core in an effort to conserve heat. There is also an inhibiting effect on the anterior hypothalamus to reduce or virtually eliminate sweating. In addition, the secretion of epinephrine and nor-epinephrine increases cellular metabolism and with it the production of heat, at the same time stimulating shivering. It should be pointed out that in most areas of the world the effects of environmental cold are modified to a significant extent by the addition of clothing, so much so that working in a cold climate sometimes becomes more a matter of heat regulation than cold. Moreover, differing environments sometimes overlap. For example, high altitude is invariably accompanied by a cold climate, so the mountain climber must be able to respond both to low ambient pressure and to the rigors of cold weather as well.

Exercise and Heat Exchange

Most athletes and many observers seem to subscribe to the notion that elevating body temperature prior to vigorous performance is a wise procedure. It has not been very well substantiated in the research literature that this protects against injury to muscles or tendons. In fact, studies on warm-up point out that injuries seldom occur to subjects in the un-warmed state. However, athletes who have suddenly pulled a muscle for little apparent reason are quick to search for a cause. Often some change in the pattern of warming up has seemed to be responsible. This will be discussed in more detail later.

If sufficient activity is generated during exercise, one can anticipate substantial increases in body temperature. This change results in the gradual increase in activity of the anterior hypothalamus, causing first of all a peripheral vasodilation. The most important response, though, is an increase in the rate of sweating, which tends to keep pace with the in-crease in temperature. One of the essential requirements for this mechanism is that a sufficient amount of water must be present, which in turn means that there has to be a sufficient intake of water. Failure to keep pace with water loss by drinking fluids may cause dehydration, which then limits the amount of sweating and consequently impairs the temperature regulation, leading to very high body temperatures. Heat stroke may well be the consequence. It seems wise, therefore, to provide water on demand for athletes exercising in a hot environment.

Iampietro and Adams[14] summarize the heat production during exercise by pointing out that it may increase twelvefold over resting values, to as high as 960 kcal/hr. This is accomplished primarily by an increased skin blood flow, amounting to 400 ml/min at rest and 1,200 ml/min during exercise. The increased blood flow to the periphery is not without its problems to the performer. The hyperemic skin, plus a widespread muscular vasodilation, cause a decrease in the amount of peripheral resistance and a loss of blood volume, contributing to an elevated heart rate and general circulatory stress.[15] In addition, the volume of sweat that is secreted falls, and its sodium and chloride content rises.

Acclimatization to Heat

Individuals unaccustomed to high temperatures usually find themselves exhausted very quickly, unable to perform at a customary level. After several days, however, the ability to perform satisfactorily has returned. This represents an *acclimatization* to heat. The principal factor accounting for it is an increase in the sweating rate.[16] Sweating seems to begin at a lower body temperature and is more profuse at all temperatures, so that the total output of sweat is greater after acclimatization. Also, the sodium and chloride content falls as the electrolyte content of the extracellular fluid is maintained.

Second, there are changes in peripheral circulation, increasing the amount of vasodilation so that it is triggered at a lower temperature, which means that it is more generalized at all levels of body temperature. Thus, there is an increase in the sensitivity of the regulatory mechanisms, so that a smaller change in temperature produces a greater correction.

Acclimatization can be hastened when performing work, since exercise itself may be responsible for some of the physical changes observed, such as a decreased heart rate, skin and rectal temperature, and increased working ability.[17] Approximately one week of chronic exposure to heat is sufficient to cause acclimatization, provided work is performed at the same

---

[14]P. F. Iampietro and Thomas Adams, "Temperature Regulation," in Harold B. Falls, ed., *Exercise Physiology* (New York: Academic Press, 1968), p. 188.

[15]D. S. Kronfeld *et al.*, "Strenuous Exercise in a Hot Environment," *Journal of Applied Physiology*, 13 (November 1958), 425.

[16]H. S. Belding, "Biophysical Principles of Acclimatization to Heat," in Mohamed Yousef, Steven M. Horvath, and Robert W. Bullard, *Physiological Adaptations: Desert and Mountain* (New York: Academic Press, 1972), p. 9.

[17]Troy S. Cleland, Steven M. Horvath and M. Phillips, "Acclimatization of Women to Heat after Training," *Int. Z. angew. Physiol.*, 27 (1969), 15.

time. Apparently little acclimatization can be expected by exposure to heat alone.[18] This obviously has important practical implications for athletics, as contests frequently are played in very warm and humid climates. One team or individual could have an advantage if habitually training at high ambient temperatures when compared with others who might be used to cooler environments.

Effects of Cold

It is interesting to note that the human body is ordinarily faced with environmental temperatures below that of the core, so it must be able to adjust to what could be considered lower thermal levels. Deep body temperature is normally 98°–99°F, skin temperature around 93°F, yet comfortable environmental temperatures are found close to 70°F. In fact, rather low temperatures can be tolerated rather comfortably, although people ordinarily don heavier clothing and seek shelter rather than be exposed to the cold for any length of time. The body also seeks to maintain a homeostatic condition by increasing its heat production in addition to protecting itself against heat loss.

One of the first physiological adjustments to cold is to increase the metabolic rate, partly by secreting adrenaline and thyroid hormones, but in great part by shivering, which releases large amounts of heat in the muscles. In addition, heat loss is minimized by vasoconstriction of the cutaneous vessels, which restricts the amount of heat transported to the surface of the body. There may be some modification of this response to the hands and feet, however, which seem to experience an increased heat distribution by the vascular system to maintain temperatures higher than the rest of the body. Similar responses are experienced in the face and ears as well.

Extreme cold can be restrictive to the exercising person, as normal movement is often impaired; rapid movement of cold extremities becomes difficult. The key to success for athletics taking place in the cold would seem to be a combination of wearing proper clothing and warming the body through preliminary exercise. Clearly, the clothing should be adapted to the environmental conditions, but this must be consistent with the dictates of mobility and weight. Thus, the use of warm-up clothing may be helpful in preliminary practice to assist in raising core and surface temperatures so that the athlete may participate in lighter, more practical attire, provided the performance is started right away. Long delays may cause a chill if sweat has begun to flow on the skin surface. Once again, the clothing worn should be able to breathe, since heavy clothing may turn exercise in a cold environment into one in which the prime consideration is heat dissipation. Cross-country skiers and skaters, for example, fully realize that during their event lightweight clothing is usually sufficient protection. Spectators, on the other hand, may experience great discomfort

[18]Iampietro and Adams, *op cit.*, p. 191.

unless moving about. In addition, runners or joggers exercising in extremely cold conditions must beware of possible ill effects of drawing very frigid air into the lungs. Breathing through a mask serves to warm the air first and helps prevent any internal tissue damage.

Cold Acclimatization

A controversy exists with respect to the occurrence of acclimatization to cold in man. One might anticipate that cold and heat would affect body fluids in opposite ways. To a limited extent this is true, although the evidence tends to show that cold affects the fluid compartments less and not as predictably as does heat. Yet, some acclimatization seems to occur, especially in hands and feet. There is an increase in metabolic heat production, due in part at least to increased thyroid secretion, resulting in distribution of heat by the vascular system to maintain temperature of the extremities at a higher level than in the unacclimatized.[19]

WARM-UP

Warm-up is usually not thought of as an environmental problem, since the emphasis is less on the ambient temperature and more on the internal temperature. However, warm-up does involve a temperature change, so it will be discussed in this chapter. Our main thrust will be to discern any differences between *metabolic* warm-up and *nonmetabolic* warm-up. The literature usually discusses this as active versus passive warm-up; the former occurs as a result of some muscular activity, such as running or swimming; the latter may be effected by means of a water bath or shower. In other words, the temperature may increase from internal cellular heat production, or the application may be made to the external body surface in expectation that it will affect the internal milieu.

Earlier it was pointed out that athletic practice usually includes the ritual of warming up, partly because it will prepare the performer and permit him to make a maximum effort. Thus, an elevated temperature has the built-in proviso, at least in the mind of the athlete, that it may help performance, while cooling may impair performance. This conviction, incidentally, makes the study of warm-up difficult, since the design of the experiment usually calls for the performer to complete a task in an unwarmed state. Worry about the consequences of going all-out without a warm-up may inhibit a full effort and thus bias the results.

No agreement seems to exist as to what constitutes appropriate warm-up, and individual performers are apt to adopt a routine that is comfortable for them, whether or not any real metabolic change occurs. Thus, the warm-up for the runner in the short dash events differs from that of the distance runner. The hurdler includes a great deal of stretching

[19]G. Malcolm Brown *et al.*, "Cold Acclimatization," *Canadian Medical Association Journal*, 70 (March 1954), 258.

in his routine, and the basketball player engages in generalized activities centered around shooting baskets. The baseball pitcher requires quite a bit of throwing, and the kicker practices kicking field goals or punting. The swimmer, like the runner, needs to warm up more for the longer distance events. In short, not only is there no unanimity as to what constitutes an appropriate warm-up, but two performers in the same event may prepare differently.

The research literature on this topic has been extensive in the past several decades, yet no definitive statement on warm-up can be made. Part of the difficulty is in the specificity of tasks, part in the fact that some of the differences found, even if favoring warm-up, are small. Of course, it might be argued that for the champion performer a small improvement may be extremely meaningful, perhaps making the difference between winning and losing a contest. The research investigator, however, must demonstrate that any difference observed between a control condition and the warm-up condition can not be attributed to *chance* occurrence, occasioned by the fact that arithmetic differences between two conditions are bound to occur. In this respect, differences that are said to be *significant* indicate that some factor is operating to cause the difference, that the observed differences are not due to the factor of chance. Obviously, practice effects must be ruled out, which means that a control group is required, so that interpretation of significant differences, if favoring the experimental (warm-up) group, can be ascribed to the treatment itself.

A complete analysis of the literature cannot be accomplished here, so the reader may wish to refer to a more definitive treatment of the subject.[20] Using a nonmetabolic (passive) heat treatment has resulted in significant improvement in some activities, although deVries[21] failed to find that hot showers improved swimming times. In fact, he found that an active (swimming) warm-up was best. In the performance of short dash events, some form of warm-up may be beneficial, as many studies reflect improvement. Unfortunately, there are notable exceptions, which makes generalizations difficult.[22] The same holds true for longer events, although some warm-up, such as provided by jogging and calisthenics, is helpful in the mile run.[23]

Jumping has received quite a bit of attention, partly, one would suppose, because the vertical jump can be measured fairly objectively, and partly because it can be obtained in the laboratory. Environmental temperature can thus be controlled, and no strategy for the performer is involved. In addition, participation in the nonwarmed state seems to pose

[20]B. Don Franks, "Physical Warm-up," in William P. Morgan, ed., *Ergogenic Aids and Muscular Performance* (New York: Academic Press, 1972), chap. 6.

[21]Herbert A. deVries, "Effects of Various Warm-up Procedures on 100-Yard Times of Competitive Swimmers," *Research Quarterly*, 30 (March 1959), 11.

[22]Donald K. Mathews and H. Alan Snyder, "Effect of Warm-Up on the 440-Yard Dash," *Research Quarterly*, 30 (December 1959), 446.

[23]Amos Grodjinovsky and John R. Magel, "Effect of Warm-Up on Running Performance," *Research Quarterly*, 41 (March 1970), 116.

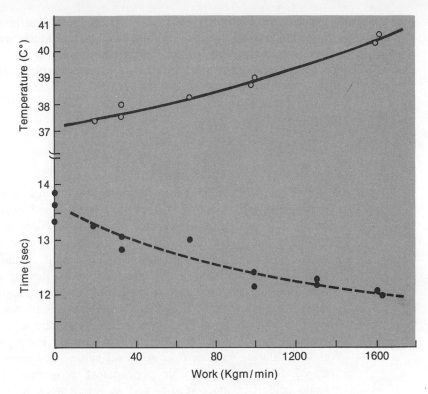

Figure 92. The Effect of Preliminary Warm-up on Short-Duration Bicycle Ergometer Sprint Times. [E. Asmussen and O. Boje, "Body Temperature and Capacity for Work," *Acta Physiologica Scandinavica*, 10 (1945), p. 13.]

little threat of injury, which should encourage all-out effort. Pacheco[24] found that three minutes of vigorous running in place produced a significant improvement. It should be noted that the warm-up was produced after a rather large amount of exercise.

The same may also be applicable to other tasks. One of the earliest formal warm-up studies was conducted by Asmussen and Boje,[25] who employed warm-up on a stationary bicycle, hot baths, radio diathermy, and massage, in addition to a no warm-up (control) condition, to observe their effects on short and long all-out bicycle ergometer rides. Also measured were rectal and muscle temperatures. It was found that massage was ineffectual, but passive warm-up did increase the capacity for work. Clearly dominant, however, were conditions of active, or metabolic, preliminary work; such improvement paralleled very closely the increased temperature of the working muscles. Both short-duration and long-duration tasks were improved as a result of warm-up. A somewhat surprising finding, shown in Figure 92, was that in one of the subjects, improvement was still being

[24]Betty A. Pacheco, "Effectiveness of Warm-Up Exercise in Junior High School Girls," *Research Quarterly*, 30 (May 1959), 202.

[25]Erling Asmussen and Ove Boje, "Body Temperature and Capacity for Work," *Acta Physiologica Scandinavia*, 10 (1945), 1.

experienced even after the preliminary exercise had reached 1,600 kgm/min. This extremely high rate should not be considered attainable by everyone, but it does emphasize that the warm-up, to be effective, must be vigorous enough to raise internal body temperatures, especially those of the appropriate muscles.

SUMMARY

The reduction in barometric pressure at high altitude reduces the partial pressure of oxygen so that the arterial blood will not be fully saturated. The density of air is decreased, so, in order to compensate, the individual may hyperventilate. Hypoxia (lack of oxygen at the tissue level) increases resting heart rate and cardiac output, pulmonary ventilation, systolic blood pressure, and blood lactic acid. Resting oxygen consumption does not change. Exercise capacity is impaired, and athletic performance involving endurance events deteriorates. Heart rate increases during exercise at altitude, although maximum heart rate is decreased, which is the pattern followed by total cardiac output. Pulmonary ventilation is elevated during exercise over sea-level values, and aerobic capacity is reduced. Short-term anaerobic performance is unaffected by altitude, but lactic acid rises more readily and at lower work loads. Acclimatization results in an increase in pulmonary ventilation, an increase in the amount of hemoglobin and number of erythrocytes, and a decrease in the alveolar-arterial gradient for oxygen.

Underwater diving exposes an individual to increased pressure, so that an additional atmosphere is experienced at 33 feet, doubling the partial pressure of oxygen. At 100 feet the individual is exposed to a total of four atmospheres of pressure. One of the hazards of breathing air under pressure is the potentiality for developing nitrogen narcosis, or "raptures of the deep," producing lethargy, euphoria, slowing of the mental processes, and other symptoms. Nitrogen dissolves into the fats of the body and the neurons. When an individual descends to a considerable depth there is the danger that the nitrogen will dissolve to a large extent in the tissues of the body. Rapid ascent could cause the formation of nitrogen bubbles in the tissues, resulting in circulatory blockage and tissue damage, a condition known as decompression sickness, or the "bends." Slow surfacing permits the nitrogen to dissolve safely into the blood to be exhaled. Breathing pure oxygen under pressure can impair tissue enzyme systems, leading to oxygen toxicity, resulting eventually in convulsions and coma. Pain in diving can be experienced in the ear and sinuses and, when sufficiently deep, about the body as well. Surfacing should be accompanied by exhalation, since the air in the lungs will expand and can cause air embolism to occur.

Heat may be lost from the body by radiation, conduction, convection, and evaporation. Continual heat loss may average 15–20 kcal/hr from diffusion of water through the skin and lungs, depending upon the humidity of the day. Sweating, the primary means of protecting the body from over-heating, occurs from eccrine and apocrine sweat glands. The onset of sweating for the lightly clothed person is 84°F. Under extreme conditions an individual can lose 1.5 l/hr, and more if acclimatized to the heat. Body temperature is regulated primarily by the anterior hypothalamus, which stimulates activity of the sweat glands and causes vasodilation of the skin blood vessels in an effort to dissipate the heat. The posterior hypothalamus protects against the cold primarily by directing blood flow toward the core of the body to preserve heat. Exercise causes a gradual increase in activity of the anterior hypothalamus to increase rate of sweating, which means that additional water intake may be required to prevent dehydration. Acclimatization results in an increased sweating rate and increased peripheral vasodilation, both of which can be hastened when the individual performs work in the heat. Acclimatization to cold may occur in the hands and feet, but this effect is not as consistently found as acclimatization to heat.

Warm-up, either metabolic (active) or nonmetabolic (passive), is practiced in some form by most athletes. Research shows some improvement by nonmetabolic means, although this is not a consistent finding. Rather, active warm-up, when fairly vigorous and extensive enough to cause elevated muscle temperature, seems best.

SELECTED REFERENCES

Adolph, E. F., "Heat Exchanges of Man in the Desert," *American Journal of Physiology*, 123 (1938), 486.

American College of Sports Medicine and the Athletic Institute, *Physiological Aspects of Sports and Physical Fitness,* "Symposium: Sport Performance in Hot Environments." Chicago: The Athletic Institute, 1968, pp. 31–52.

Asmussen, Erling, and Ove Boje, "Body Temperature and Capacity for Work," *Acta Physiologica Scandinavica*, 10 (1945), 1.

Balke, Bruno, "Variation in Altitude and its Effects on Exercise Performance," In Harold B. Falls, *Exercise Physiology*. New York: Academic Press, 1960, p. 246.

Brouha, L., *et al.*, "Physiological Reactions of Men and Women during Muscular Activity and Recovery in Various Environments," *Journal of Applied Physiology*, 16 (January 1961), 133.

Brown, G. Malcolm, *et al.*, "Cold Acclimatization," *Canadian Medical Association Journal*, 70 (March 1954), 258.

Franks, B. Don, "Physical Warm-Up," in William P. Morgan, ed., *Ergogenic Aids and Muscular Performance*. New York: Academic Press, 1972, chap. 6.

Goddard, Roy F., ed., *The Effects of Altitude on Physical Performance*. Chicago: The Athletic Institute, 1967.

Iampietro, P. F., and Thomas Adams, "Temperature Regulation," in Harold B. Falls, ed., *Exercise Physiology*. New York: Academic Press, 1968, p. 188.

Mathews, Donald K., and Edward L. Fox, *The Physiological Basis of Physical Education and Athletics*. Philadelphia: W. B. Saunders Company, 1971, chap. 6.

Scholander, P. F., *et al.*, "Circulatory Adjustments in Pearl Divers," *Journal of Applied Physiology*, 17 (March 1962), 184.

Yousef, Mohamed K., Steven M. Horvath, and Robert W. Bullard, eds., *Physiological Adaptations: Desert and Mountain*. New York: Academic Press, 1972.

Shephard, Roy J., *Alive Man! The Physiology of Physical Activity*. Springfield, Ill.: Charles C. Thomas, 1972.

physiology of physically handicapping conditions

Society today seems more sensitive to the medical aspects of sports, what with the emerging emphasis on sports medicine and the whole area of adapted physical education. Considerable publicity has been given to injuries and deaths in athletics, and a great deal of discussion has centered on prevention and treatment of such accidents. In addition, concern for increasing the active lifespan has stimulated an interest in the role of endurance exercise in protecting the cardiovascular system. Clinics and exercise-stress evaluation centers are emerging in substantial numbers, based on the belief that the heart and blood vessels can be protected and the vascular integrity can be upheld by systematic stressful exercise continued over a long period.

Programs of adapted physical education have been inaugurated in public schools to provide special instruction in physical activities, including adapted sports, in an effort to assist in overcoming handicapping conditions and achieve other benefits of regular exercise. These programs have their corollaries in physical rehabilitation clinics in hospitals and elsewhere for the immediate treatment of physical handicaps. Once the student is able to return to school there is still an obligation to provide adapted programs tailored to individual specifications dictated by the residual dysfunction. In many cases these programs are temporary, and the student develops the strength and endurance to return to regular physical education classes. In other cases the time in adapted classes may be extended. Both situations demand that the teacher be knowledgeable with respect to the disability so that an intelligent program can be developed and appropriate activities provided.

The responsibility for adequate care of adapted students rests heavily on the teacher. It is not enough simply to know how to adapt activities or how to administer exercise, important as they are. A key element is to know something of the medical history, including the prognosis and treatment of residual handicaps. Moreover, since many of the students qualifying for such programs have conditions that involve disturbances of some of the physiological mechanisms described in this text, it would seem important to focus attention, however briefly, on some of these conditions. The descriptions must be considered primarily as summaries, since it is beyond the scope of this chapter to attempt anything really definitive. Obviously, too, space limitations require that medical diagnosis and pre-

scription of treatment with the specific application to adapted programs be discussed elsewhere.[1] Within such a framework, then, we shall consider the relevant physiological aspects of physically handicapping conditions.

NEUROMUSCULAR CONDITIONS

Some of the most serious of the physically handicapping conditions are those that interrupt nerve transmission and muscle contraction. Annually, quite a number of accidents occur to young people, and others contract some debilitating disease which may have long-term residual effects. While the prognosis in some cases may be grave, many of these individuals become rehabilitated, or their condition stabilizes for a period of time, and they are able to attend school.

Multiple Sclerosis

Multiple sclerosis is a neurological disease, chronic in nature, that strikes young adults primarily between the ages of 20 and 40 years. Its course is unpredictable, and in fact resembles other related neuromuscular diseases, although multiple sclerosis is probably the most widely known and, indeed, most prevalent of the demyelinating diseases. It is characterized by destruction of the myelin sheath which covers the axon, creating what is known as "placques" scattered about the central nervous system. The demyelination interrupts the nerve impulse, either wholly or in part, resulting in impairment of muscle function and motor control. The prognosis is somewhat unpredictable, but individuals apparently achieve declining levels of disability, followed by periods of partial recovery, a sequence that may go on for a number of years.

Muscular Dystrophy

Several forms of *muscular dystrophy* exist, including the Duchenne (pseudohypertrophic) form, the type most widely encountered in young children, frequently occurring by six years of age. The term pseudohypertrophic refers to "false swelling," as fat deposition among muscles early in the disease gives the individual an appearance of being quite well developed. Fat infiltrates between individual muscle fibers, while the muscles themselves atrophy and gradually become weaker. There is a diminished concentration of creatine phosphate and potassium in the muscle, along with other clinical changes. Frequent falling, waddling gait, and signs of trunk weakness characterize this form of muscular dystrophy. The prognosis is grave, as the disease is progressive, few patients surviving beyond adolescence.

[1]H. Harrison Clarke and David H. Clarke, *Developmental and Adapted Physical Education* (Englewood Cliffs, N.J.: Prentice-Hall, Inc., 1963).

Myasthenia Gravis

Myasthenia gravis is a chronic neuromuscular disease characterized by the development of excessive weakness when performing voluntary muscle activity. This is a result of defective transmission of the action potential at the myoneural junction, either as the result of failure to produce sufficient acetylcholine, or because of excessive destruction of acetylcholine by cholinesterase. At any rate, activity brings about rapid fatigue and an exaggerated and prolonged recovery period. Most often affected are muscles of the eyes and those that control facial expression, mastication, and swallowing. Later, muscles of the neck, trunk, and limbs may become involved. Treatment with the drug Prostigmin (neostigmine), an anticholinesterase agent, may reverse the defect of neuromuscular transmission.

Anterior Poliomyelitis

Poliomyelitis in epidemic proportions has been essentially eliminated with the advent of the Salk vaccine, although on a global basis there may still be concern over whether it can be eliminated entirely. Poliomyelitis is caused by a filterable virus that may eventually reach the central nervous system. It is apt to cause gray matter damage, particularly in the anterior horn cells of the spinal cord. These lesions involve destruction of the neurons, with consequent loss, either wholly or partially, of motor function of the muscles. Over the twelve months following the acute episode maximal motor function will return, although in some individuals residual deficiencies may persist to become chronic handicaps.

Paraplegia

Paraplegia, a paralysis of the legs and lower portion of the body, is but one of the paralyzing conditions that may be caused by lesion of the spinal cord. When the cord is affected in the cervical region to affect both arms and legs as well as most of the trunk, it is termed *quadriplegia;* when the lesion occurs in one side of the brain and affects function on one side of the body only, it is called *hemiplegia*. The latter is a frequent result of a cerebral vascular accident (stroke).

Paraplegia is usually thought to occur as a result of some trauma to the spinal cord, such as would occur with a broken back accompanied by severance of the cord. Injury of this sort includes loss of motor control and sensory feedback and can be considered permanent. Complete flaccid paralysis ensues. The loss of normal motor and sensory control causes certain metabolic changes to occur after a short time. A loss in control of protein breakdown may occur, and certain blood changes leading to anemia may develop, disturbing normal water and electrolyte balance in the body.

In addition, lack of nervous control disturbs the heat regulating and sweat mechanisms and impairs sexual functions. For the quadriplegic with a high cord lesion, there is the additional difficulty that the motor control for pulmonary ventilation may be impaired.

The oxygen-uptake ability of the paraplegic is hindered when it comes to ambulation because of the great loss of muscle bulk, coupled with the fact that now the arms and shoulders must support on crutches the entire mass of the body. Since the lower extremities and perhaps the lower trunk must be supported by heavy braces, the metabolic cost of crutch walking can be severe. The $\dot{V}O_2$ max depends on metabolizing tissue; clearly, the paraplegic is at a major disadvantage at such times when moving about with crutches.

Peripheral Nerve Injuries

Injuries to peripheral nerves may occur as a result of some accident which interrupts the normal flow of action potentials and results in paralysis of the designated musculature. Careful muscle testing, therefore, can tell just which nerve is involved, and the site of the insult will determine the distance from the muscles that the injury has occurred. A completely severed peripheral nerve has some ability to repair itself. Schwann cells and fibroblasts from the central portion attempt to bridge the gap to the distal end of the nerve, where they may enter the neurilemmal tubes leading to the peripheral terminals. The rate of growth is normally considered to be 1 to 2 mm per day, so if the distance to be covered is long, the duration of regeneration is appropriately lengthened. Therapeutic treatment should include electrical stimulation applied directly to the involved muscles to prevent atrophy due to disuse. During this time electromyography may prove useful in evaluating the time course of return of function, since the action potentials may be detected before noticeable contraction can be seen. As pointed out in Chapter 1, fibers of the brain and spinal cord will not regenerate in this way.

METABOLIC DISORDERS

A number of disturbances of normal metabolism exist; we shall discuss here those conditions most appropriate to the field of adapted physical education. In this context we shall consider diabetes mellitus and the effects of extended bed rest.

Diabetes Mellitus

Diabetes is more prevalent in the adult population over 50 years of age than during younger years and is among the leading causes of death in the United States. It is a complex metabolic disease, apparently transmitted as a recessive genetic characteristic. Thus, mating of diabetics to either nondiabetics or diabetics is likely to produce the disease in the first or second generation. It is caused by a diminished or ineffective production of insulin secreted by the beta cells of the islets of Langerhans of the pancreas. Insulin is concerned primarily with the metabolism of carbohydrates but also of some protein and fat. It helps to maintain normal levels of blood glucose, regardless of a high or low caloric diet. Insulin is required to increase the rate of glucose transport through the membranes of most cells of the body. In the nondiabetic, ingestion of excessive carbohydrates causes the secretion of an abundance of insulin and consequently accelerates glucose transport. The reduction of insulin in the diabetic reduces glucose transport and impairs glycogen storage in skeletal muscle. Thus, the excess sugar accumulation in the blood is eliminated from the body in the urine.

The classical treatment for diabetes is the administration of insulin to provide the amount not provided by the pancreas. Since a great percentage of diabetics have had a history of obesity, there must also be a rigid control of the diet. The amount of exercise undertaken by the individual must also be calculated, and because exercise may help in the transport of glucose into the muscle cells, it may be an important adjunct to treatment. In fact, a balance among these three factors provides the best management of the diabetic. Many successful athletes have had diabetes, which attests to the fact that when the physician prescribes them, exercise and sports may be a part of the daily activities of such individuals.

Hypokinetic Disease (Bed Rest)

The concept of *hypokinetic disease* was developed at length by Kraus and Raab[2] in an effort to describe the widely ranging derangements resulting from a lack of physical activity. Many of these ill effects can be considered metabolic, but clearly there is a relationship with cardiovascular conditions, which will be discussed in the next section. The early use of ambulation by physicians following medical and surgical treatment is well established and constitutes essential therapy in hospitals. Unnecessary and excessive bed rest is considered debilitating, often leading to complications and delaying recovery. For the physical educator, reversal of the loss of physical conditioning caused by extended illness or disability constitutes a real challenge.

Bed rest increases the possibility of phlebothrombosis in the veins of the lower extremities and pulmonary embolism, both complications that can largely be avoided with exercise and by adopting an upright posture. In addition, decreased bowel activity leads to constipation, muscle atrophy leads to a loss of lean body mass and a reduction in nitrogen, potassium, and phosphorus from body tissues. Another problem of extended bed rest

[2]Hans Kraus and Wilhelm Raab, *Hypokinetic Disease* (Springfield, Ill.: Charles C. Thomas, 1961).

is the loss of calcium associated with atrophy of bone, along with a loss of vasomotor tone and blood volume, leading to hypotension and tachycardia.

A number of circulatory changes were noted by Saltin *et al.*[3] in subjecting male volunteers to a 20-day period of bed rest. The $\dot{V}o_2$ max declined by 27 percent, from 3.3 l/min to 2.4 1/min. At a standard work load (600 kgm/min) the stroke volume decreased 25 percent, from 116 to 88 ml, while at the same time the heart rate rose about 19 percent, from 129 to 154 beats per minute. Because the arteriovenous difference for oxygen increased slightly, the cardiac output fell from 14.4 to 12.4 1/min. Maximal running caused the cardiac output to fall by 26 percent, from 20.0 1/min to 14.8 1/min. Since the maximal heart rate did not change, the drop in cardiac output was attributed to a reduction in stroke volume.

CARDIOVASCULAR CONDITIONS

The category of cardiovascular conditions contains all those factors associated with diseases of the heart and blood vessels. The study of exercise physiology is properly concerned with the seemingly well person, but unfortunately, so many thousands annually become victims of coronary heart disease, that it becomes not only a significant health problem but also a matter for prevention as well. The overwhelming majority of medical reports from many countries points out the role played by inactivity and sedentary living in the incidence of heart disease. Moreover, the treatment in the recovery period following survival of an initial attack ordinarily includes an exercise regimen designed to provide some protection against future attacks. Thus, the spectrum of adapted physical education, especially for the older individual, should include concern for the cardiovascular domain.

CORONARY HEART DISEASE

The present discussion will center on coronary heart disease (CHD), which encompasses a host of symptoms and manifestations accompanying complications caused by narrowing or blockage of the coronary arteries. Loss of blood supply to the myocardium, causing the muscle in that region to die, is called a *myocardial infarction* or, more popularly, a heart attack. The immediate cause of an occlusion of this sort may be a blood clot, or *thrombus*, which blocks the artery. When the blockage occurs in one of the major avenues of the coronary artery network, the attack may be considered "massive," since there is likely to be a wholesale restriction of blood to the heart. If the obstruction is further along, the result may be milder, with only a few symptoms of circulatory insufficiency.

[3]Bengt Saltin *et al.*, "Response to Exercise after Bed Rest and after Training," *Circulation*, 38, Supplement 7 (November 1968), 1.

The term *atherosclerosis* refers to a disease of the large arteries in which deposits of lipid appear on the subintimal layer. These *atheromatous placques* are especially high in cholesterol. When they occur in the coronary arteries, the rate of blood flow and the amount of blood going to the heart are reduced, gradually increasing the probability of a coronary heart attack. In later life these degenerative areas may be infiltrated with fibroblasts, causing progressive sclerosis of the arteries. When calcium reacts with the lipids, calcified placques occur, the arteries become quite hard, and a condition called *arteriosclerosis* occurs. The loss of distensibility means that they are more easily ruptured, and the roughened inner surface may cause the formation of blood clots. Should one break off and enter the circulation, it could lodge in a coronary artery. An additional problem associated with arteriosclerosis is the increase in blood pressure that occurs because the arteries have become less elastic, which itself puts greater pressure on a vascular system already less capable of coping with such circumstances.

The factors identified as contributing to CHD are numerous, including high blood pressure (hypertension), smoking, obesity, heredity, blood lipid abnormalities. electrocardiographic (ECG) abnormalities, and other problems. Also mentioned by most cardiologists concerned with this matter is a general lack of exercise that seems to predispose a person to coronary heart disease. Fox, Naughton, and Haskell[4] point out that while there may be a presumption that progressive inactivity is a major contributing factor to CHD, clear proof is still lacking. Moreover, it is not necessarily assured that increasing activity will forever reverse the risk of CHD. In fact, because many of the predisposing factors are somewhat interrelated, isolating one factor would not be very appropriate. Until the longitudinal studies clearly show a cause-and-effect relationship, we must be tentative in such generalizations. Be that as it may, however, there is considerable evidence that inactivity is at least *associated* with the occurrence of coronary heart disease.

A complete review of studies concerned with physical activity and coronary heart disease is beyond the scope of this text, although a review is available from a publication of the President's Council on Physical Fitness and Sports.[5] Studies indicate that individuals engaged in physically strenuous occupations tend to have less incidence of CHD and overall a reduction in mortality. This is not to say that all research is in agreement, but the trend is strongly in this direction. Some of the difficulties encountered involve first of all finding a suitable sample of individuals who are habitually physically active. The next thing is to make sure that some selection factor has not made one group different than another, so that the sedentary group does not contain all those who for one reason or another were unable to perform in the active occupation. Further, it is

[4]S. M. Fox, J. P. Naughton, and W. L. Haskell, "Physical Activity and the Prevention of Coronary Heart Disease," *Annals of Clinical Research*, 3 (1971), 404.

[5]"Physical Activity and Coronary Heart Disease," *Physical Fitness Research Digest*, April, 1972.

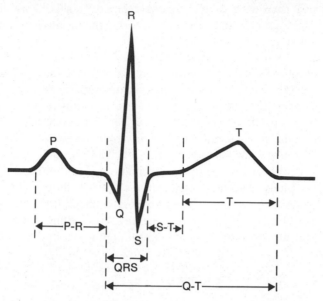

Figure 93. The Electrocardiogram.

important to try and rule out other factors, if possible, that might be a cause of CHD. At any rate, there is every reason to be optimistic about the role that regular exercise may play in the prevention and treatment of coronary heart disease.

Cardiac Abnormalities

It would be presumptuous and unwise to attempt a major description of cardiac abnormalities, since it would of necessity be incomplete. The typical electrocardiogram (ECG) was discussed in Chapter 10, and it might be helpful to review the normal ECG once again. Part of a medical examination involves the monitoring of heart sounds, in an effort to detect disease of the valves. Improperly functioning valves give rise to *murmurs*. However, the electrocardiogram is a more helpful tool in diagnosing CHD, especially since many manifestations appear as irregularities (Figure 93).

The P-R interval is the elapsed time between the beginning of atrial excitation to the start of ventricular excitation, and any lengthening of this interval would signify abnormality in the A-V conduction system. Similarly, extending the time of the QRS complex would suggest abnormality in depolarization of the ventricles. A meaningful observation can come with an *S-T segment depression.* Such an occurrence signifies myocardial ischemia,[6] a reduced blood supply to the heart, and might suggest exces-

---

[6]Robert A. Bruce, "Comparative Prevalence of Segmental S-T Depression after Maximal Exercise in Healthy Men in Seattle and Taipei," in Martti J. Karvonen and Alan J. Barry, eds., *"Physical Activity and the Heart* (Springfield, Ill.: Charles C. Thomas, 1967).

sive narrowing of the coronary blood vessels. This condition often produces pain, called *angina pectoris*, that may develop from physical or emotional factors.

A *premature ventricular systole*, or premature ventricular contraction, occurs when the ventricular myocardium discharges out of phase with the regular rhythm. This originates from some independent source, known as *ectopic foci*, and is followed by a compensatory pause that actually lengthens the normal cardiac cycle. Extrasystoles are fairly common but become more serious should *ventricular fibrillation* occur. Here the ventricles are contracting in an irregular and ineffectual way, so that blood is not effectively pumped. Fibrillation, if not stopped immediately, is fatal. Hospitals and emergency stations are usually equipped with an electronic defibrillator which delivers an electric shock directly over the heart to stop the fibrillation and return the regular rhythm. External cardiac massage may also be employed for the same purpose.

Exercise Stress Testing

It is generally conceded that the resting electrocardiogram may not provide sufficient information to judge the fitness of the cardiovascular system to withstand stresses such as exercise. In fact, an individual with a normal ECG at rest could have abnormal signs during exercise. For this reason, it is increasingly recommended that medical examinations include an exercise stress test. This is essential for adults who contemplate beginning an exercise program, and it is an excellent adjunct to a program for a postcardiac patient.

The stress test is designed to monitor the electrocardiogram and blood pressure as the individual is taken through a series of progressive work loads, each lasting for a few minutes, until a steady state at that work level is obtained. If everything is satisfactory, the next level is started, and thus the various stages become progressively more severe as the subject is taken to the last intended work load. The exercise stress test is not designed to be maximal; in fact at least 85 percent of the age-adjusted maximum heart rate is usually chosen prior to the test. Thus, the test is terminated when this predetermined heart rate has been reached, or earlier if signs or symptoms of distress are noted. A more complete stress test would also include measures of $\dot{V}o_2$ and $\dot{V}e$, providing information on aerobic capacity and pulmonary ventilation.

It should be pointed out that the exercise stress test used as a diagnostic tool must be supervised by a physician, preferably one trained to interpret the data from such an examination, and conducted by someone designated by him who has been properly trained to critically observe test results. Any indication of cardiac difficulty would mean an immediate termination of the test and referral to a physician. This is the usual procedure to be followed in testing an apparently healthy adult. More stringent precautions must be taken if coronary heart disease is already suspected, or if the individual has had such a history.

It is beyond our present scope to set forth all of the types of exercise programs that could be employed to result in fitness gains and CHD protection. It does seem reasonably clear that extended endurance work of a running or jogging nature leads to the sorts of changes in circulation and aerobic capacity that are needed, as compared with weight lifting and short-term activities. The well-rounded fitness program, though, would make use of both forms of exercise. The usual treatment of the postcardiac patient, once the acute episode has passed and rehabilitation has begun, is to increase the level of activity gradually over a period of time, so that he enlarges his exercise capacity enough as to permit a normal life style with some reserve for emergencies. Ordinarily this will mean adopting exercise as a part of the daily routine, striving to improve cardiovascular endurance. Since the motivation may well be high, such persons schedule exercise just as conscientiously as any other important event. It is interesting to note that occasionally, former cardiac patients have actually developed such high states of fitness that they have been able to compete without difficulty in age-group distance running events.

SUMMARY

The appearance of programs of adapted physical education has brought a concern for an understanding of the medical disabilities associated with handicapping conditions. Multiple sclerosis, characterized by destruction of the myelin sheath covering the axon, creates placques widely scattered about the central nervous system. This interrupts normal motor control. Muscular dystrophy of the Duchenne form results in the infiltration of fat between individual muscle fibers and a gradual atrophy and weakening of the muscles. Myasthenia gravis results from defective transmission of action potentials at the myoneural junction, either from an insufficient production of acetylcholine or from an excessive destruction of acetylcholine by cholinesterase. This brings about rapid fatigue and prolonged recovery from exercise. Anterior poliomyelitis is caused by a filterable virus that results in damage to the anterior horn cells of the spinal cord, destroying the neurons and thus the motor function of muscles. Paraplegia usually occurs as a result of some injury to the spinal cord, leading to loss of motor and sensory control of muscles below that level. A number of metabolic disturbances follows. Peripheral nerve injuries may regenerate because of the presence of Schwann cells, which are lacking in the central nervous system itself.

Diabetes mellitus is a complex metabolic disease caused by an insufficient secretion of insulin by the pancreas. Insulin helps in maintaining normal levels of blood glucose and is required to increase the rate of glucose transport through cell membranes. The diabetic has an impairment in muscle glycogen storage. Bed rest leads to a number of metabolic consequences, including phlebothrombosis, pulmonary embolism, decreased bowel activity, muscle atrophy, and reductions in nitrogen, potassium, phosphorus, and calcium, as well as a loss of vasomotor tone and blood volume. The aerobic capacity declines considerably, as do cardiac output and circulation.

Coronary heart disease encompasses those symptoms accompanying reduction in blood supply to the heart muscle due to narrowing or blockage of the coronary arteries. Atherosclerosis results in a deposition of lipid on the subintimal layer of arteries; the deposit is especially high in cholesterol. When the arteries become hardened, the condition is known as arteriosclerosis. Coronary heart disease is precipitated by such factors as high blood pressure, smoking, obesity, electrocardiographic abnormalities, and others, including lack of exercise. Of particular significance on the electrocardiogram is an S-T segment depression, which signifies myocardial ischemia, a condition that often causes angina pain. Diagnosis of cardiac abnormality can best be made by employing an exercise stress test, and then prevention can include a progressive, well-rounded fitness program.

SELECTED REFERENCES

Alpers, Bernard J., and Elliott L. Mancall, *Clinical Neurology*, 6th ed. Philadelphia: F. A. Davis Company, 1971.

Clarke, H. Harrison, and David H. Clarke, *Developmental and Adapted Physical Education*. Englewood Cliffs, N.J.: Prentice-Hall, Inc., 1963.

Cooper, Kenneth H., "Guidelines in the Management of the Exercising Patient," *Journal of the American Medical Association*, 211 (March 9, 1970), 1663.

Fox, S. M., J. P. Naughton, and W. L. Haskell, "Physical Activity and the Prevention of Coronary Heart Disease," *Annals of Clinical Research*, 3 (1971), 404.

Hamwi, George J., and T. S. Danowski, *Diabetes Mellitus: Diagnosis and Treatment*, Vol. II. New York: American Diabetes Association, Inc., 1967.

Karvonen, Martti, and Alan J. Barry, eds., *Physical Activity and the Heart*. Springfield, Ill.: Charles C. Thomas, 1967.

Kraus, Hans, and Wilhelm Raab, *Hypokinetic Disease*. Springfield, Ill.: Charles C. Thomas, 1961.

Parmley, Loren F., *et al.*, eds., "Proceedings of the National Workshop on Exercise in the Prevention, in the Evaluation, in the Treatment of Heart Disease," *Journal of the South Carolina Medical Association*, 65, Supplement 1 (December 1969), 1.

"Physical Activity and Coronary Heart Disease," *Physical Fitness Research Digest*, April 1972; "Exercise and Blood Cholesterol," *Physical Fitness Research Digest*, July 1972; "Effects of Exercise on Risk Factors Associated with Coronary Heart Disease," *Physical Fitness Research Digest*, October 1972.

Saltin, Bengt, *et al.*, "Response to Exercise after Bed Rest and after Training," *Circulation*, 38, Supplement 7 (November 1968), 1.

measurement and evaluation

The field of exercise physiology comes alive when one can begin to apply knowledge through measurement of performance. Just as the athlete wants to know how fast he is running, so the exercise physiologist wants to know why. Time on the stopwatch is the result, the aerobic capacity is the cause. Superficially, contests are won by best times, but the reason is closely interwoven with the physiological events that support individual effort. The premise that underlies the study of exercise physiology is that the individual, his teacher, and his coach should understand the mechanisms that form the foundation for physical performance, and should also understand their measurement.

It is customary for undergraduate students to have a course in measurement and evaluation, where they learn the fundamentals of testing as well as the method of treating test scores. Usually some stress is placed upon tests of physical or physiological fitness, emphasizing the applicability to the physical education class—and the more practical the test the better. In fact, if it can be self-administered, or done by students in pairs, it seems to be favored. Since some of the widely known field tests require little equipment and minimal facilities, they tend to be used more extensively; however, most of them provide but limited insight into the underlying physiological mechanisms, and they become simply performance measures.

The use of fitness tests is not being criticized, for they can play an important role in total program development. This chapter, however, will attempt to expand measurement and evaluation into the physiological realm, which will call for some tests requiring extensive and technical equipment that would be available only in fairly well-equipped laboratories or clinics. This seems justifiable, since the trend in colleges and universities is to provide such facilities for advanced undergraduate and graduate work in physical education. Moreover, the increase in stress testing as an adjunct to adult fitness has meant an increase in instrumentation. Equipment manufacturers have become sensitive to these trends, and the growth in laboratory hardware reflects these developments.

Another current trend in undergraduate exercise physiology is an increased emphasis on laboratory experiences. Students are now exposed to regular laboratory experiments dealing with the underlying physiological mechanisms, so that many of the ideas expressed in lecture can be observed in practice. Moreover, some of the equipment and facilities might be available so that the student can gain experience in administering the tests. The reader is encouraged to become familiar with measurement and evaluation in exercise physiology and to make use of as many of the tests as possible.

MUSCULAR STRENGTH AND ENDURANCE

Strength Tests

Tests of muscular strength are among the oldest of objective measurements. Development of muscular force was a requirement in earlier civilizations where survival depended upon the ability to protect one's life and to provide food and shelter. According to Hunsicker and Donnelly,[1] the first scientific study of the measurement of strength was conducted in 1699 by a French scientist, De La Hire, who compared the strength of men with that of horses in lifting weights and carrying loads. In the nineteenth century instruments called *dynamometers* appeared, which were the forerunners of those in use today.

Cable-Tension Strength Tests

The reader will be acquainted with many of the devices that can serve to measure maximum strength. Single isolated tests, however, do not necessarily reflect the strength of the body as a whole. What is needed are representative tests of appropriately selected muscle groups. The cable tensiometer allows for testing of a variety of such groups; in fact, instructions are available for thirty-eight tests involving the following joints: fingers, thumb, wrist, forearm, elbow, shoulder, neck, trunk, hip, knee, and ankle.[2] Recently, the use of a battery of these tests as an overall indicator of body strength has proven successful. In fact, such batteries are available for both boys and girls at the upper elementary, junior high school, and college levels.[3]

Test Instructions. It would not be appropriate to give all of the instructions for each of the tests mentioned above, but since those for boys were the same at each level, they are illustrated in Figure 94. Some special equipment is needed to administer these tests. First of all, depending upon the strength of the subject, more than one tensiometer[4] is likely to be required. The tensiometer with a capacity of 200 lb is the most useful one for testing upper arm and shoulder movements, and it is used for all tests

[1]Paul A. Hunsicker and Richard J. Donnelly, "Instruments to Measure Strength," *Research Quarterly*, 26 (December 1955), 408.

[2]H. Harrison Clarke and David H. Clarke, *Developmental and Adapted Physical Education* (Englewood Cliffs, N.J.: Prentice-Hall, Inc., 1963), pp. 73–96.

[3]H. Harrison Clarke and Richard A. Monroe, *Test Manual: Oregon Cable-Tension Strength Test Batteries for Boys and Girls from Fourth Grade through College* (Eugene, Oregon: University of Oregon, 1970).

[4]Manufactured by Pacific Scientific Co., Inc., Anaheim, California 92803.

BOYS	GIRLS

Upper Elementary School

BOYS	GIRLS
Shoulder extension	Shoulder extension
Knee extension	Hip extension
Ankle plantar flexion	Trunk flexion

Junior High School

BOYS	GIRLS
Shoulder extension	Shoulder extension
Knee extension	Hip extension
Ankle plantar flexion	Trunk flexion

Senior High School

BOYS	GIRLS
Shoulder extension	Shoulder flexion
Knee extension	Hip flexion
Ankle plantar flexion	Ankle plantar flexion

College

BOYS	GIRLS
Shoulder extension	Shoulder flexion
Knee extension	Hip flexion
Ankle plantar flexion	Ankle plantar flexion

at the elementary school level. A 400-lb tensiometer will be needed for some junior high school boys and for boys and girls at the senior high school and college levels. An 800-lb tensiometer will be needed for senior high school boys and college men.

A testing table is necessary, as well as an assortment of appropriate straps and cables. In addition, a goniometer is necessary for measuring joint angles.

Scoring. In each instance the total score, called the *Strength Composite* (SC), is the sum of the three strength tests in pounds. The *Strength Quotient* (SQ) is found by dividing the achieved SC by the normal SC and mutiplying by 100.

Norms. Norms for the Strength Composite are shown in Tables A–1 to A–6 of the Appendix, based on age and weight separately for boys and girls from upper elementary school through senior high school. For college men and women (Tables A–7 and A–8) two scoring scales are used: (1) a double-entry table based on arm and abdominal girths for men, and arm girth and sitting height for women; and (2) a Strength Composite T scale.

Muscular Endurance

As brought out in Chapter 3, some performances under the guise of muscular strength are in reality measures of muscular endurance. The number of push-ups or sit-ups indicates endurance rather than strength. Yet it

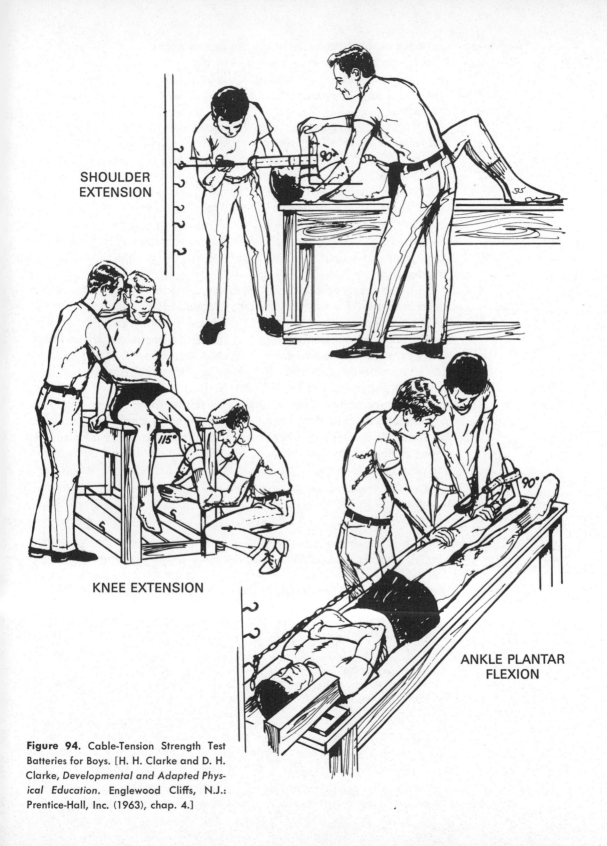

SHOULDER EXTENSION

KNEE EXTENSION

ANKLE PLANTAR FLEXION

Figure 94. Cable-Tension Strength Test Batteries for Boys. [H. H. Clarke and D. H. Clarke, *Developmental and Adapted Physical Education*. Englewood Cliffs, N.J.: Prentice-Hall, Inc. (1963), chap. 4.]

may be desirable to know an individual's endurance capacity in rather specific muscle groups. In this case it would be necessary to isolate the body segment and measure its performance. Even so, there has been very little standardization of procedure, and comprehensive norms are not as yet available.

The term "ergograph" was first defined in 1890 by Mosso,[5] who performed a series of experiments in which a weight was raised and lowered as a finger was flexed and extended. Various modifications of this *weight-loaded* device have been made over the years; some of the most widely used have been the Kelso-Hellebrandt ergographs,[6] originally designed for disability evaluation. The subject must raise and lower weights according to an established rhythm and usually at a percentage of maximum strength. Shaver[7] found that young male subjects could manage about 35 percent of strength in elbow flexion at a cadence of 30 repetitions per minute.

A more recent device has been the California *spring-loaded* ergograph employed for studying muscular fatigue of the hand-gripping muscles.[8] Each individual contraction of the hand is made against the spring of the Smedley hand dynamometer, so when it is connected to a variable-speed kymograph a continuous record can be obtained of the entire endurance performance. Some laboratories are becoming equipped with special strain gauges or force transducers to permit just as wide a testing of muscle groups as would be allowed with tensiometers. These are usually connected to special laboratory recorders[9] so that a continuous record can be obtained. Interesting laboratory experiments can be conducted comparing rhythmic (isotonic) bouts of differing cadences with static (isometric) exercise.

CARDIOVASCULAR VARIABLES

A number of cardiovascular variables can be measured, but those that require the most extensive calculations involve the assessment of oxygen uptake. Energy expenditure may be approached either directly or indirectly. The direct method of calorimetry requires a body calorimeter to measure the heat given off by the body, but since this device is seldom

[5]Angelo Mosso, *Fatigue*, trans. M. and W. B. Drummond (New York: G. P. Putnam's Sons, 1906).

[6]F. A. Hellebrandt, Helen V. Skowland, and L. E. A. Kelso, "New Devices for Disability Evaluation: Hand, Wrist, Radioulnar, Elbow and Shoulder Ergographs," *Archives of Physical Medicine*, 29 (January 1948), 21.

[7]Larry G. Shaver, "Maximum Isometric Strength and Relative Muscular Endurance Gains and Their Relationships," *Research Quarterly*, 42 (May 1971), 194.

[8]David H. Clarke and H. Harrison Clarke, *Research Processes in Physical Education, Recreation, and Health* (Englewood Cliffs, N.J.: Prentice-Hall, Inc., 1970), pp. 271–272.

[9]David H. Clarke, "The Influence on Muscular Fatigue Patterns of the Intercontraction Rest Interval," *Medicine and Science in Sports*, 3 (Summer 1971), 83.

found in laboratories of exercise physiology, the method will not be considered further here. Indirect calorimetry, on the other hand, is the most common method employed in determining the energy cost of activity, and consists of either the *closed-circuit* or the *open-circuit* method.

Closed-Circuit Method

The simplest of the two methods of assessing $\dot{V}o_2$, the closed-circuit method, simply requires the subject to inhale oxygen from a closed source, a spirometer, and exhale back into the system. The expired air passes through a canister of soda lime which absorbs the carbon dioxide and readmits the oxygen. As successive breaths are taken, the cylinder rises and falls, but since some of the oxygen is being used for purposes of metabolism, the cylinder gradually settles lower and lower. Respirometers of this sort are equipped with an ink-writing unit with variable-speed kymograph so that a breath-by-breath record is obtained (Figure 95).

The estimated trend of the respiratory line is used to compute the oxygen utilization. When steady-state conditions prevail, the trend will be linear, so it is usually possible to draw a line that represents that trend. Knowing the volume characteristics given on the kymograph paper allows us to calculate $\dot{V}o_2$. As shown in Figure 96, the first portion is the subject at rest, the second is the steeper exercise trend, and the third is a recovery from exercise. According to the theory established in Chapter 6, a slight deficit would occur as the subject began exercise. This can be seen in Figure 96, where a short time was required before the steady state is achieved. The work load was rather modest (750 kgm/min), so during the major portion of exercise steady-state conditions prevailed, as indicated by the fact that the respiratory line was linear. Note the increase in respiration rate and depth during this time. Note also that slight increments in single breaths do not significantly affect the trend line. Also according to theory, the immediate postexercise interval should be given to paying off any alactic or lactic debt incurred during this exercise. Notice the repayment period during the first minute or so of recovery, until resting conditions are once again reestablished. It is not unusual to find this portion of rest elevated slightly over the preexercise value. This incomplete recovery represents some sort of ergogenic shift in the resting level, perhaps brought about by changes in cellular temperatures. For present purposes the oxygen debt may be calculated as the difference in recovery from exercise over and above that which would have occurred at rest. In this case it would seem permissible to use the later portion of recovery as an estimate of resting rate. It should be mentioned that it is appropriate to correct all measures to standard temperature and pressure dry (STPD), since we have learned that a volume of gas will vary according to the temperature and pressure to which it is exposed. More will be said about these corrections later, when we discuss open-circuit calorimetry.

Respiratory rate can be determined by counting the number of breaths per minute, and $\dot{V}_E$ can be calculated by measuring the volume of

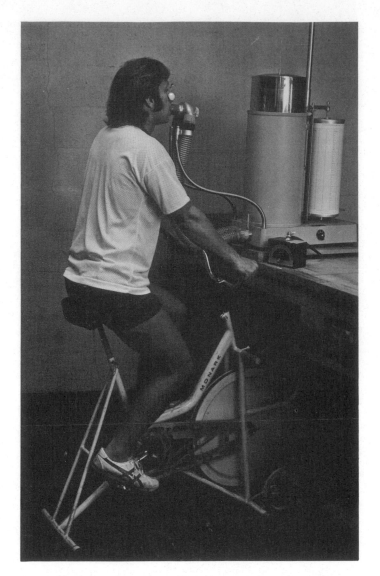

Figure 95. Closed-Circuit Method of Obtaining Oxygen Uptake.

each breath over a given period. Since no value for carbon dioxide production is available, the respiratory exchange ratio is not known. Moreover, there is an additional limitation in the use of closed-circuit devices during heavy exercise, since extensive movement of the subject may make measurement very difficult. Not only that, but a limitation in the oxygen capacity of the respirometer may make heavy work loads impossible. In fact, even with low work loads it may be necessary at certain times to refill the canister to avoid having to stop the subject or interrupt the experiment.

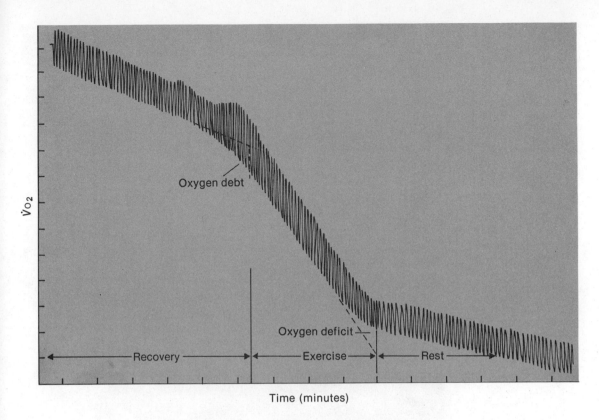

Figure 96. Measurement of the Closed-Circuit Record.

Open-Circuit Method

The open-circuit method is preferred in obtaining energy-cost data because it is ordinarily more accurate and is not affected by subject movement and variations in respiratory rate. What makes it an open circuit is the fact that the individual inhales atmospheric air, the composition of which is known, and exhales into a collection receptacle, the composition of which must be determined. The difference in composition between the two will reflect the energy cost as the body uses oxygen and produces carbon dioxide. The equipment is more extensive than used in the closed-circuit method, and the measurements more exacting, and consequently more valid for all ranges of work loads.

The subject is equipped with a three-way high-velocity valve and mouthpiece which permits inhalation of atmospheric air and exhalation into the collection assembly. The use of Douglas bags to collect the expired air permits the separation of periods of rest, exercise, and recovery; or a single large gasometer may suffice (Figure 97). At any rate, there must be available sufficient accessories, including nose clip, hoses, and four-way or five-way valves to direct the expired air to appropriate bags when used.

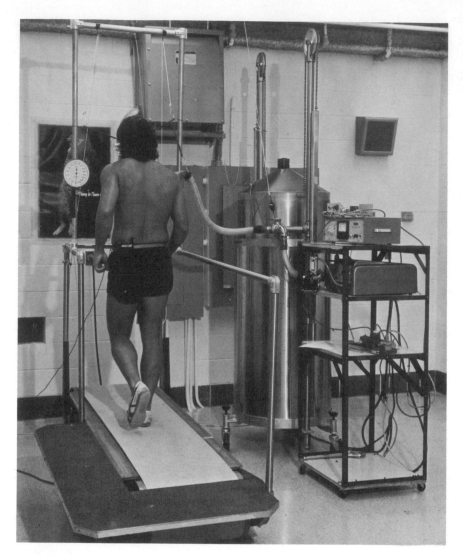

Figure 97. Open-Circuit Method of Obtaining Oxygen Uptake.

Following the collection, the volume of air in each bag must be measured by passing the contents through a dry gas meter. In addition, the concentration of oxygen and carbon dioxide must be determined. We can do this by withdrawing a small sample of expired air and subjecting it to analysis by means of a Haldane or Scholander gas analyzer. This procedure is eminently satisfactory, but great precision is required not only in making the actual measurement but in preparing the apparatus with proper chemicals in the first place. The alternative is to use a continuous automatic recorder and have the air drawn through by a vacuum pump. Not only can the content of the air be analyzed, but if the air is first drawn through a gas meter, the volume can be obtained at the same time. Remember to note the temperature of the gas and the total barometric pressure, so that appropriate corrections may be made later to the volume of gas.

Calculations. A number of calculations are required to complete the analysis of $\dot{V}_{O_2}$ from open-circuit data. The use of automatic analyzers help in the area of data acquisition, but there is still quite a bit of work to do to finally achieve the end result, and this work must be repeated for all collection bags. For those who may contemplate making such calculations routinely, or who have ready access to a computer, a program for data of this sort has been prepared.[10] The following calculations are required:

1. Volume of ventilation per minute, ambient temperature and pressure, saturated ($\dot{V}_E$ ATPS).

$$\dot{V}_E \text{ ATPS} = \dot{V}_E \times \frac{60}{ct},$$

where $\dot{V}_E$ = volume of expired gas as measured.
ct = collection time in seconds.
60 = conversion of volume from seconds to minutes.

2. The $\dot{V}_E$ ATPS is converted to volume of ventilation per minute, body temperature and pressure, saturated ($\dot{V}_E$ BTPS), as follows:

$$\dot{V}_E \text{ BTPS} = \dot{V}_E \text{ ATPS} \times \frac{310}{273 + T} \times \frac{P_B - P_{H_2O} \text{ at } T}{P_B - 47},$$

where T = temperature in degrees centigrade,
P_B = barometric pressure in mm Hg,
P_{H_2O} = water-vapor tension.

Water-vapor tension at the designated temperature (T) can be obtained by consulting the values in Table 14–1. The value 47 is the alveolar P_{H_2O} in mm Hg; 310 is the average respiratory tract temperature in deg K; 273 is the temperature at absolute zero in deg K.

3. The oxygen consumption per minute (BTPS) can be calculated from knowledge of the proportion (fraction, F) of the oxygen and carbon dioxide expired, along with the known values of both gases in the inspired air, as follows:

$$\dot{V}_{O_2} \text{ BTPS} = \dot{V}_E \text{ BTPS} \times \frac{F_{I_{O_2}} (1 - F_{E_{CO_2}}) - F_{E_{O_2}} (1 - F_{I_{O_2}})}{(1 - F_{I_{O_2}} - F_{I_{CO_2}})}.$$

where $F_{I_{O_2}}$ = proportion of oxygen inspired (.2093).
$F_{E_{O_2}}$ = proportion of oxygen expired.
$F_{I_{CO_2}}$ = proportion of carbon dioxide inspired (.004).
$F_{E_{CO_2}}$ = proportion of carbon dioxide expired.

[10]Jay T. Kearney and G. Alan Stull, "A Fortran Program for the Reduction of Open-Circuit Data," *Research Quarterly*, 42 (May 1971), 223.

Table 14–1. Values for Water Vapor Tension at Various Temperatures

Temp. (C)	P_{H_2O} (mm Hg)	Temp. (C)	P_{H_2O} (mm Hg)
20	17.54	31	33.70
21	18.65	32	35.66
22	19.83	33	37.73
23	21.07	34	39.90
24	22.38	35	42.18
25	23.76	36	44.56
26	25.21	37	47.07
27	26.74	38	49.69
28	28.35	39	52.44
29	30.04	40	55.32
30	31.82		

4. The $\dot{V}_{O_2}$ BTPS is converted to STPD, according to the following:

$$\dot{V}_{O_2}\,\text{STPD} = \dot{V}_{O_2}\,\text{BTPS} \times \frac{273.0}{310.0} \times \frac{P_B - 47}{760}$$

5. The $\dot{V}_{CO_2}$ BTPS may be calculated by using the following formula:

$$\dot{V}_{CO_2}\,\text{BTPS} = \dot{V}_E\,\text{BTPS} \times \frac{F_{ECO_2}\,(1 - F_{IO_2}) - F_{ICO_2}\,(1 - F_{EO_2})}{(1 - F_{IO_2} - F_{ICO_2})}.$$

6. $\dot{V}_{CO_2}$ STPD is calculated as follows:

$$\dot{V}_{CO_2}\,\text{STPD} = \dot{V}_{CO_2}\,\text{BTPS} \times \frac{273.0}{310.0}\;\frac{P_B - 47}{760}.$$

7. The Respiratory Exchange Ratio (R) is calculated as:

$$R = \frac{\dot{V}_{CO_2}\,\text{STPD}}{\dot{V}_{O_2}\,\text{STPD}}$$

(see Chapter 7).

Example. Barry, a 170-lb male, ran on a treadmill at 7 mph on a 7 percent grade for 2 minutes and collected expired air for the last minute. The following data were obtained:

Percent O_2 expired: 16.05
Percent CO_2 expired: 4.75
Percent N_2 expired: 79.20 (which makes the total 100 percent)
Temperature (deg C): 26.0
Barometric pressure (mm Hg): 751
Collection time (sec): 60
$\dot{V}_E$ (liters): 99.8

1. $\dot{V}_E \text{ ATPS} = 99.8 \left(\dfrac{60}{60}\right) = 99.8 \text{ l/min.}$

2. $\dot{V}_E \text{ BTPS} = 99.8 \left(\dfrac{310}{273+26.0}\right) \left(\dfrac{751-25.21}{751-47}\right) = 106.70 \text{ l/min.}$

3. $\dot{V}_{O_2} \text{ BTPS} = 106.70 \times \dfrac{.2093(1-.0475)-.1605(1-.0003)}{(1-.2093-.0003)}$
$= 5.25 \text{ l/min.}$

4. $\dot{V}_{O_2} \text{ STPD} = 5.25 \times \dfrac{273.0}{310.0} \times \dfrac{751-47}{760} = 4.278 \text{ l/min.}$

5. $\dot{V}_{CO_2} \text{ BTPS} = 106.70 \times \dfrac{.0475(1-.2093)-.0003(1-.1605)}{(1-.2093-.0003)} = 5.026.$

6. $\dot{V}_{CO_2} \text{ STPD} = 5.026 \times \dfrac{273.0}{310.0} \times \dfrac{751-47}{760} = 4.098 \text{ l/min.}$

7. $R = \dfrac{4.098}{4.278} = .958.$

TESTS OF CARDIOVASCULAR FITNESS

Quite a number of cardiovascular tests are available to be employed in exercise physiology, from those that measure aerobic capacity to those that only estimate it. The first section will deal with procedures for the determination of maximum oxygen uptake ($\dot{V}_{O_2}$ max), while the second section will present various submaximal tests.

Maximal

The exercise physiologist has shown a fondness for the assessment of $\dot{V}_{O_2}$ max, since aerobic capacity seems to be of value as a measure of physical fitness. In research there can be no doubt that the capacity of the individual to utilize oxygen is important. The $\dot{V}_{O_2}$ max test can be performed in a number of ways, but it is usual to have the subject first warm up by walking on a treadmill (say, 3.5 mph, 10 percent grade) and then begin the first work load. According to Taylor et al.[11] the warm-up is followed by a 5-minute rest and then the first work load is administered. This would be running on the treadmill for 3 minutes at 7 mph, 0 percent grade, with a one-minute gas-collection period between 1 minute 45 second and 2 minutes 45 seconds. The second stage would follow on a second visit to the laboratory, but if one desired to complete the entire test in one session, a rest period of 5 to 10 minutes would be appropriate

[11]Henry L. Taylor, Elsworth Buskirk, and Austin Henschel, "Maximal Oxygen Intake as an Objective Measure of Cardio-Respiratory Performance," *Journal of Applied Physiology*, 8 (July 1955), 73.

between stages.[12] The second stage, then, would last 3 minutes at 7 mph and 2.5 percent grade, gas collection being accomplished after 1 minute 45 seconds. Likewise, additional stages would be employed, keeping the speed constant, but increasing the grade by 2.5 percent on each occasion. The test is terminated when the oxygen uptake for successive work loads fails to increase by more than 150 ml/min, or 2.1 ml/kg/min. This is the $\dot{V}O_2$ max. It may help in administering this test if some prior information is obtained on the fitness of the subject, since well-conditioned individuals can justifiably by-pass the early stages.

The procedures may be altered to fit individual requirements, but most investigators seem to agree that a succession of increasingly heavy work loads is needed, that they should be separated by a period of rest, and that the exercise at each stage should probably be of sufficient duration to insure steady-state conditions. It may actually be desirable, therefore, for the exercise to last for 5 minutes at each stage. Additional variables such as heart rate, blood pressure, and blood lactate may also be obtained during exercise when needed. Moreover, the $\dot{V}O_2$ max test may employ a bicycle ergometer rather than a treadmill, but in this case it may be preferable to extend the test to two days or more.[13]

Submaximal

Efforts spanning a number of years have sought a means for estimating maximal oxygen uptake from submaximal efforts. Such a test has obvious practical benefits because the individual is asked to work at lower levels, thus making it more readily usable, especially for subjects who are not used to more strenuous activity. To achieve this end, most of the tests make use of heart rate and thus eliminate the more expensive laboratory instruments needed for gas analysis.

Physical Work Capacity (PWC$_{170}$)

Very simply, the PWC$_{170}$ test requires the subject to exercise in two successive bouts on a bicycle ergometer for six minutes each. The loads selected should be such that heart rates between 140 and 170 bpm are elicited. Theoretically at least, heart rates between these values are generally linear with increasing work loads. Thus, the PWC$_{170}$ test requires the heart rates to be plotted against work load and a straight line drawn through them. The score is the work load (kgm/min) that corresponds with the line as it intersects the heart rate at 170 bpm.

[12]Victor F. Froelicker, Jr., *et al.*, "A Comparison of Three Maximal Treadmill Exercise Protocols," *Journal of Applied Physiology*, 36 (June 1974), 720.

[13]Per-Olof Åstrand and Kaare Rodahl, *Textbook of Work Physiology* (New York: McGraw-Hill Book Company, 1970), pp. 615–616.

Astrand-Ryhming Test

Making use of the above principle, researchers have constructed a nomogram to score a single work test on a bicycle ergometer, a bench-stepping task, or running on a treadmill.[14, 15] Best results are obtained when exercise produces heart rates between 125 and 170. Consultation with the nomogram, shown in Figure 98, will permit estimation of the $\dot{V}_{O_2}$ max. When bench-stepping is used (33 cm for women, 40 cm for men, at a cadence of 22.5 complete steps per minute for 5 minutes), body weight is lined up against exercise heart rate and the $\dot{V}_{O_2}$ max is read from the diagonal line. When the bicycle ergometer is employed, work load (kpm/min) is lined up with exercise heart rate; with the treadmill, it is heart rate vs. $\dot{V}_{O_2}$ at a submaximal work rate. The authors report approximately 6 percent error for two-thirds of the subjects in this test when the results are compared with the actual determination of $\dot{V}_{O_2}$ max. When subjects above 27 years of age are tested, it is necessary to apply an age-correction factor.[16]

Stress Testing

An adjunct to medical practice that is rapidly gaining endorsement as greater reliance is placed on the preventive aspects of medicine is the *exercise stress test*. There is growing awareness that the resting electrocardiogram is not sufficient to evaluate the ability of the heart to withstand exercise. In fact, it is not uncommon for the resting ECG to appear perfectly normal, but for signs of abnormality to appear during a moderate exercise bout. The heart may be receiving an adequate coronary blood supply at rest, but symptoms of ischemia may become evident during stress. The exercise stress test is designed to permit observation of signs of abnormality and to assess the functional capacity of the heart and cardiovascular system. For the healthy person it may serve as assurance that an exercise program may be inaugurated without immediate concern.

The purpose of this discussion is not to encourage diagnosis of abnormal electrocardiograms. That would be impossible in a text of this sort, but the administration of the stress test itself should be understood by the exercise physiologist and physical educator. In fact, the entire medical community should be aware of the test as a diagnostic tool and move

---

[14]Per-Olof Åstrand and Irma Ryhming, "A Nomogram for Calculation of Aerobic Capacity (Physical Fitness) from Pulse Rate During Submaximal Work," *Journal of Applied Physiology*, 7 (September 1954), 218.

[15]Irma Åstrand, "Aerobic Work Capacity in Men and Women with Special Reference to Age," *Acta Physiologica Scandinavica*, 49, Supplement 169 (1960).

[16]W. Von Döbeln, I. Åstrand, and A. Bergström, "An Analysis of Age and Other Factors Related to Maximal Oxygen Uptake," *Journal of Applied Physiology*, 22 (1967), 934.

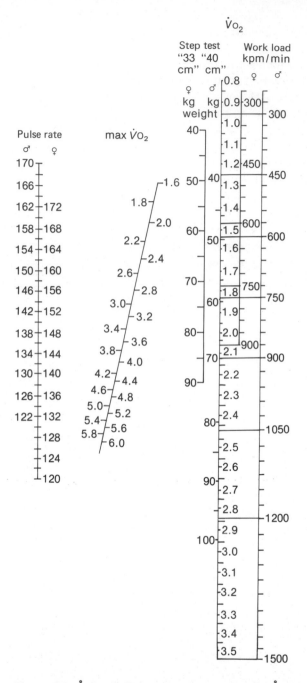

Figure 98. Åstrand-Ryhming Nomogram. [P. O. Åstrand and Irma Ryhming, "A Nomogram for Calculation of Aerobic Capacity (Physical Fitness) from Pulse Rate During Submaximal Work," *Journal of Applied Physiology*, 1 (September 1954), p. 219.]

toward endorsement and support for the development of such centers. Of particular importance is the requirement for medical consultation and overall supervision of the testing, including the training of testing personnel, the reading of the electrocardiogram, and the follow-up procedures in the event of an abnormal ECG. Moreover, the establishment of a safe testing protocol must be uppermost in the minds of all concerned, so there must be a clear understanding of emergency procedures. The individual in charge, therefore, should be well trained in the preliminary diagnosis of potential cardiac abnormality so that he knows when to terminate the test before any serious difficulty arises. It is then appropriate to refer the individual to his physician for a more complete physical examination.

The exercise stress test may be extensive or it may be brief. The simplest form involves monitoring the exercise ECG and blood pressure during various stages of treadmill running; more advanced forms include the data for oxygen uptake as well, and of course a complete fitness appraisal would also include strength, agility, speed, and other factors. The discussion here will be limited to the cardiovascular variables.

The specific procedures vary among stress-testing centers, but the usual objective is to arrive at the number of METS equivalent to a given heart rate achieved in the multistage submaximal treadmill exercise (Chapter 6). To accomplish this end, it is necessary to decide first of all what will be the target heart rate. Since this is a submaximal exercise, a typical stress test would employ a heart rate of 85 percent of maximum, or even 70 percent. The maximum heart rate would not be known for each subject, so it is necessary to consult a table that reflects the decline in heart rate with age (Table 14–2) and terminate the stress test when this selected heart rate is achieved. For example, a 45-year-old man would have a predicted value for 85 percent of maximum of 150 bpm (in which case maximum would be predicted at 176). The number of METS achieved for various treadmill speeds and grades when the criterion heart rate is reached can then be estimated from values in Table 14–3.

Table 14–2. Heart Rate as a Function of Age

Age	70% of Max.	85% of Max.	Max.
25	140	170	200
30	136	165	194
35	132	160	188
40	128	155	182
45	124	150	176
50	119	145	171
55	115	140	165
60	111	135	159
65	107	130	153

Table 14–3. VO_2 and METS Achieved at Various Speeds and Grades of Treadmill Running

Speed	3.4 3.0	3.4 3.0	3.4 3.0	3.4 3.0	3.4 3.0	3.4 3.0	3.4 3.0	3.4 3.0	3.4 3.0	3.4 3.0	3.4 3.0	3.4	3.4	3.4
Grade	0 0	2 2.5	4 5	6 7.5	8 10	10 12.5	12 15	14 17.5	16 20	18 22.5	20 25	22	24	26
METS	3	4	5	6	7	8	9	10	11	12	13	14	15	16
VO_2 (ml/kg)	10.5	14.0	17.5	21.0	24.5	28.0	31.5	35.0	38.5	42.0	45.5	49.0	52.5	56.0

Thus, the testing sequence can be seen as follows: The subject reports to the stress testing center usually with written permission from his physician, which should mean that a resting ECG or at least some cardiac evaluation has been made to clear him for the exercise task. The subject is then given resting ECG and blood-pressure measurements prior to the test, and if they both appear normal he may then proceed to a preliminary warm-up phase (sometimes called an *accommodation* period), at which time an evaluation is made concerning his fitness for further stress. It is acceptable to use a 0 percent grade and treadmill speed of 2 mph for this portion of the test, which may last for only 2 minutes, or until the heart rate stabilizes.

The successive stages include a number of options. Taking all subjects through each possible level could result in a rather prolonged test for some. The well-conditioned young person would be expected to go through a number of stages in reaching his target heart rate, while the out-of-condition older person would reach his final stage much sooner. Thus, some judgment may be exercised concerning the starting stage to be adopted. At any rate, with the speed constant at 3.0 mph, the first stage would be at 0 percent grade, and each successive stage would increase the grade by 2.5 percent. The length of time at each level would be 3 to 5 minutes, or long enough for steady-state conditions to be established. Blood pressures should be taken every 1½ minutes and heart rate monitored continuously via oscilloscope. Rhythm strips of the ECG should be obtained during the steady-state portion of each work level, and of course the heart rate itself determined so that a decision to continue to the next stage can be made. As stated earlier, any abnormal sign is an indication to terminate the test.

The "Abnormal" Normal ECG

The physical educator and coach should be aware that the electrocardiogram of well-trained endurance athletes can sometimes mimic that of the diseased heart. Heart sounds may also appear different, so some of the aberrations exhibited by highly fit individuals may actually be normal for them. In other words, the results of intense physical training which lead to measurable changes in cardiac output and other cardiovascular effects may cause other subtle changes to occur that could lead to a diagnosis of cardiac pathology. Obviously any suggestion of abnormality must be thoroughly investigated, but frequently an erroneous diagnosis is made when the athlete is compared with the typical normal individual. The danger here is that such a situation may cause the subject undue concern and at the same time end his athletic endeavors. It would seem reasonable for him to seek consultation with a cardiologist familiar with sports medicine, and especially one who has had experience with long-distance runners.

Measurement of human performance is a natural outgrowth of programs that seek a change in physical fitness. While a number of tests exist, those that emphasize muscular strength and endurance and cardiovascular endurance are extremely important to the exercise physiologist. Muscular strength can be evaluated by use of various cable-tension strength-test batteries designed for boys and girls at designated ages, and muscular endurance can be tested employing an ergograph.

Cardiovascular endurance can be assessed by either submaximal or maximal means. Metabolism itself will require either closed-circuit or open-circuit calorimetry. Closed-circuit procedures involve inhaling from a closed container containing oxygen, then exhaling into the canister while the carbon dioxide is absorbed as it passes through a container of soda lime. The change in the amount of oxygen is a measure of the metabolism for a given period of time. The open-circuit system involves inhaling atmospheric air and collecting all the expired air, which is then subjected to analysis for its oxygen and carbon dioxide content. The difference between the composition of this sample and that of atmospheric air gives a measure of the metabolic activity. Tests of maximal oxygen uptake usually involve a stepwise increment in work load until the point is reached where an insignificant increase in $\dot{V}O_2$ occurs. Submaximal tests are usually designed to predict $\dot{V}O_2$ max from such submaximal variables as heart rate.

The exercise stress test involves monitoring the electrocardiogram and other cardiovascular variables as the individual is taken through a multistage submaximal treadmill test. The test is usually employed for diagnostic purposes, so the ECG and blood pressure are monitored continuously during each stage as the subject reaches the criterion level. This level is usually based on some value of heart rate, such as 85 percent of maximum. From the level of exercise reached the number of METS achieved may be determined.

S E L E C T E D   R E F E R E N C E S

Åstrand, Per-Olof, and Kaare Rodahl, *Textbook of Work Physiology*. New York: McGraw-Hill Book Company, 1970.

Åstrand, P.-O., and Irma Ryhming, "A Nomogram for Calculation of Aerobic Capacity (Physical Fitness) from Pulse Rate During Submaximal Work," *Journal of Applied Physiology*, 7 (September 1954), 218.

Auchincloss, J. Howland, and Robert Gilbert, "Estimation of Maximum Oxygen Uptake with a Brief Progressive Stress Test," *Journal of Applied Physiology*, 34 (April 1973), 525.

Clarke, David H., and H. Harrison Clarke, *Research Processes in Physical Education, Recreation, and Health*. Englewood Cliffs, N.J.: Prentice-Hall, Inc., 1970.

Clarke, H. Harrison, and David H. Clarke, *Developmental and Adapted Physical Education*. Englewood Cliffs, N.J.: Prentice-Hall, Inc., 1963.

Clarke, H. H., and Richard A. Monroe, *Test Manual: Oregon Cable-Tension Strength Test Batteries for Boys and Girls from Fourth Grade Through College*. Eugene, Oregon: University of Oregon, 1970.

Cooper, Kenneth H., *The New Aerobics*. New York: Bantam Books, 1970.

Cureton, Thomas K., "Improvements in Oxygen Intake Capacity Resulting from Sports and Exercise Training Programs: A Review," *American Corrective Therapy Journal*, 23 (September–October 1969), 144.

Fox, Edward L., "A Simple, Accurate Technique for Predicting Maximal Aerobic Power," *Journal of Applied Physiology*, 35 (December 1973), 914.

Froelicher, Victor F., *et al.*, "A Comparison of Three Maximal Treadmill Exercise Protocols," *Journal of Applied Physiology*, 36 (June 1974), 720.

Girandola, Robert N., Frank I. Katch, and Franklin M. Henry, "Prediction of Oxygen Intake from Ventilation, and Oxygen Intake and Work Capacity from Heart Rate During Heavy Exercise," *Research Quarterly*, 42 (December 1971), 362.

Hermiston, R. T., and J. A. Faulkner, "Prediction of Maximal Oxygen Uptake by a Stepwise Regression Technique," *Journal of Applied Physiology*, 30 (June 1971), 833.

Hurzeler, Philip A., William S. Gualtiere, and Lenore R. Zohman, "Time-Saving Tables for Calculating Oxygen Consumption and Respiratory Quotient," *Research Quarterly*, 43 (March 1972), 121.

Kearney, Jay T., and G. Alan Stull, "A Fortran Program for the Reduction of Open-Circuit Data," *Research Quarterly*, 42 (May 1971), 223.

Metz, Kenneth F., and John F. Alexander, "Estimation of Maximal Oxygen Intake from Submaximal Work Parameters," *Research Quarterly*, 42 (May 1971), 187.

Taylor, Henry L., Elsworth Buskirk, and Austin Henschel, "Maximal Oxygen Intake as an Objective Measure of Cardio-Respiratory Performance," *Journal of Applied Physiology*, 8 (July 1955), 73.

strength composite
norms
and
T scales

All tables in this Appendix are adapted from H. Harrison Clarke and Richard A. Monroe, *Test Manual: Cable-Tension Strength Test Batteries for Boys and Girls from Fourth Grade through College* (Eugene, Oregon: University of Oregon, 1970).

Table A–1. Strength Composite Norms for Age and Weight
Upper Elementary School Boys

AGE (yrs-mos)	9-0 9-5	9-6 9-11	10-0 10-5	10-6 10-11	11-0 11-5	11-6 11-11
WEIGHT (lbs) 149						538
148						534
147						531
146						527
145						524
144						520
143					530	517
142					526	514
141					522	510
140					518	507
139				495	514	503
138				491	510	500
137				487	506	496
136				484	502	493
135				480	499	490
134			477	476	495	486
133			473	473	491	483
132			470	469	487	479
131			466	465	483	476
130			463	462	479	472
129			459	458	475	469
128			455	454	471	465
127			452	451	467	462
126			448	447	464	459
125			445	443	460	455
124		437	441	440	456	452
123		433	437	436	452	448
122		430	434	432	448	445
121		426	430	429	444	441
120		423	427	425	440	438
119		420	423	421	436	434
118		416	419	418	432	431
117		413	416	414	429	428
116		409	412	410	425	424
115		406	409	407	421	421

AGE (yrs-mos)	9-0 9-5	9-6 9-11	10-0 10-5	10-6 10-11	11-0 11-5	11-6 11-11
WEIGHT						
(lbs) 114	401	402	405	403	417	417
113	397	399	401	399	413	414
112	394	395	398	396	409	410
111	390	392	394	392	405	407
110	386	389	390	388	401	404
109	383	385	387	385	397	400
108	379	382	383	381	394	397
107	376	378	380	377	390	393
106	372	375	376	374	386	390
105	368	371	372	370	382	386
104	365	368	369	366	378	383
103	361	364	365	363	374	379
102	358	361	362	359	370	376
101	354	357	358	355	366	373
100	350	354	354	352	362	369
99	347	351	351	348	359	366
98	343	347	347	344	355	362
97	340	344	344	341	351	359
96	336	340	340	337	347	355
95	332	337	336	333	343	352
94	329	333	333	330	339	348
93	325	330	329	326	335	345
92	322	326	325	322	331	342
91	318	323	322	319	327	338
90	314	320	318	315	324	335
89	311	316	315	311	320	331
88	307	313	311	308	316	328
87	304	309	307	304	312	324
86	300	306	304	300	308	321
85	296	302	300	297	304	<u>318</u>
84	293	299	297	293	300	314
83	289	295	293	289	296	311
82	286	292	289	286	292	307
81	282	288	286	282	<u>289</u>	304
80	278	285	282	278	285	300

Table A–1. (Continued)

AGE (yrs-mos)	9-0 9-5	9-6 9-11	10-0 10-5	10-6 10-11	11-0 11-5	11-6 11-11
WEIGHT						
(lbs) 79	275	282	279	<u>275</u>	281	297
78	271	278	275	271	277	293
77	268	275	261	267	273	290
76	264	271	268	263	269	287
75	260	268	264	260	265	283
74	257	264	<u>261</u>	256	261	280
73	253	261	257	252	257	276
72	250	257	253	249	253	273
71	246	254	250	245	250	269
70	242	<u>251</u>	246	241	246	266
69	239	247	242	238	242	262
68	235	244	239	234	238	259
67	232	240	235	230	234	256
66	228	237	232	227	230	252
65	224	233	228	223	226	249
64	221	230	224	219	222	245
63	217	226	221	216	218	242
62	<u>214</u>	223	217	212	215	238
61	210	219	214	208	211	235
60	206	216	210	205	207	232
59	203	213	206	201		
58	199	209	203	197		
57	196	206	199	194		
56	192	202	196	190		
55	188	199	192	186		
54	185	195	188	183		
53	181	192	185	179		
52	178	188	181	175		
51	171	185	177	172		
50	170	182	174	168		
49	167	178				
48	163	175				
47	160	171				
46	156	168				
45	152	164				
	*3.60	3.45	3.61	3.67	3.89	3.44

*Weight deviation multipliers.
Note: Underlined scores constitute the median Strength Composite score at median weight for each half-year age interval.

Table A–2. Strength Composite Norms for Age and Weight
Junior High School Boys

AGE (yrs-mos)	12-0 12-5	12-6 12-11	13-0 13-5	13-6 13-11	14-0 14-5	14-6 14-11	15-0 15-5	15-6 15-11
WEIGHT								
(lbs) 174						784	787	795
173						779	783	790
172						774	778	785
171						769	773	781
170						764	768	776
169				725	763	759	764	771
168				720	758	753	759	766
167				716	752	748	754	762
166				711	747	743	750	757
165				706	742	738	745	752
164				702	736	733	740	747
163				697	731	728	735	743
162				692	726	722	731	738
161				687	720	717	726	733
160				683	715	712	721	728
159			680	678	710	707	717	724
158			675	673	704	702	712	719
157			670	668	699	697	707	714
156			666	664	694	692	702	709
155			661	659	688	686	698	705
154			656	654	683	681	693	700
153			651	650	678	676	688	695
152			647	645	672	671	683	690
151			642	640	667	666	679	686
150			637	635	662	661	674	681
149		549	633	631	656	656	669	676
148		546	628	626	651	650	665	671
147		543	623	621	646	645	660	667
146		539	618	617	640	640	655	662
145		536	614	612	635	635	650	657
144		533	609	607	630	630	646	652
143		529	604	602	624	625	641	648
142		526	600	598	619	619	636	643
141		523	595	593	614	614	632	638
140		519	590	588	608	609	627	633

280

AGE (yrs-mos)	12-0 12-5	12-6 12-11	13-0 13-5	13-6 13-11	14-0 14-5	14-6 14-11	15-0 15-5	15-6 15-11
WEIGHT								
(lbs) 139	504	516	585	584	603	604	622	<u>629</u>
138	500	513	581	579	598	599	617	624
137	497	509	576	574	592	594	613	619
136	494	506	571	569	587	589	608	614
135	490	503	567	565	582	583	603	610
134	487	499	562	560	576	578	<u>599</u>	605
133	484	496	557	555	571	573	594	600
132	480	493	553	550	566	568	589	595
131	477	489	548	546	560	563	584	591
130	474	486	543	541	555	558	580	586
129	470	483	538	536	550	<u>553</u>	575	581
128	467	479	534	532	544	547	570	576
127	464	476	529	527	539	542	565	572
126	460	473	524	522	534	537	561	567
125	457	469	520	517	528	532	556	562
124	454	466	515	513	523	527	551	557
123	450	463	510	508	518	522	547	553
122	447	460	505	503	<u>513</u>	516	542	548
121	444	456	501	499	507	511	537	543
120	440	453	496	494	502	506	532	538
119	437	450	491	489	497	501	528	534
118	434	446	487	484	491	496	523	529
117	430	443	482	480	486	491	518	524
116	427	440	477	475	481	486	514	519
115	424	436	472	470	475	480	509	515
114	420	433	468	<u>466</u>	470	475	504	510
113	417	430	463	461	465	470	499	505
112	414	426	458	456	459	465	495	500
111	410	423	454	451	454	460	490	496
110	407	420	449	447	449	455	485	491
109	404	416	444	442	443	450	481	486
108	400	413	439	437	438	444	476	481
107	397	410	435	432	433	439	471	477
106	394	406	430	428	427	434	466	472
105	390	403	425	423	422	429	462	467

AGE (yrs-mos)	12-0 12-5	12-6 12-11	13-0 13-5	13-6 13-11	14-0 14-5	14-6 14-11	15-0 15-5	15-6 15-11
WEIGHT								
(lbs) 104	387	400	421	418	417	424	457	462
103	384	396	416	414	411	419	452	458
102	380	393	411	409	406	413	447	453
101	377	390	<u>407</u>	404	401	408	443	448
100	374	386	402	399	395	403	438	443
99	370	383	397	395	390	398	433	439
98	367	380	392	390	385	393	429	434
97	364	<u>377</u>	388	385	379	388	424	429
96	360	373	383	381	374	383	419	424
95	357	370	378	376	369	377	414	420
94	354	367	374	371	363	372	410	415
93	350	363	369	366	358	367	405	410
92	347	360	364	362	353	362	400	405
91	<u>344</u>	357	359	357	347	357	396	401
90	340	353	355	352	342	352	391	396
89	337	350	350	348	337			
88	333	347	345	343	331			
87	330	343	341	338	326			
86	327	340	336	333	321			
85	323	337	331	329	315			
84	320	333	326	324	310			
83	317	330	322	319	305			
82	313	327	317	314	299			
81	310	323	312	310	294			
80	307	320	308	305	289			
79	303	317	303	300				
78	300	313	298	296				
77	297	310	293	291				
76	293	307	289	286				
75	290	303	284	281				
74	287	300	279	277				
73	283	297	275	272				
72	280	294	270	267				
71	277	290	265	263				
70	273	287	260	258				
	*3.34	3.32	4.71	4.72	5.33	5.15	4.72	4.75

*Weight deviation multipliers.
Note: Underlined scores constitute the median Strength Composite score at median weight for each half-year age interval.

Table A–3. Strength Composite Norms for Age and Weight
Senior High School Boys

AGE (yrs-mos)	16-0 16-5	16-6 16-11	17-0 17-5	17-6 17-11	18-0 18-5	18-6 18-11
WEIGHT						
(lbs) 199					1020	1011
198					1013	1005
197					1007	999
196					1001	994
195					995	988
194				1036	989	982
193				1029	983	977
192				1022	977	971
191				1015	971	965
190				1007	965	959
189				1000	958	954
188				993	952	948
187				986	946	942
186		964	973	979	940	937
185		957	966	971	934	931
184		950	959	964	928	925
183		944	952	957	922	920
182		937	945	950	916	914
181		930	938	943	910	908
180		924	931	935	903	902
179		917	924	928	897	897
178		910	917	921	891	891
177		904	911	914	885	885
176	852	897	904	907	879	880
175	847	890	897	899	873	874
174	841	884	890	892	867	868
173	835	877	883	885	861	863
172	830	870	876	878	855	857
171	824	863	869	871	848	851
170	818	857	862	863	842	845
169	812	850	855	856	836	840
168	807	843	848	849	830	834
167	801	837	841	842	824	828
166	795	830	834	835	818	823
165	790	823	827	827	812	817

AGE (yrs-mos)	16-0 16-5	16-6 16-11	17-0 17-5	17-6 17-11	18-0 18-5	18-6 18-11
WEIGHT						
(lbs) 164	784	817	820	820	806	811
163	778	810	813	813	800	<u>806</u>
162	773	803	806	806	<u>794</u>	800
161	767	797	799	799	787	794
160	761	790	792	791	781	788
159	756	783	785	784	775	783
158	750	776	778	777	769	777
157	744	770	771	770	763	771
156	738	763	764	<u>763</u>	757	766
155	733	756	757	755	751	760
154	727	750	750	748	745	754
153	721	743	743	741	739	749
152	716	736	<u>737</u>	734	732	743
151	710	730	730	727	726	737
150	704	723	723	719	720	731
149	699	716	716	712	714	726
148	693	710	709	705	708	720
147	687	703	702	698	702	714
146	682	696	695	691	696	709
145	676	<u>690</u>	688	683	690	703
144	670	683	681	676	684	697
143	<u>665</u>	676	674	669	677	692
142	659	669	667	662	671	686
141	653	663	660	655	665	680
140	647	656	653	647	659	674
139	642	649	646	640	653	669
138	636	643	639	633	647	663
137	630	636	632	626	641	657
136	625	629	625	619	635	652
135	619	623	618	611	629	646
134	613	616	611	604	622	640
133	608	609	604	597	616	635
132	602	603	597	590	610	692
131	596	596	590	583	604	623
130	591	589	583	575	598	617

AGE (yrs-mos)	16-0 16-5	16-6 16-11	17-0 17-5	17-6 17-11	18-0 18-5	18-6 18-11
WEIGHT						
(lbs) 129	585	582	576	568	592	612
128	579	576	569	561	586	606
127	573	569	563	554	580	600
126	568	562	556	547	574	595
125	562	556	549	539	567	589
124	556	549	542	532	561	583
123	551	542	535	525	555	578
122	545	536	528	518	549	572
121	539	529	521	511	543	566
120	534	522	514	503	537	560
119	528	516	507			
118	522	509	500			
117	517	502	493			
116	511	495	486			
115	505	489	479			
114	499	482	472			
113	494	475	465			
112	488	469	458			
111	482	462	451			
110	477	455	444			
109	471					
108	465					
107	460					
106	454					
105	448					
104	443					
103	437					
102	431					
101	426					
100	420					
	*5.69	6.69	6.96	7.20	6.11	5.70

*Weight deviation multipliers.

Note: Underlined scores constitute the median Strength Composite score at median weight for each half-year age interval.

Table A-4. Strength Composite Norms for Age and Weight
Upper Elementary School Girls

AGE (yrs-mos)	9-0 9-5	9-6 9-11	10-0 10-5	10-6 10-11	11-0 11-5	11-6 11-11	12-0 12-5	12-6 12-11	13-0 13-5
WEIGHT (lbs)									
155						332	335	345	346
154						330	333	343	344
153						327	331	340	342
152						325	329	338	340
151						323	326	336	337
150					340	321	324	334	335
149					338	318	322	331	333
148					335	316	319	329	330
147					333	314	317	327	328
146					330	311	315	324	326
145					327	309	312	322	324
144					325	307	310	320	321
143					322	304	308	317	319
142					320	302	306	315	317
141					317	300	303	313	314
140					314	298	301	311	312
139					312	295	299	308	310
138					309	293	296	306	307
137					307	291	294	304	305
136					304	288	292	301	303
135					301	286	289	299	301
134					299	284	287	297	298
133					296	281	285	294	296
132					294	279	283	292	294
131					291	277	280	290	291
130					288	274	278	288	289
129					286	272	276	285	288
128					283	270	273	283	284
127					281	268	271	281	282
126					278	265	269	278	280
125					275	263	266	276	278
124					273	261	264	274	275
123					270	258	262	271	273
122					268	256	260	269	271
121					265	254	257	267	268
120					262	252	255	265	266
119					260	249	253	262	264
118					257	247	250	260	261
117					255	245	248	258	259
116					252	242	246	255	257

Table A–4. *(Continued)*

AGE (yrs-mos)	9-0 9-5	9-6 9-11	10-0 10-5	10-6 10-11	11-0 11-5	11-6 11-11	12-0 12-5	12-6 12-11	13-0 13-5
WEIGHT (lbs)									
115					249	240	243	253	255
114					247	238	241	251	252
113					244	235	239	248	250
112					242	233	237	246	248
111					239	231	234	244	245
110	220	221	237	231	236	229	232	242	243
109	218	219	235	229	234	226	230	239	241
108	216	217	232	226	231	224	227	237	238
107	214	214	230	224	229	222	225	235	236
106	212	212	227	221	226	219	223	232	234
105	210	210	225	219	223	217	220	230	232
104	208	208	222	216	221	215	218	228	229
103	206	206	220	214	218	212	216	225	227
102	204	204	217	211	216	210	214	223	225
101	201	202	215	209	213	208	211	221	222
100	199	200	212	206	210	206	209	219	<u>220</u>
99	197	198	210	204	208	203	207	216	218
98	195	196	207	201	205	201	204	214	215
97	193	193	205	199	203	199	202	212	213
96	191	191	202	196	200	196	200	209	211
95	189	189	200	194	197	194	197	<u>207</u>	209
94	187	187	197	191	195	192	<u>195</u>	205	206
93	185	185	195	189	192	189	193	202	204
92	183	183	192	186	190	187	191	200	202
91	180	181	190	184	187	185	188	198	199
90	178	179	187	181	184	183	186	196	197
89	176	177	185	179	182	180	184	193	195
88	174	175	182	176	179	178	181	191	192
87	172	172	180	174	177	176	179	189	190
86	170	170	177	171	174	173	177	186	188
85	168	168	175	169	<u>171</u>	171	174	184	186
84	166	166	172	166	169	169	172	182	183
83	164	164	170	164	166	166	169	179	181
82	162	162	167	161	164	164	168	177	179
81	159	160	165	<u>159</u>	161	162	165	175	176

Table A–4. (Continued)

AGE (yrs-mos)	9-0 9-5	9-6 9-11	10-0 10-5	10-6 10-11	11-0 11-5	11-6 11-11	12-0 12-5	12-6 12-11	13-0 13-5
WEIGHT									
(lbs) 80	157	158	162	156	158	160	163	173	174
79	155	156	160	154	156	157	161	170	172
78	153	154	157	151	153	155	158	168	169
77	151	151	155	149	151	153	156	166	167
76	149	149	152	146	148	150	154	163	165
75	147	147	150	144	145	148	151	161	163
74	145	145	<u>147</u>	141	143	146	149	159	160
73	143	143	145	139	140	143	147	156	158
72	141	141	142	136	138	141	145	154	156
71	138	<u>139</u>	140	134	135	139	142	152	153
70	136	137	137	131	132	137	140	150	151
69	134	135	135	129	130	134	138	147	149
68	132	133	132	126	127	132	135	145	146
67	<u>130</u>	130	130	124	125	130	133	143	144
66	128	128	127	121	122	127	131	140	142
65	126	126	125	119	119	125	128	138	140
64	124	124	122	116	117				
63	122	122	120	114	114				
62	120	120	117	111	112				
61	117	118	115	109	109				
60	115	116	112	106	106				
59	113	114	110	104	104				
58	111	112	107	101	101				
57	109	109	105	99	99				
56	107	107	102	96	96				
55	105	105	100						
54	103	103	97						
53	101	101	95						
52	99	99	92						
51	96	97	90						
50	94	95	87						
49	92	93	85						
48	90								
47	88								
46	86								
	*2.1	2.1	2.5	2.5	2.6	2.3	2.3	2.3	2.3

*Weight deviation multipliers.
Note: Underlined scores constitute the median Strength Composite score at median weight for each half-year age interval. Figures for ages 9-5, 12-11, and 13-5 were derived by extrapolation.

Table A–5. Strength Composite Norms for Age and Weight
Junior High School Girls

AGE (yrs-mos)	11-6 11-11	12-0 12-5	12-6 12-11	13-0 13-5	13-6 13-11	14-0 14-5	14-6 14-11	15-0 15-5	15-6 15-11	16-0 16-5
WEIGHT										
(lbs) 195				450	456	476	514	553	591	628
194				448	454	473	511	549	586	623
193				445	451	470	508	545	582	619
192				443	448	467	504	541	578	614
191				440	446	464	501	537	574	609
190				438	443	462	498	534	569	604
189				435	441	459	494	530	565	599
188				433	438	456	491	526	561	595
187				430	435	453	488	522	556	590
186				428	433	450	485	518	552	585
185				425	430	448	481	515	548	580
184				423	428	445	478	511	543	575
183				420	425	442	475	507	539	571
182				418	422	439	471	503	535	566
181				415	420	436	468	499	531	561
180				413	417	434	465	496	526	556
179				410	415	431	461	492	522	551
178				408	412	428	458	488	518	547
177				405	409	425	455	484	513	542
176				403	407	422	452	480	509	537
175				400	404	420	448	477	505	532
174				398	402	417	445	473	500	527
173				395	399	414	442	469	496	523
172				393	396	411	438	465	492	518
171				390	394	408	435	461	488	513
170				388	391	406	432	458	483	508
169				385	389	403	428	454	479	503
168				383	386	400	425	450	475	499
167				380	383	397	422	446	470	494
166				378	381	394	419	442	466	489
165				375	378	392	415	439	462	484
164				373	376	389	412	435	457	479
163				370	373	386	409	431	453	475
162				368	370	383	405	427	449	470
161				365	368	380	402	423	445	465

Table A–5. (Continued)

AGE (yrs-mos)	11-6 11-11	12-0 12-5	12-6 12-11	13-0 13-5	13-6 13-11	14-0 14-5	14-6 14-11	15-0 15-5	15-6 15-11	16-0 16-5
WEIGHT										
(lbs) 160				363	365	378	399	420	440	460
159				360	363	375	395	416	436	455
158				358	360	372	392	412	432	451
157				355	357	369	389	408	427	446
156				353	355	366	386	404	423	441
155				350	352	364	382	401	419	436
154				348	350	361	379	397	414	432
153				345	347	358	376	393	410	427
152				343	344	355	372	389	406	422
151				340	342	352	369	385	402	417
150				338	339	350	366	382	397	412
149				335	337	347	362	378	393	407
148				333	334	344	359	374	389	403
147				330	331	341	356	370	384	398
146				328	329	338	353	366	380	393
145	325	326	328	325	326	336	349	363	376	388
144	323	324	325	323	324	333	346	359	371	383
143	320	321	323	320	321	330	343	355	367	379
142	318	319	320	318	318	327	339	351	363	374
141	315	316	317	315	316	324	336	347	359	369
140	312	313	315	313	313	322	333	344	354	364
139	310	311	312	310	311	319	329	340	350	359
138	307	308	310	308	308	316	326	336	346	355
137	305	306	307	305	305	313	323	332	341	350
136	302	303	304	303	303	310	320	328	337	345
135	299	300	302	300	300	308	316	325	333	340
134	297	298	299	298	372	305	313	321	328	335
133	294	295	297	295	295	302	310	317	324	331
132	292	293	294	293	292	299	306	313	320	326
131	289	290	291	290	290	296	303	309	316	321
130	286	287	289	288	287	294	300	306	311	316
129	284	285	286	285	285	291	296	302	307	311
128	281	282	284	283	282	288	293	298	303	307
127	279	280	281	280	279	285	290	294	298	302
126	276	277	278	278	277	282	287	290	<u>294</u>	297

AGE (yrs-mos)	11-6 11-11	12-0 12-5	12-6 12-11	13-0 13-5	13-6 13-11	14-0 14-5	14-6 14-11	15-0 15-5	15-6 15-11	16-0 16-5
WEIGHT (lbs) 125	273	274	276	275	274	280	283	287	289	<u>292</u>
124	271	272	273	273	272	277	280	283	285	287
123	268	269	271	270	269	274	277	279	281	283
122	266	267	268	268	266	271	273	<u>275</u>	277	278
121	263	264	265	265	264	268	270	271	273	273
120	260	261	263	263	261	266	<u>267</u>	268	268	268
119	258	259	260	260	259	263	264	264	264	263
118	255	256	258	258	256	260	260	260	260	259
117	253	254	255	255	253	<u>257</u>	257	256	255	254
116	250	251	252	253	251	254	254	252	251	249
115	247	248	250	250	<u>248</u>	252	251	249	247	244
114	245	246	247	248	246	249	247	245	242	239
113	242	243	245	245	243	246	244	241	238	235
112	240	241	242	243	240	243	241	239	234	230
111	237	238	239	240	238	240	237	233	230	225
110	234	235	237	238	235	238	234	230	225	220
109	232	233	234	<u>235</u>	233	235	231	226	221	215
108	229	230	232	233	230	232	227	222	216	211
107	227	228	229	230	227	229	224	218	212	206
106	224	225	226	228	225	226	221	214	208	201
105	221	222	<u>224</u>	225	222	224	218	211	204	196
104	219	220	221	223	220	221	214	207	199	191
103	216	217	219	220	217	218	211	203	195	187
102	214	215	216	218	214	215	208	199	191	182
101	211	212	213	215	212	212	204	195	187	177
100	208	209	211	213	209	210	201	192	182	172
99	206	207	208	210	207	207	198	188	178	167
98	203	204	206	208	204	204	194	184	174	163
97	201	202	203	205	201	201	191	180	169	157
96	198	199	200	203	199	198	188	176	165	153
95	195	196	198	200	196	196	185	173		
94	193	<u>194</u>	195	198	194	193	181	169		
93	190	191	193	195	191	190	178	165		
92	188	189	190	193	188	187	175			
91	<u>185</u>	186	187	190	186	184	171			

AGE (yrs-mos)	11-6 11-11	12-0 12-5	12-6 12-11	13-0 13-5	13-6 13-11	14-0 14-5	14-6 14-11	15-0 15-5	15-6 15-11	16-0 16-5
WEIGHT										
(lbs) 90	182	183	185	188	183	182	168			
89	180	181	182	185	180	179	165			
88	177	178	180	183	178	176	161			
87	175	176	177	180	175	173	158			
86	172	173	174	178	173	170	155			
85	*169	170	172	175	170	168	152			
84	167	168	169	173	168	165	148			
83	164	165	167	170	165	162	145			
82	162	163	164	168	162	159	142			
81	159	160	161	165	160	156	138			
80	156	157	159	163	157	154	135			
79	154	155	156	160	155	151	132			
78	151	152	154	158	152					
77	149	150	151	155	149					
76	146	147	148	153	147					
75	143	144	146	150	144					
74	141	142	143	148	142					
73	138	139	141	145	139					
72	136	137	138	143	136					
71	133	134								
	*2.6	2.6	2.6	2.5	2.6	2.8	3.3	3.8	4.3	4.8

*Weight deviation multipliers.

Note: Underlined scores constitute the median Strength Composite score at median weight for each half-year age interval. Figures for ages 11-6, 15-6, and 16-0 were derived by extrapolation.

Table A–6. Strength Composite Norms for Age and Weight
Senior High School Girls

AGE (yrs-mos)	14-6 14-11	15-0 15-5	15-6 15-11	16-0 16-5	16-6 16-11	17-0 17-5	17-6 17-11	18-0 18-5	18-6 18-11	19-0 19-5	19-6 19-11
WEIGHT (lbs)											
200	761	763	767	763	715	682	653	660	641	631	624
199	756	759	762	759	711	679	650	657	638	627	621
198	751	754	758	754	707	676	647	654	635	624	618
197	747	749	753	749	703	672	644	650	632	621	615
196	742	744	748	744	699	669	641	647	628	618	612
195	737	739	743	740	695	665	637	643	625	615	608
194	732	735	738	735	691	662	634	640	622	611	605
193	727	730	734	730	687	658	631	637	618	608	602
192	723	725	729	726	683	655	628	633	615	605	599
191	718	721	724	721	679	652	625	630	612	602	596
190	713	716	719	716	675	648	622	626	608	599	592
189	708	712	714	712	671	645	619	623	605	595	589
188	703	707	710	707	667	641	616	620	602	592	586
187	699	702	705	702	663	638	613	616	599	589	583
186	694	697	700	697	659	635	610	613	595	586	580
185	689	692	695	693	655	631	606	609	592	583	576
184	684	688	690	688	651	628	603	606	589	579	573
183	679	683	686	683	647	624	600	603	585	576	570
182	675	678	681	679	643	621	597	599	582	573	567
181	670	673	676	674	639	618	594	596	579	570	564
180	665	668	671	669	635	614	591	592	575	567	560
179	660	664	666	665	631	611	588	589	572	563	557
178	655	659	662	660	627	607	585	586	569	560	554
177	651	654	657	655	623	604	582	582	566	557	551
176	646	649	652	650	619	601	579	579	562	554	548
175	641	644	647	646	615	597	575	575	559	551	544
174	636	640	642	641	611	594	572	572	556	547	541
173	631	635	638	636	607	590	569	569	552	544	538
172	627	630	633	632	603	587	566	565	549	541	535
171	622	625	628	627	599	584	563	562	546	538	532
170	617	620	623	622	595	580	560	558	542	535	528
169	612	616	618	618	591	577	557	555	539	531	525
168	607	611	614	613	587	573	554	552	536	528	522
167	603	606	609	608	583	570	551	548	533	525	519
166	598	601	604	603	579	567	548	545	529	522	516
165	593	596	599	599	575	563	544	541	526	519	512
164	588	592	594	594	571	560	541	538	523	515	509
163	583	587	590	589	567	556	538	535	519	512	506
162	579	582	585	585	563	553	535	531	516	509	503
161	574	577	580	580	559	550	532	528	513	506	500

AGE (yrs-mos)	14-6 14-11	15-0 15-5	15-6 15-11	16-0 16-5	16-6 16-11	17-0 17-5	17-6 17-11	18-0 18-5	18-6 18-11	19-0 19-5	19-6 19-11
WEIGHT (lbs)											
160	569	572	575	575	555	546	529	524	509	503	496
159	564	568	570	571	551	543	526	521	506	499	493
158	559	563	566	566	547	539	523	518	503	496	490
157	555	558	561	561	543	536	520	514	500	493	487
156	550	553	556	556	539	533	517	511	496	490	484
155	545	548	551	552	535	529	513	507	493	487	480
154	540	544	546	547	531	526	510	504	490	483	477
153	535	539	542	542	527	522	507	501	486	480	474
152	531	534	537	538	523	519	504	497	483	477	471
151	526	529	532	533	519	516	501	494	480	474	468
150	521	524	527	528	515	512	498	490	476	471	464
149	516	520	522	524	511	509	495	487	473	468	461
148	511	515	518	519	507	505	492	484	470	465	458
147	507	510	513	514	503	502	489	480	467	461	455
146	502	505	508	509	499	499	486	477	464	458	452
145	497	500	503	505	495	495	482	473	460	455	449
144	492	496	498	500	491	492	479	470	457	452	446
143	487	491	494	495	487	488	476	467	454	449	442
142	483	486	489	491	483	485	473	463	450	445	439
141	478	481	484	485	479	482	470	460	447	442	436
140	473	476	479	481	475	478	467	456	444	439	433
139	468	472	474	477	471	475	464	453	440	436	430
138	463	467	470	472	467	471	461	450	437	433	426
137	459	462	465	467	463	468	458	446	434	429	423
136	454	457	460	462	459	465	455	443	431	426	420
135	449	452	455	458	455	461	451	439	427	423	417
134	444	448	450	453	451	458	448	436	424	420	414
133	439	443	446	448	447	454	445	433	421	417	<u>410</u>
132	435	438	441	444	443	451	442	429	<u>417</u>	<u>413</u>	407
131	430	432	436	439	439	448	439	426	<u>414</u>	<u>410</u>	404
130	425	428	431	434	435	444	436	<u>422</u>	411	407	401
129	420	424	426	430	431	441	433	<u>419</u>	407	404	398
128	415	419	422	425	427	437	<u>430</u>	416	404	401	394
127	411	414	417	420	423	434	<u>427</u>	412	401	397	391
126	406	409	<u>412</u>	415	<u>419</u>	431	424	409	398	394	388
125	401	404	407	<u>411</u>	415	<u>427</u>	420	405	394	391	385
124	396	400	402	<u>406</u>	411	424	417	402	391	388	382
123	391	395	398	401	407	420	414	399	388	385	378
122	387	<u>390</u>	393	397	403	417	411	395	384	381	375
121	382	385	388	392	399	414	408	392	381	378	372

AGE (yrs-mos)	14-6 14-11	15-0 15-5	15-6 15-11	16-0 16-5	16-6 16-11	17-0 17-5	17-6 17-11	18-0 18-5	18-6 18-11	19-0 19-5	19-6 19-11
WEIGHT (lbs)											
120	377	380	383	387	395	410	405	388	377	375	368
119	372	376	379	383	391	407	402	385	374	371	365
118	367	371	374	378	387	403	399	382	371	368	362
117	363	366	369	373	383	400	396	378	368	365	359
116	358	361	364	368	379	397	393	375	364	362	356
115	353	356	359	364	375	393	389	371	361	359	352
114	348	352	355	359	371	390	386	368	358	355	349
113	343	347	350	354	367	386	383	365	354	352	346
112	339	342	345	350	363	383	380	361	351	349	344
111	334	337	340	345	359	380	377	358	348	346	340
110	329	332	335	340	355	376	374	354	344	343	336
109	324	328	331	336	351	373	371	351	341	339	333
108	319	323	326	331	347	369	368	348	338	336	330
107	315	318	321	326	343	366	365	344	335	333	327
106	310	313	316	321	339	363	362	341	331	330	324
105	305	308	311	317	335	359	358	337	328	327	320
104	300	304	307	312	331	356	355	334	325	323	317
103	295	299	302	307	327	352	352	331	321	320	314
102	291	294	297	303	323	349	349	327	318	317	311
101	286	289	292	298	319	346	346	324	315	314	308
100	281	284	287	293	315	342	343	320	311	311	304
99	276	280	283	289	311	339	340	317	308	307	301
98	271	275	278	284	307	335	337	314	305	304	298
97	267	270	273	279	303	332					
96	262	265	268	274	299	329					
95	257	260	263	270	295						
94	252	256	259	265	291						
93	247	251	254	260	287						
92	243	246	249								
91	238	241	244								
	*4.8	4.8	4.8	4.7	4.0	3.4	3.1	3.4	3.3	3.2	3.2

*Weight deviation multipliers.
Note: Underlined scores constitute the median Strength Composite score at median weight for each half-year age interval. Figures for ages 14-6, 15-0, 18-6, 19-0, and 19-6 were derived by extrapolation.

Table A–7. T Scale for Cable-Tension Strength Composites
College Men

T Score	Strength Composite (Pounds)	T Score	Strength Composite (Pounds)
86	1105	49	755
83	1095	49	745
74	1085	48	735
73	1075	48	725
72	1065	47	715
71	1055	45	705
71	1045	45	695
70	1035	44	685
69	1025	44	675
69	1015	43	665
68	1005	43	655
68	995	42	645
67	985	41	635
66	975	40	625
65	965	39	615
64	955	39	605
64	945	38	595
63	935	37	585
62	925	37	575
61	915	36	565
60	905	35	555
59	895	34	545
59	885	34	535
58	875	33	525
57	865	33	515
56	855	32	505
55	845	32	495
54	835	32	485
54	825	31	475
54	815	30	465
53	805	29	455
52	795	29	445
51	785	28	435
51	775	27	425
50	765	26	415
		23	405

Table A–8. T Scale for Cable-Tension Strength
College Women

Strength Score	T Score	Strength Score	T Score
625	80	405	57
615	78	395	56
605	77	385	54
595	76	375	53
585	76	365	52
575	74	355	51
565	73	345	50
555	72	335	48
545	72	325	47
535	72	315	45
525	71	305	43
515	70	295	42
505	69	285	41
495	68	275	39
485	67	265	37
475	66	255	35
465	64	245	33
455	63	235	32
445	61	225	30
435	60	215	29
425	59	205	26
415	58	195	20
		185	20

index